Assistive Technology

Assistive Technology

Matching Device and Consumer for Successful Rehabilitation

Marcia J. Scherer
Editor

American Psychological Association
Washington, DC

First Printing November 2001
Second Printing December 2003

Published by
American Psychological Association
750 First Street, NE
Washington, DC 20002
www.apa.org

To order
APA Order Department
P.O. Box 92984
Washington, DC 20090-2984
Tel: (800) 374-2721;
    Direct: (202) 336-5510
Fax: (202) 336-5502;
    TDD/TTY: (202) 336-6123
Online: www.apa.org/books/
E-mail: order@apa.org

In the U.K., Europe, Africa, and the
Middle East, copies may be ordered from
American Psychological Association
3 Henrietta Street
Covent Garden, London
WC2E 8LU England

Typeset in Goudy by World Composition Services, Inc., Sterling, VA

Printer: Phoenix Color Corp., Hagerstown, MD
Cover Designer: Ramona Hutko, Bethesda, MD
Technical/Production Editor: Emily I. Welsh

The opinions and statements published are the responsibility of the authors, and
such opinions and statements do not necessarily represent the policies of the
American Psychological Association.

Library of Congress Cataloging-in-Publication Data

Assistive technology : matching device and consumer for successful rehabilitation / edited
by Marcia J. Scherer.
        p. cm.
    Includes bibliographical references and indexes.
    ISBN 1-55798-840-4
    1. Rehabilitation technology. 2. Medical rehabilitation—Psychological aspects.
    I. Scherer, Marcia J. (Marcia Joslyn), 1948-

    RM950.A874 2001
    617'.03'019—dc21   2001041249

British Library Cataloguing-in-Publication Data
A CIP record is available from the British Library.

Printed in the United States of America

To you, upon whom the future of both assistive technology and rehabilitation psychology depend

CONTENTS

CONTRIBUTORS

Rochelle Balter, PhD, Private Practice, New York

Serenella Besio, PhD, SIVA, Fondazione Don Carlo Gnocchi, Milano, Italy

Denise L. Brown-Triolo, MS, Department of Educational Foundations and Special Services, Kent State University, OH

Michele N. Carroll, PsyD, Region 1 Mental Health, Clarksdale, MS

Albert M. Cook, PhD, Faculty of Rehabilitation Medicine, University of Alberta, Edmonton, Alberta, Canada

Gerald Craddock, B.Eng, Hdip, Client Technical Services, Central Remedial Clinic, Dublin, Ireland

Chandra M. Donnell, PhD, Department of Counseling, Educational Psychology, and Research, University of Memphis, TN

Timothy R. Elliott, PhD, Department of Physical Medicine and Rehabilitation, University of Alabama–Birmingham

Martin Forchheimer, MPP, Department of Physical Medicine and Rehabilitation, University of Michigan, Ann Arbor

Heather Roberts Fox, PhD, Science Directorate, American Psychological Association, Washington, DC

Jan C. Galvin, CEO, The Galvin Group, LLC, Tucson, AZ

Laura N. Gitlin, PhD, Community and Homecare Research Division, Thomas Jefferson University, and Senior Health Institute, Jefferson Health System, Philadelphia, PA

Robert L. Glueckauf, PhD, Center for Research on Telehealth and Healthcare Communications, Department of Clinical and Health Psychology, and the VA Brain Rehabilitation Research Center, University of Florida, Gainesville

Allen W. Heinemann, PhD, Northwestern University Medical School and Rehabilitation Institute of Chicago

Mark Jensen, PhD, Department of Rehabilitation Medicine, Harborview Medical Center, Seattle, WA

Monica Kurylo, PhD, Rehabilitation Psychology, OSF Saint Francis Medical Center, Peoria, IL

Aimee J. Luebben, EdD, Occupational Therapy Program, University of Southern Indiana, Evansville

Steven Mendelsohn, Esq., Lawyer and Advocate, New York

David W. Nickelson, PhD, Practice Directorate, American Psychological Association, Washington, DC

Theresa Louise-Bender Pape, Dr PH, MA, Rehabilitation Institute of Chicago and Edward Hines Jr. Veterans Administration Hospital, Hines, IL

David R. Patterson, PhD, Department of Rehabilitation Medicine, Harborview Medical Center, Seattle, WA

Barth Riley, PhD, Department of Disability and Human Development, University of Illinois at Chicago

Diana Hopkins Rintala, PhD, Department of Physical Medicine and Rehabilitation, Baylor College of Medicine, Houston, TX

Caren L. Sax, EdD, Interwork Institute, San Diego State University, CA

Marcia J. Scherer, PhD, Institute for Matching Person & Technology, Webster, NY, and University of Rochester Medical Center, Rochester, NY

Denise G. Tate, PhD, ABPP, Department of Physical Medicine and Rehabilitation, University of Michigan, Ann Arbor

Rhoda Weiss-Lambrou, Professor, School of Rehabilitation, Faculty of Medicine, Université de Montréal, Canada

Jeffrey D. Whitton, BSW, Center for Research on Telehealth and Healthcare Communications, Department of Clinical and Health Psychology, University of Florida, Gainesville

ACKNOWLEDGMENTS

Much gratitude is due the Rehabilitation Engineering and Assistive Technology Society of North America and Division 22, Rehabilitation Psychology, of the American Psychological Association (APA), for their support of this book. In return, each of these two organizations will share the royalties from its sales. It is my fondest hope that the monies received will be used to encourage and foster continued efforts in the overarching theme and subject matter the authors have presented herein. I also hope that these two organizations will continue to collaborate in the future.

Susan Reynolds, Acquisitions Editor, and Ed Meidenbauer, Development Editor, both of APA Books, receive my appreciation and accolades for their unswerving belief in this project and their dedication and hard work in seeing it through to successful publication.

Finally, I extend thanks to all my former educators and mentors, my spouse, colleagues, and past and present consumers, each of whom has taught me valuable lessons in better listening, helping, and reaching out to and working with others.

Assistive Technology

INTRODUCTION

MARCIA J. SCHERER

Rehabilitation professionals have a long and rich history of coordinating their services to help individuals with disabilities achieve lifestyles that maximize their physical functioning, independence, employment, and quality of life (QOL). This "rehabilitation team" has traditionally comprised physicians specializing in physical medicine and rehabilitation (physiatrists), rehabilitation psychologists, rehabilitation nurses, vocational rehabilitation counselors, occupational therapists, physical therapists, social workers, and other specialists, depending on need.

In 1990, it was not unusual for a person with a new and significant disability receiving acute rehabilitation services to stay in rehabilitation for months, and the rehabilitation team would have the opportunity for many collaborative discussions regarding the person's treatment course and rehabilitation plan. More than a decade later, a person with a new disability may receive acute rehabilitation services for only a few weeks, with ongoing rehabilitation being provided on discharge to one's home or other community setting. The emphasis now is on minimizing the length of stay in rehabilitation without reducing the quality of rehabilitation. To many rehabilitation providers, this often seems an impossible goal.

The need to contain health care costs and to help the people who arrive to rehabilitation "quicker and sicker" have placed a strain on both the system and the providers and consumers who must operate within it. Today's consumers, who in general are better educated and more assertive than consumers of even 10 years ago, may perceive an adversarial relationship between them and providers when requests for services go unanswered or are only partially addressed. Rehabilitation providers, trained to help people achieve independent and satisfying post-illness or –injury lives, often feel frustrated when having to keep cost containment in such close focus.

A new rehabilitation paradigm is in operation today, one that emphasizes expanded spheres of involvement while often failing to provide essential supports necessary to succeed.

HELPING PEOPLE WITH DISABILITIES LIVE ACTIVE, COMMUNITY LIVES

A person with very poor or no eyesight can read almost any printed material independently today. Twenty, even 10 years ago, such a person would likely have required the services of another person to read materials to him or her, thus resulting in loss of privacy. A person with little or no hearing can converse and interact in real time with anyone in the world by means of the printed word as delivered through the Internet or text telephones. People who cannot independently walk have more means to travel independently than ever before.

Because a great many people with disabilities can now lead more independent lives in their communities, attend regular schools, and seek professional careers than ever before in history, a plea is being heard to move away from the medical model of rehabilitation, which focuses on the disability and the limitation of its effects, to a social model, which emphasizes the person and his or her participation in society at large—for example, beyond the provision of prosthetic limbs to the consideration of how such limbs affect where that person can walk and the goals that can be achieved once he or she arrives there. This expansion of rehabilitation's sphere of concern and involvement has meant an evolution from a philosophy of normalization (people with disabilities should strive to be like people without disabilities) to empowerment (people with disabilities have the right to be self-determining and to make their own choices about their lives and to achieve the QOL each believes is personally best). As much—or more—emphasis is to be placed on community (re)integration as on physical rehabilitation and functional capabilities. One practical example of this change is the newly revised *International Classification of Functioning, Disability and Health*, also known as ICF (World Health Organization, 2001), in which a disability is seen as a consequence of efforts to interact and participate within a variety of environments. Thus, rehabilitation attention is now to include a focus on the built and attitudinal features of environments that impede a person's participation. This has tremendous implications for all rehabilitation professionals and the services they provide. A key service that will be given increased attention as a result is *assistive technology* (AT).

To function more independently at home, school, work, and throughout the community, people with physical disabilities often require assistance. This assistance may come from another person, such as a family member or paid personal assistant, or from an AT device.

AT devices are tools for enhancing the independent functioning of people who have physical limitations or disabilities. They range from low-tech devices, such as built-up handles on eating utensils, to high-tech ones, such as computerized communication systems for people with speech disabilities and battery-powered wheelchairs for people with mobility limitations (e.g. Galvin & Scherer, 1996). Examples of commonly used devices are listed in Table I.1.

Every piece of federal legislation enacted since 1988 regarding people with disabilities has explicitly referred to AT devices and services, a term initially defined in the Technology-Related Assistance for Individuals With Disabilities Act of 1988 (known popularly as "the Tech Act," which was reauthorized in 1998 as the Assistive Technology Act). An AT device is "any item, piece of equipment, or product system, whether acquired

TABLE I.1
Examples of Assistive Technologies Within Major Product Categories

Category	Examples
Recreation—These products enable people to participate in social activities, team sports, and other forms of indoor and outdoor recreation	• Adapted games • Gardening aids • Sports wheelchairs
Sensory disabilities—Devices in this category assist people with vision or hearing loss	• Tactile and auditory mobility aids • Auditory signaling devices • Print and computer screen magnification devices • Audiotapes • Vibrating pagers and alarm clocks
Communication—Products for communication center on the ability to send and receive messages in spoken and written form	• Adapted telephones • Captioned television • Voice-controlled computer input • Writing aids • Speech output devices
Personal care—These devices enable independence in such fundamental areas as grooming, bathing, dressing, eating, and accessing home appliances	• Eating utensils with angled or built-up handles • Razor holders • Reachers • Nonslip placemats under dinner plates • Bath sponges • Book holders • Transfer boards • Commode chairs
Mobility—Devices in this category provide support for people to get around in their environments of choice	• Walkers • Canes • Crutches • Manual and powered wheelchairs, scooters • Portable ramps

Note. These product categories represent only a partial list from the ABLEDATA classification system. ABLEDATA is a compilation of more than 26,000 assistive devices organized by functional activities. See http://www.abledata.com

commercially off the shelf, modified, or customized, that is used to increase, maintain, or improve functional capabilities of individuals with disabilities" (Scherer, 2000, p. 37). From the above definition, one can see how broad a scope the term *assistive technology devices* covers. Basically, an AT is any product that is useful to a person's enhanced functioning and participation. Key to an individual obtaining such devices is the availability of AT providers and services. An AT service is

> Any service that directly assists an individual with a disability in the selection, acquisition, or use of an assistive technology device, including . . . evaluation of the needs of an individual . . .; Purchasing, leasing, or otherwise providing for the acquisition by an individual with a disability of an assistive technology device; Selecting, designing, fitting, customizing, adapting, applying, maintaining, repairing, or replacing assistive technology devices; . . . Training and technical assistance. (Scherer, 2000, p. 185)

Today, because of legislation like the Tech Act and advances in technology, a person with control over just his or her arms and shoulders and above can live alone, travel, and work in a competitive job. It can generally be said that individuals with the most severe disabilities require the most customized, computerized, complex devices to achieve enhanced independent functioning. In fact, if these technologies were not available, many individuals with severe or multiple disabilities would not be able to attend school and work.

There are more than 26,000 AT devices available, making the process of choosing the most appropriate device for a particular user more complex and time consuming.

MOVING FROM A MEDICAL TO A SOCIAL MODEL OF SERVICE PROVISION

There are two opposing forces in rehabilitation today: (a) people with disabilities who want more comprehensive care and (b) the realities of the need to contain costs and deliver services in the most cost-efficient manner possible. Although it may be tempting to rely heavily on ATs to help consumers become more independent in their functioning, more than ever people with disabilities say they need and want more comprehensive rehabilitation—especially rehabilitation that acknowledges and works with their feelings, moods, and attitudes; helps them to become more self-determining, to have choices and to exercise choice; and facilitates community participation. Rehabilitation psychologists are uniquely qualified to assist in all of these areas.

Rehabilitation psychology has traditionally embraced coping with and adjustment to disability, yet rehabilitation psychologists have been late in assessing and understanding the contribution ATs can make to a person's enhanced sense of well-being. While always focusing on QOL, the key role ATs play in the achievement of a high QOL has been largely ignored by psychologists until very recently. Thus, a major purpose of this book is to discuss a variety of realms related to AT use in which rehabilitation psychologists have a tremendous amount to contribute; I also hope it will point out to professionals in other disciplines involved with AT areas in which rehabilitation psychology can provide valuable support and assistance.

Regardless of one's primary discipline, rehabilitation professionals can expect to see changes in how they work with consumers and deliver their services as they increasingly move from a medical to a social model of rehabilitation. If you are an educational, developmental, health, clinical, counseling, or rehabilitation psychologist, this book has been put together with you in mind. If you are an occupational or physical therapist, a rehabilitation engineer, a speech–language therapist, or a special educator, this book has also been created for you. Figure I.1 depicts three essential areas in the new rehabilitation paradigm around which the topics in this book have been organized and that will affect all rehabilitation providers as they strive to provide people with disabilities with the best possible services. I discuss these three areas, and the substantive contributions offered by experts in these areas who graciously agreed to author chapters, in turn below.

Larger Society

Disability is no longer considered to be merely a reflection or result of an individual's developmental or medical condition but a situation that arises from a societal perspective of what it means to have a limitation in one or more aspects of expected functioning. Therefore, rehabilitation now must address societal (or social) and cultural views of disability as well as the personal meaning (or construction) of disability.

The physical–architectural, legislative–political, and attitudinal–cultural environments in which AT services are provided and in which consumers live and work will be affected by legislation and changes in health care policies. Accessible transportation will need to be provided throughout an entire community (central city and suburbs). AT use in school, the home, workplace, and community will all receive increasing attention.

The first chapter in this book sets the larger stage on which the subsequent chapters are based. AT is a young field that exists within society at large, which means it reacts to and acts on changes in legislation, public

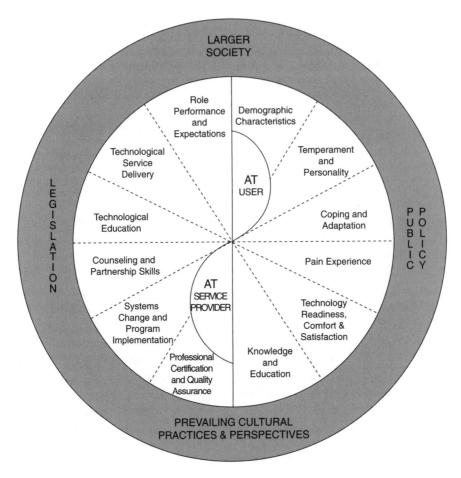

Figure I.1. Primary factors comprising the assistive technology (AT) service process.

policy and societal priorities, and attitudes toward people with disabilities and the rehabilitation delivery system. In chapter 1 Steve Mendelsohn and Heather Roberts Fox trace the development of the field of AT and rehabilitation in the context of civil rights; barriers in the built environment; shifting emphases in social policy; and various pieces of legislation, such as the Rehabilitation Act of 1973, the Individuals With Disabilities Education Act, the Americans With Disabilities Act, and the Assistive Technology Act.

The Individual AT User

AT users differ as much personally as they do functionally. Each potential user brings to the AT evaluation and selection process a unique set of needs and expectations. Adding to the complexity of matching users with the most appropriate AT is a variety of attitudinal and environmental influences on the use of AT—the factors that impinge on the rehabilitation and AT matching process from society at large.

Individuals vary in their attraction to AT use and their readiness for use. As rehabilitation professionals strive to help people with disabilities achieve their self-determined goals and inclusion in all aspects of community and society, it is imperative that personal preferences are addressed when matching a person with an AT device. The assessment of individual preferences, ways to help individuals articulate their goals and dreams, and methods for combating obstacles to personal growth are major areas of expertise that rehabilitation psychologists can offer the AT field. In chapter 2, by Denise Brown-Triolo, factors influencing a person's readiness for and use of AT are reviewed, with an emphasis on identifying those factors early in the rehabilitation and device evaluation process. It is hoped that attention to these factors will reduce the underutilization rate for ATs.

Psychological readiness, or lack of readiness, for technology use is a strong determinant of use, nonuse, or less-than-optimal use. For many users of ATs, their devices become an extension of the self, not just to themselves but also to other people. The device, then, is incorporated into the individual's identity. However, this process can be difficult for some, thus leading to underutilization or nonuse of ATs. In chapter 3 the importance of personality and its assessment is discussed in the context of person–technology matching by Timothy Elliott, Monica Kurylo, and Michele Carroll.

Another influence on decisions to use or not use an AT has to do with pain as it is subjectively experienced. Pain must be assessed, and in chapter 4 David Patterson addresses many options for accomplishing this, including the use of AT as an assessment tool.

Pain may also be an outcome of AT use. Once an AT device is obtained and used, the matching process is not over. It is important to assess the user's physical and psychological comfort with a device and his or her level of satisfaction with use in various environments. This is the focus of chapter 5, by Rhoda Weiss-Lambrou.

Rehabilitation professionals are concerned about the QOL of individuals with disabilities and how ATs can positively affect an individual's QOL. QOL has been described as life satisfaction, subjective well-being, and a positive general affect. In addition to these global constructs it is associated with satisfaction in specific areas of life, such as work, social relationships, and being able to go where one wishes beyond the mere physical capability to do so. To comprehensively address QOL, rehabilitation professionals need to attend to many areas of life functioning as well as background and demographic factors (including gender, age, and race–ethnicity). Although rehabilitation professionals have traditionally tried to control for these factors in rehabilitation research, chapters 6 and 7, by Diana Rintala and Laura Gitlin, respectively, embrace such differences and advocate making them an important part of matching the person with the most appropriate technology for his or her use.

The successful integration of an AT device into a user's lifestyle ideally results in a higher QOL for that person. The psychosocial aspects of achieving this are reviewed and discussed by Allen Heinemann and Theresa Louise-Bender Pape in chapter 8.

Successful integration of AT use into a person's lifestyle also depends heavily on the acceptance of AT by family members and the willingness to adjust customary routines to accommodate use. In chapter 9, Jan Galvin and Chandra Donnell discuss many issues that need to be considered when educating consumers, their families, and caretakers about the effective use of AT. Next, in chapter 10, Denise Tate, Barth Riley, and Martin Forchheimer discuss ways rehabilitation psychologists can help people with disabilities and their families and caregivers examine the benefits of technology even in a challenging arena of shorter lengths of inpatient stays and restrictive health care financing.

The AT Service Provider

As indicated in Figure I.1, AT users and service providers have unique characteristics and roles, yet they will increasingly need to form a partnership and share responsibilities. More than ever, consumers will "partner" with providers in product evaluation and selection as rehabilitation providers strive to individualize services, help people achieve their self-determined goals, and be included in all aspects of community life. To achieve a good match of person and technology it is important that the potential technology user be paired with a well-informed provider.

The field of AT is only about 20 years old, yet the existence of AT undergraduate programs and interdisciplinary graduate programs in rehabilitation science makes it imperative that the field incorporate diverse perspectives and focus on collaborative initiatives—especially in this challenging health care climate. In chapter 11 Rochelle Balter discusses future roles for rehabilitation professionals in light of consumer empowerment, diversity, and lifelong learning.

The majority of people who use assistive devices are older than age 65, which reflects the higher prevalence of impairments in this population. The push to keep aging people home and out of hospitals or nursing care facilities for as long as possible means that more health care and rehabilitation services will move into consumers' homes. As Robert Glueckauf, Jeffrey

Whitton, and Dale Nickelson discuss in chapter 12, future rehabilitation services will increasingly be delivered outside of rehabilitation facilities, and telecommunications technologies will play a role in the actual delivery of rehabilitation services.

Many individuals, however, show an aversion to replacing more and more interpersonal interactions with technologies, something that can be overcome by understanding the particular user and providing appropriate training in the use of those technologies. Providers will have to become user centered and not technology centered.

Professionals will face the need to address a number of constituencies and stakeholders and will need to inform a variety of publics about the availability and benefits of AT in ways that can reach them easily and in an understandable, personalized way. More information about specific devices will be available on the Internet, and the use of information technologies for narrowing down product options and ordering devices will proliferate. In addition, the education of consumers and caretakers will be done by means of distance learning and use of the Internet. Caren Sax, a pioneer of instruction in AT delivered by distance-learning technologies, discusses in chapter 13 the value of this approach in educating AT providers and consumers in diverse settings and geographic locations.

Improvements will continue in the design and availability of technologies. To keep the focus on the user of these products and services, providers must play a key role in assessing user preferences and predispositions to the use of particular technologies and must assess the outcomes of those products and services provided. In chapter 14 Serenella Besio, a rehabilitation psychologist and AT specialist, discusses how the evaluation and selection of ATs can be facilitated by a user-centered counseling process. Next, in chapter 15, Gerald Craddock discusses how a user-centered AT service delivery process can be implemented throughout an entire region—in this case, the Republic of Ireland. His model program has effectively resulted in systems change and the empowerment and involvement of consumers in rehabilitation research and the delivery of AT services.

AT is a new field and one in which credentialing of practitioners is only a few years old. A push for quality assurance and for providers of rehabilitation and AT services to demonstrate competency in their areas of specialization is at present well under way. In the near future, continuing professional development in AT, as well as the education and training of new practitioners in the field, will be addressed in tandem. The delivery of instruction and continuing education will be accomplished more by distance learning than in traditional classrooms. In the appendix, Aimee Luebben provides a model from the field of occupational therapy as relevant for similar efforts in the field of AT.

Finally, by way of tying together many of the book's themes, Al Cook, a past president of the Rehabilitation Engineering and Assistive Technology Society of North America, contributes in chapter 16 his thoughts on what the future for ATs and rehabilitation is likely to be like. He discusses both current trends as well as issues looming on the horizon.

CONCLUDING THOUGHTS

Rehabilitation professionals associated with the American Psychological Association's Science Directorate and Division 22 (Rehabilitation Psychology) and with the Rehabilitation Engineering and Assistive Technology Society of North America, have contributed chapters to this book with the goal of providing a forum for the discussion of key influences on the delivery of AT and other rehabilitation services in the context of today's health care system and societal priorities. This book thus aims to present a multidisciplinary set of chapters of relevance to students, practitioners, and researchers and to appeal to rehabilitation engineers; occupational, physical, and speech–language therapists; rehabilitation, clinical, counseling, and developmental psychologists; special educators and faculty training the aforementioned in university-based courses; people affiliated with independent living centers and organizations for people with disabilities and their families.

The shared perspective of this volume—consumer-centered service delivery with a goal of attainment of QOL beyond the mere enhancement of physical capability—can also be said to be its bias. Authors were invited to contribute chapters based on their practices, which in some cases collaboratively involved myself, and readers will definitely note a distinctive trend for the authors to reference one another's work. If this is a limitation, then it needs to be pointed out as such. Readers should also keep in mind that several colleagues were asked to contribute but had to decline because of the nature of the demands on their time. Thus, the omission of any particular contributor cannot be assumed to mean lack of agreement with the book's fundamental premises.

AT is a field for the future. Professionals in AT and rehabilitation psychology who are enthusiastic about maximizing the potential of individuals with disabilities will benefit tremendously by obtaining a good working knowledge of the many varieties of AT products and services involved and various ways to involve and partner with the technology user. Although it is difficult today to have all the benefits of an interdisciplinary rehabilitation team, this book aims to provide perspectives from a variety of disciplines to help guide readers into more informed AT evaluation and selection.

REFERENCES

Galvin, J. C., & Scherer, M. J. (Eds.). (1996). *Evaluating, selecting and using appropriate assistive technology*. Gaithersburg, MD: Aspen.

Scherer, M. J. (2000). *Living in the state of stuck: How technology impacts the lives of people with disabilities* (3rd ed.). Cambridge, MA: Brookline Books.

World Health Organization. (2001, May). *ICF: International classification of functioning, disability and health, final draft* [On-line]. Retrieved from http://www.who.int/icidh

I

THE CONTEXT OF
ASSISTIVE TECHNOLOGY
SERVICE DELIVERY

1

EVOLVING LEGISLATION AND PUBLIC POLICY RELATED TO DISABILITY AND ASSISTIVE TECHNOLOGY

STEVEN MENDELSOHN AND HEATHER ROBERTS FOX

Technology has long been a key component of rehabilitation. One needs only to reflect on the widely held notion of "rehabilitation" as physical rehabilitation, involving treatment and training after illness or injury, to appreciate the long and implicit relationship between these two subjects.

The term *assistive technology* (AT) was coined in the Technology-Related Assistance for Individuals With Disabilities Act of 1988 (P.L. 100-407), but the concept, under a variety of names or under no particular name at all, long predates that legislation. Elsewhere in this book is discussed the shift in thinking about technology from the medical to the social model. Suffice it to say here that although wheelchairs, hearing aids, Braille watches, and other traditional devices were often provided under medical auspices, their function as AT devices is now clear and indisputable. It is not the source of a device or the affiliations of a third-party funder that defines its nature as AT. The device's function does that.

Even within rehabilitation programs the prevalence of the medical model left little room for consumer choice in services or for consumer involvement in decision making regarding the extent and content of those services. It was not until the emergence of the independent-living movement in the 1960s and its first statutory embodiment in 1973 (Rehabilitation Act of 1973, P.L. 93-112) that the right of consumers to have choice in services and devices began to gain legitimacy and attention.

EMERGENCE OF A CIVIL RIGHTS PERSPECTIVE

The modern era of U.S. disability policy dates from the 1970s and is epitomized by the enactment within a span of 7 years of four major statutes incorporating all the paradigms, as well as contradictions, in our nation's disability policy: (a) the Architectural Barriers Act of 1968 (P.L. 90-480, which created the requirement that buildings and facilities constructed with federal funds be designed to be "accessible" to individuals with disabilities); (b) the Social Security Act Amendments of 1972 (42 U.S.C. Sec. 1382 et seq., which established the Supplemental Security Income program and in other respects defined the scope of income maintenance programs); (c) the Rehabilitation Act of 1973 (P.L. 93-112, which established the modern program of federal–state partnership in the provision of vocational rehabilitation [VR] services to individuals with disabilities but which also created the first national civil rights protections against discrimination on the basis of "handicap" and created federally funded independent-living concepts for the first time); and (d) the Education of All Handicapped Children Act of 1975 (P.L. 94–142), now the Individuals With Disabilities Education Act.

Whether these laws ignited a social revolution or merely betokened one that had already occurred is beyond the scope of this chapter. What can be said is that they created the major policy themes that have emerged, and battled for primacy, in most legislative debates that followed. They established the notion that people with disabilities have a civil rights interest, not only in the services they receive but also in the treatment they receive from society as a whole. They also created (albeit inadvertently) a complex web of work disincentives that continue to stifle many people with disabilities in their efforts, including their efforts through the use of technology, to achieve independence, autonomy, and self-sufficiency. They gave structure to the kinds of federal–state relationships that have likewise characterized most programs that have followed on their heels. Also, they created the notion of universal design, as a legal principle, by requiring that in light of the difficulties and expense associated with retrofitting, facilities paid for with federal funds be designed with accessibility features in mind from the outset.

Although the legislative mandates covered in the next sections are broad, our goal is to describe more fully the language that protects individuals with disabilities in educational and work environments. In these summaries we do not attempt to incorporate interpretations of the law based on case law decisions rather, the summaries of the statutes are supplemented with information on federal government programs and implementing agency regulations. Readers are encouraged to investigate refinements of the legislation that has resulted from legal action and from future regulatory guidance that attempts to clarify or strengthen any of these legislative provisions.

Rehabilitation Act of 1973, as Amended

The first significant piece of federal legislation to protect the civil rights of people with disabilities was the Rehabilitation Act of 1973, the purpose of which as it has evolved over the years is to

1. assist States in operating a coordinated, comprehensive, effective, accountable (VR) program designed to assess, plan, develop and implement VR services in order for individuals with disabilities to prepare for and engage in gainful employment (Sec. 100[a][2]);
2. empower individuals with disabilities to maximize employment, economic self-sufficiency, independence, and inclusion and integration into society through: (a) comprehensive and coordinated state-of-the-art programs of (VR); (b) independent-living centers and services; (c) research; (d) training; (e) demonstration projects; and (f) the guarantee of equal opportunity; and,
3. ensure that the Federal Government plays a leadership role in promoting the employment of individuals with disabilities, especially individuals with severe disabilities, and in assisting States and providers of services in fulfilling the aspirations of such individuals with disabilities for meaningful and gainful employment and independent-living of individuals with disabilities, especially those with severe disabilities. (Sec. 2 [b] [1][2])

Sections 501, 503, and 504 contain the primary language that fosters the Act's general goal to "promote and expand employment opportunities in the public and private sector for handicapped individuals." Specifically, Section 501 requires federal agencies to implement affirmative action programs within the federal civil service to advance opportunities for individuals with disabilities. In addition, Section 503 required federal contractors receiving contracts over specified amounts to go beyond nondiscrimination and take affirmative action to employ and advance in employment qualified handicapped individuals.

Section 504 of the Rehabilitation Act, in perhaps the most sweeping effect of the act, states that

> No otherwise qualified individual with a disability shall, solely by reason of his or her disability, be excluded from the participation in, be denied

the benefits of, or be subjected to discrimination under any program or activity receiving Federal financial assistance. (29 U.S.C. 794[a])

The provisions of Section 504 apply to a federally funded program or agency, a private organization that receives federal financial assistance, all public elementary and secondary education programs, and the vast majority of public and private institutions of higher education. The provisions of Section 504 and its regulations are designed to ensure equal opportunities for individuals with disabilities to "benefit" from any aid, benefit, or service and to participate in employment and other life activities without discrimination.

The enforcement provisions of the act have been progressively strengthened by each successive amendment, including those of 1992, which brought the law into compliance with the Americans With Disabilities Act of 1990 (described later). The 1992 amendments and, more recently, the Rehabilitation Act Amendments of 1998, place emphasis on serving individuals with severe (now referred to as *significant*) disabilities. The criteria for individuals who meet this qualification must be established by each state and must be based on the statutory definition of the term.

In 1998 Congress significantly restructured the VR system by incorporating the Rehabilitation Act into the Work Force Investment Act (P.L. 105-220) and linking the VR system to the new federal–state job training and placement system operating through the "one-stop" centers and related modalities. An eligible individual is now seen as a collaborating partner with the qualified rehabilitation counselor in the development, monitoring, implementation, and evaluation of the individualized plan of employment (IPE). Consistent with the integration of VR into the broader national labor force development effort, the 1998 Rehabilitation Act amendments also encourage greater cooperation between the VR and special education systems. These amendments strengthen in several ways the provisions for the planning and coordinating of "transition services" for youths as they prepare to leave school.

Individuals With Disabilities Education Act

In 1975, Congress passed a law to require that states "ensure that all children with disabilities have available to them a free appropriate public education that emphasizes special education and related services designed to meet their unique needs and prepare them for employment and independent-living" (P.L. 94-142). The law, now known as the Individuals With Disabilities Education Act (IDEA), has been amended several times and was most recently reauthorized in June 1997 (P.L. 105-17).

IDEA attempts to guarantee that the rights of children with disabilities and their parents are protected. The act has been extended to help states implement a coordinated and comprehensive system for early intervention for infants and toddlers with disabilities. Because IDEA deals with children and youth, while VR provides adult services, the need for interagency collaboration in managing the transition from educational to community-based services is great. The services involved in this process are "transitional services" and are dealt with in both the Rehabilitation Act and IDEA.

In many respects, the protections afforded by IDEA are identical to those of Section 504 in the Rehabilitation Act; however, some students with disabilities are not covered under IDEA but are covered by Section 504. Students with disabilities who do not meet the standard for receipt of special education services are not covered by IDEA or most analogous state laws but still qualify for a Section 504 accommodation plan, which is intended to help the institution avoid discriminatory practices. A student qualifies for special education and "related services" only if an educational deficit can be identified to which the services are responsive, or when the services are needed to enable the student to participate in educational activities. Thus, existence of a definable sensory, physical, mental, or cognitive impairment is not the test of eligibility for special education. Equally though, by reason of Section 504, students have civil rights protections going beyond those set forth in IDEA.

IDEA sets out detailed procedures by which children are evaluated and appropriate programs of special education are developed. For a program to be "appropriate" it must be based on and responsive to the child's individualized educational needs as identified in the evaluation process. IDEA requires extensive parental involvement in the child's evaluation and the planning of the child's program. IDEA requires a written individual education program (IEP) to be developed for the student with a disability. Among the variety of services authorized under IDEA, assistive technology devices and services are especially important. Depending on the context, they may be special education or related services. Their greatest significance lies in their critical role in facilitating the central goal of IDEA: to provide children with disabilities a mainstream education in the "least restrictive environment" as a matter of course.

Americans With Disabilities Act

The Americans with Disabilities Act (ADA) of 1990 (P.L. 101-336) is the United States' landmark disability civil rights law. The purpose of the ADA is "to provide a clear and comprehensive national mandate for the elimination of discrimination against individuals with disabilities and to provide clear, strong, consistent, enforceable standards addressing discrimination against individuals with disabilities." The ADA defines *disability* as a physical or mental impairment that substantially limits one or more major life activities, a record of such impairment, or being regarded as having such an impairment.

Also protected under the ADA are those discriminated against on the basis of their "association" with people who have a disability and those subjected to retaliation for assisting individuals with disabilities to assert their rights under the law.

Major life activities include seeing, hearing, walking, caring for oneself, learning, breathing, and working. The ADA prohibits discrimination against people with disabilities in the areas of employment, public services of state and local government, and public accommodations provided by private entities. While the employment provisions of the ADA apply to employers of 15 employees or more, the public-accommodations provisions apply to all sizes of business, regardless of the number of employees. Responsibility for enforcing the ADA is divided among a number of federal agencies, including most notably the Equal Employment Opportunity Commission (EEOC), the Department of Justice, and the Department of Transportation.

Title I of the law addresses discrimination in employment and is regulated by the EEOC; it draws heavily on two earlier pieces of legislation: Section 504 of the Rehabilitation Act of 1973 and Title VII of the Civil Rights Act of 1964. The ADA applies to all aspects of employment: hiring, promotions and transfers, training, compensation, employee benefits, layoffs, and terminations. In particular, certain steps in the hiring process that may serve to intentionally or unintentionally screen out candidates with disabilities (e.g., employment testing, medical examinations, or interview questions) are highly regulated. Employers cannot inquire if someone has a disability. Employers are permitted, at any time, to ask the candidate or employee about his or her ability to perform job-related functions.

The ADA requires employers to make reasonable accommodations that do not cause "undue hardship," so that a qualified individual with a disability can perform the job's essential job functions. The EEOC released enforcement guidance in 1999 explaining an employer's legal obligations regarding reasonable accommodation and undue hardship. There are a number of typical reasonable accommodations that an employer may have to provide in connection with modifications to the work environment or adjustments in how and when a job is performed. These include making existing facilities accessible; job restructuring; part-time or modified work schedules; acquiring or modifying equipment; changing tests, training materials, or policies; providing qualified readers or interpreters; and reassignment to a vacant position.

Title II of the law addresses public services of state and local government. Public services and programs must be equally accessible to people with or without disabilities.

Title III of the law requires that all new construction and modifications must be accessible to individuals with disabilities. For existing facilities, barriers to access, including barriers to effective communications, must be removed if this is readily achievable. Public accommodations include a broad range of organizations and facilities that affect commerce, such as restaurants, hotels, retail stores, private educational institutions, and recreational facilities. Titles I and III also require the entities they cover to provide auxiliary aids and services necessary to enable people who have sensory or other communication impairments to participate in the program. The business may choose among various alternatives as long as the result is effective communication. Title AND of the ADA, although not a civil rights statute in the same sense as the earlier three titles, mandates the provision of key telecommunications relay services to facilitate use of the telephone system by people who have severe hearing impairments or are deaf (and for people with speech disabilities as well). To the degree that such access to the telecommunications network is basic to full participation in society, these services may also be regarded as civil rights.

Assistive Technology Act of 1998

On November 13, 1998, President Clinton signed into law the Assistive Technology Act of 1998 (AT Act; P.L. 105-394), which affirms the importance placed on the role of technology to improve the lives of people with disabilities. The AT act extends for three years the funding of the 50 states and 6 U.S. territories that had received funding under an earlier version of the statute addressing AT.

Congress formally recognized the value of AT devices and services for individuals with disabilities when it enacted the Technology-Related Assistance for Individuals with Disabilities Act of 1988 (P.L. 100-218) and when it reauthorized the "Tech Act" upon its first sunset (P.L. 103-218). Like the Tech Act before it, the AT Act authorizes a variety of activities related to making ATs available to individuals of all ages. Among the modalities used in the Tech and AT Acts are capacity-building in state government, community outreach activities, public awareness efforts, technical assistance and information provision, barrier identification and removal, and other strategies. Most recently, the 1998 legislation provided funding to implement an AT loan program, which is now in operation in six states. The AT Act, as the Tech Act before it, also established national programs of technical assistance. Current programs coming under this rubric emphasize technical assistance to state AT projects and outreach to various other stakeholder communities.

One important element of the AT Act, dating back to the 1994 amendments to the Tech Act, is its support of funding for individualized legal advocacy in connection with AT by state-based protection and advocacy (P & A) legal services agencies. Under the AT Act, state protection and advocacy agencies receive funding directly from the National Institute on Disability and Rehabilitation Research, the administrating agency for the AT programs.

Our primary task in following these legislative and policy strands is to understand how they have affected the development of the profession of rehabilitation psychology. However, to the degree that we are particularly concerned with the interplay between technology policy and rehabilitation psychology, our inquiry must give some attention to parallel changes in the nature and role of technology itself.

THE MOVE TO INTEGRATED DEVICES

No technology exists in isolation from the general trends in materials, design, and aesthetics that prevail at any given time. Once electricity came into common use, a variety of household appliances were invented. The advent of the microchip made possible a variety of new devices and capabilities but also led to the redesign, through incorporation of microchips, of almost every familiar consumer device, ranging from the television to the automobile. AT, in tandem with technology as a whole, has passed through several generations or iterations within our lifetimes. These generations are defined not only by predominant engineering principles and materials but also by functional features, assumptions about the people and environments in which they were designed to function, and fundamentally important precepts about the nature of society itself. To understand these assumptions is to know a great deal about how rehabilitation practice, if not philosophy, has evolved over the past two generations.

The period from the end of World War II to about 1970 can be characterized as the era of self-contained technology. Devices designed for or purchased for use by people with disabilities could be bought and used in relative isolation. A wheelchair could be fitted and maintained without regard to the personal needs or preferences of the individual. Certainly the destinations to which one wanted to travel were not ordinarily a consideration in their prescription. Indeed, few choices in size or design were available. In the stand-alone character of devices, technology for the mainstream consumer and business market paralleled technology for people with disabilities during this postwar period. The phonograph was not purchased separately from speakers, turntables, or compact disc changers. The typewriter, manual or electric, did not come with modular keyboards, detachable printers, or other add-on component options. Consumers might have had a great deal of choice in some products, but that choice was exercised when selecting a brand and model. Nor were few disability-related issues often confronted in the design of mainstream technology. If visual displays were added to telephones, or audible reminders to cars, or if the number of steps on a city bus was increased or decreased, the rationale had little to do with the concerns of consumers with disabilities. Indeed, the notion of people with disabilities as a defined class of patrons or customers would not have been on the minds of most urban planners or automobile designers. The idea of incorporating technical breakthroughs into products for people with disabilities was practically unheard of until only a short time ago.

People may argue long and hard over the legacy of the 1960s for society, but for people with disabilities one unquestioned result of that decade was a promotion of disability as a social phenomenon more than a medical one and that a given physical condition could be more or less disabling, depending on the environment in which it occurred. If a building had a ramp by which an individual who used a wheelchair could enter and leave it, the wheelchair user was more autonomous, much less disabled than he or she would be if the building did not have such a ramp. It would be difficult to overstate the implications of the shift in the nature of technology and the nature of attitudes. Suddenly, disability was converted from an absolute to a relative phenomenon, capable of being functionally greater or lesser depending on the design, accommodation, and other decisions that society made. Suddenly, issues of mainstream public policy inevitably affected people with disabilities, and decisions made about disability policy in a vacuum were likely to be narrow and poorly considered. So it is that while we have continued to enact legislation that purports to deal specifically with disability issues, such as the acts reviewed in this chapter, people with disabilities and their issues have steadily made their way into mainstream legislation as well. From such key provisions of the Internal Revenue Code as the architectural barriers removal deduction of 1976 (Internal Revenue Code Sec. 190), to key and controversial features of the Telecommunications Act of 1996, such as Section 255, which creating accessibility requirements for the telephone system (P.L. 104-104, Sec. 255), disability policy and other areas of public policy can no longer be separated and addressed apart. Nor should they be. Today technology is increasingly best described in terms of integrated design. As this feature of the mainstream technology and information environment relates to AT, it means that unless a device or system is designed with accessibility features built in from the beginning, their potential accessibility to and usability by individuals with disabilities is substantially, and in many cases totally, nullified.

This is true of what may be called the *technology infrastructure* as well. Consider the case of closed captioning. Without reservation in the TV spectrum of a line or wavelength for the transmission of the captions, the captions could not be made available to consumers. Absence of a secondary audio channel from television receivers or on VCRs would likewise preclude the mandating of audio description or descriptive video services for people with visual impairments, no matter how strongly public policy might support its availability.

It should come as no surprise that in a society where the capabilities of people without disabilities are increasingly measured by what their technology can do, the extent to which people are disabled has likewise become more relative, more a function of technology and the overall interface between individual and environment, than ever before. Yet it is perhaps more our understanding of this interface more than any of its actual characteristics that have changed most.

AT CATEGORIES

Federal law may be said to include five major categories of AT policy. These are best described as (a) the research and development/technology transfer mode, (b) the design specification mode, (c) the reasonable accommodation mode, (d) the technical assistance mode, and (e) the service delivery mode. Although no statistics are available, let alone consensus criteria for determining how much AT would be enough, there are grounds for believing that the rehabilitation system has not made nearly the use of AT that many advocates would deem appropriate. Owing to our concern here with rehabilitation, let us examine some of the issues specific to the rehabilitation system's response to technology.

Many of the key variables that have determined the VR system's response to AT appear to derive less from rehabilitation theory than from organization science; that is, internal organizational factors, ranging from the commitment of agency leadership to technology, to the availability of expert resources to do technology assessments, to the add-on system costs associated with adding major technology initiatives to the traditional range of goods and services provided with program funds. Variables such as these are presumably not specific to VR, but the VR system's response to the demands and opportunities posed by technology are also unique. For example, in recent years the VR system has attempted to implement principles of consumer responsiveness and even consumer direction at various levels. This has included greatly enhanced consumer participation in (and approval of) their own individualized service plans. However, applying these precepts of consumer involvement to the use and provision of technology presents some vexing problems. Consumers may have technology aspirations that transcend the increasingly artificial barriers between vocational and nonvocational pursuits. After all, to say that a computer can be used to access only work-related information on the Internet is arbitrary and all but unenforceable. To deny technology to an individual because it exceeds his or her immediate needs for job placement, even when the capabilities and functions in question are likely to become necessary in the near future, represents the height of bureaucratic rigidity in the view of many. Yet when rehabilitation agencies define their mission as assisting people into entry-level employment, this is precisely the sort of determination they frequently are obliged to make. Such distinctions have little to do with technology but much to do with the requirements of current law. Finally, the current emphasis on consumer choice often collides with the historic role of experts—medical, psychological, and others—who are looked to for various assessments, evaluations, and recommendations, or who in some cases are delegated legal authority for making key recommendations, in some instances including recommendations of the appropriate AT. Just as the most skilled rehabilitation engineers cannot be expected to encompass all the variables that go into an individual's technology preferences and choices, so too is the most sensitive professional unlikely to know the individual's situation well enough to understand fully why nuanced distinctions among devices or service providers may make a huge difference to the ultimate outcome.

Efforts to integrate the consumer-choice or customer-satisfaction model with the traditional expert-decisionmaker approach varied in their success and impact. As a service delivery system, rehabilitation has always focused on identifying and meeting the needs of the individual. Although this for-the-good-of-the-client concept has accorded VR agencies considerable discretion, it may also have led to an undue focus on exhaustive eligibility determinations, diagnosis and assessment of needs and deficiencies as the predicate for developing service plans, and contention between agencies and service recipients, framed often in legal terms, over who has the ultimate right and power to make decisions about what the scope and content of services will be. However it may be that technology could or should be a vehicle for linking the policy choices made in VR with the priorities of the broader society, there is little evidence (particularly in light of the exemption of VR for people with disabilities from the broad reform of labor policy in this country under the Workforce Investment Act of 1998) that this linkage has taken place.

A final issue in this connection relates to the question of what modalities are in fact rehabilitative. Established providers have historically rendered specified services and furnished a reasonably well-established range of devices. In an age of integrated technology, the distinction between mainstream and AT has greatly blurred. What becomes of the traditional rehabilitation provider in such an environment? Also, to the degree that professional expertise remains a jurisdictional prerequisite for decision making, who is qualified to conduct the key evaluations and make binding recommendations?

CONCLUSION

The statutes described in this chapter have profound implications for individuals with disabilities and their families as well as for the professionals in the field who provide services to people with disabilities. Because many children and adults benefit from disability policies, rehabilitation services, and AT, it is critical that stakeholders continue to advocate for strong legislation, increases in funding, greater access to technology and services, and consumer-directed choice. Community efforts to heighten public awareness and recognition from policymakers will help to eliminate the barriers to successful educational, employment, and social outcomes for people with disabilities.

Advocacy can yield many benefits in terms of systems change and heightened resources. But without a thorough analysis of the legal, organizational, and theoretical premises upon which rehabilitation is based, the impact of successful advocacy may be seriously compromised.

REFERENCES

Albertson's, Inc. v. *Kirkingburg,* Docket No. 98-0591.

Murphy v. *United Parcel Service, Inc.,* Docket No. 97-1992.

Sutton v. *United Airlines,* Docket No. 97-1943.

II

THE USER OF ASSISTIVE
TECHNOLOGY DEVICES
AND SERVICES

2

UNDERSTANDING THE PERSON BEHIND THE TECHNOLOGY

DENISE L. BROWN-TRIOLO

The field of assistive technology (AT) encompasses many professions, each with its own disciplinary understanding of the client. Many take a medical viewpoint, some take a biomechanical stance, whereas others view individuals from a psychosocial perspective. One commonality among all AT professionals is their focus on increasing independence and attaining the personal goals in the day-to-day life of an individual with a disability. The delivery of the technology is not an end in and of itself; the processes involved in ensuring adequate attention to the finer points of technology integration include a unique understanding of the person with a disability. Professional efforts to deliver the targeted technology can be successful only if attention is given to the needs of the individual. This chapter summarizes the contemporary perspectives of AT services with a focus on evaluating the individual behind the technology. An overview of AT assessment issues is provided, followed by two case examples of AT service delivery in which the personal characteristics of the recipients were and were not taken into consideration. Finally, current trends and issues in assessing people for ATs are examined.

UNDERSTANDING THE PERSON BEHIND THE TECHNOLOGY

Rehabilitation professionals have just recently begun to seriously study the issues of who uses assistive devices and why they use them. This may seem counterintuitive, but it is the truth: Only since researchers began to focus on the reasons for abandonment of technology have they looked beyond the technology to the users. This section examines assessment of individual users of AT.

Use and Abandonment From the User's Perspective

Most research related to AT use and abandonment has looked at a multitude of factors, such as costs of devices, physical skills necessary for use, demographics, and device reliability and safety (Brooks, 1991; Heinemann, Magiera-Planey, Schiro-Geist, & Gimines, 1987; Phillips & Zhao, 1993). When factors associated with the person with a disability are included, the data are typically combined with environmental, technological, and disability-specific determinants (Brooks, 1991; Phillips & Zhao, 1993; Scherer, 1988). For instance, Phillips and Zhao (1993) reported an abandonment rate of 29.3% for assistive devices and found four factors that significantly related to nonuse. The factors of (a) change in user needs, (b) easy attainment of the device, (c) poor performance of the device, and (d) lack of consideration of the user's opinion during selection were related to abandonment of assistive devices among users with various disabilities. Only one of these predictors of abandonment relates directly to the technology itself (factor [c], above), and one relates to the process of attainment (factor [b]). In Phillips and Zhao's study two of the primary factors that significantly predicted abandonment are related to the person using the technology (factors [a] and [d], above). Even though the results of this study and those like it report the importance of personal characteristics of technology integration and positive match, rehabilitation professionals may fail to address these issues during the assessment process.

For AT professionals who work with younger populations the scene is not that much different. A few studies have investigated AT device use by pediatric populations (Caudrey & Seeger, 1983; McGrath et al., 1985). McGrath et al. reported on the device use and satisfaction of families in Canada. Use rates of such devices as hearing aids, wheelchairs, seating and positioning devices, prostheses, and respiratory equipment ranged from 77% to 100%. Respondents were the children themselves, a parent, or another family representative. Even though 70% of the respondents said they felt the devices were somewhat or very attractive, the devices kept some of the children (8.3%) from performing activities they thought were important; for example, a positioning device curtailing movement. In McGrath et al.'s study even though an AT was well matched cosmetically it could still be in the way. For children with disabilities, use and abandonment of AT devices are often influenced by other people in their lives, more so than for older individuals. High usage rates of newly prescribed equipment among children with disabilities were determined to be attributable to forced compliance by parents, teachers, and therapists in one study (Caudrey & Seeger, 1983). Problems of AT abandonment have led to work on more appropriate matching of assistive devices to their potential users prior to actual service delivery.

Multidimensional Models Incorporating Persons With Disabilities

AT research infrequently goes beyond identification of percentages and reasons for abandonment and usage-related factors and seeks to determine causal factors and person-centered aspects of technology use. In a qualitative study of individuals with spinal cord injury and cerebral palsy, Scherer (1988) found a dynamic relation among technology use, temperament, personal characteristics, and quality of life. Scherer linked successful device use to beliefs in personal benefits. Technology use was found to be influenced by factors associated not only with the user's environment and characteristics of the technology but also with the characteristics and nature of the purpose of use and to cognitive, personality, and temperament characteristics of the user. Longitudinal support for Scherer's (1988) findings was found in a follow-up investigation (Scherer, 1990). In Scherer's (1990) study the original 10 persons with disabilities—5 with spinal cord injuries and 5 with cerebral palsy—who had been interviewed for the 1988 study were again interviewed, observed, and then asked to complete a functional–personal capacities questionnaire and an assessment of temperament. Two additional participants with recent spinal cord injuries were also added. The follow-up design allowed for natural changes in the participants' lives to be catalogued and critically analyzed through a comparative case study design.

From this research Scherer developed a model for use in matching persons with appropriate technological interventions (Scherer, 1997). The matching person and technology (MPT) model states that the characteristics of the person, the milieu, and the technology need to be considered when using a given technical intervention (Scherer Associates, 1991; Scherer & McKee, 1991). Assessment instruments and processes based on this model are available for children with disabilities and their families through the Matching Assistive Technology and CHild (MATCH) system (Scherer, 1997) and for adolescents through adults through the Survey of Technology Use and the Assistive Technology Device Predisposition Assessment (Scherer, 1994; see Table 2.1). In most MPT instruments the degree of consumer and technology match is evaluated through the comparison of professional and client–consumer subscores in the areas of personality and temperament, technology, and environment. The Assistive Technology Device Predisposition Assessment (ATD PA) consists of a set of tools that guide professionals and AT device users in considering relevant use and nonuse issues during the selection of needed technologies. The ATD PA produces scores in four areas that have been shown to influence use and nonuse of an assistive device: (a) assistive device characteristics, (b) temperament and personality of the user, (c) disability factors, and (d) the psychosocial arena or environments of use (Scherer, 1994). The tools associated with the MPT model have utility in AT service delivery, research, and

TABLE 2.1
Assistive Technology (AT) Assessments With a Person Focus

Instrument	Purpose	Model/Basis	Scores
Matching Assistive Technology and CHild (MATCH; Scherer, 1997)	For infants through 5-year-olds • Selecting appropriate ATs • Identifying areas for further assessment	MPT	None—requires face value interpretation
Survey of Technology Use (Scherer, 1994)	For infants through adults: • Identifying a sense of well-being and self-esteem around technology	MPT	• Experiences with current technologies • Perspectives on technologies • Typical activities • Personal–social characteristics
Assistive Technology Device Predisposition Assessment (Scherer, 1994)	For adolescents through adults • Ensure consumer input in AT match process • Consideration of influences on AT use • Communication of perspectives	MPT	• Assistive device characteristics • Temperament and personality characteristics • Disability factors • Psychosocial arena–environment
Psychosocial Impact of Assistive Devices Scale (Day & Jutai, 1996)	*No age range specified by authors • Provide psychosocial outcomes of ATs • Prediction of AT use • Aid in research and design of ATs	• Self-efficacy • Competence • Quality of life	• Competence • Adaptability • Self-esteem
Quebec User Evaluation of Satisfaction With Assistive Technology (Demers, Weiss-Lambrou & Ska, 1996)	*No age range specified by authors • Evaluating personal satisfaction • Outcomes data for reimbursement • Justification of ATs	• MPT • Multidimensional satisfaction	• Satisfaction with milieu • Satisfaction with person • Satisfaction with the technology

Note. MPT = matching person and technology model.

clinical practice (Rehabilitation Engineering and Assistive Technology Society of North America [RESNA], 1998). The assessment process is meant to aid in attaining individualized information about the person and the assistive device, to assist in identifying obstacles to successful use, and to reduce abandonment. Scherer (1997) cautioned that the model and its accompanying tools are "not designed to predict use or non-use of a technology."

Psychosocial Methods

In other research focused on the person behind the technology, Day and Jutai (1996) developed the Psychosocial Impact of Assistive Devices Scale (PIADS; see Table 2.1). Specifically, the PIADS measures the AT device's impact on the user's quality of life, in areas such as self-efficacy, self-confidence, competence, and self-esteem. The PIADS contains three subscales: (a) Competence, which includes efficiency, quality of life, and independence; (b) Adaptability, which includes perceived well-being, abilities in new situations, and willingness to take chances; and (c) Self-Esteem, which includes happiness, embarrassment, sense of control, and self-confidence. The PIADS has been used in evaluating the outcomes of use of certain ATs in clients with amyotrophic lateral sclerosis (Jutai & Gryfe, 1998). Results show an overall positive psychosocial impact of assistive devices on the users. Jutai and Gryfe (1998) suggested that the PIADS be used to measure psychosocial outcomes of assistive devices, shed light on patterns of use and nonuse of technologies, aid in prediction and justification of technology applications, and assist in research and development of assistive devices in daily living and vocational arenas.

Person-Focused Satisfaction

Interest in user or consumer perspectives by rehabilitation and AT professionals has been an emerging trend (Brooks, 1991; Gjøderum, 1994; Reswick, 1994; Simon & Patrick, 1997; Walker, 1995). One specific area of interest is in consumer satisfaction. Simon and Patrick (1997) referred to three functions of satisfaction: (a) a global or unidimensional response; (b) a multidimensional response to service experiences, which is generally affective in nature; and (c) a stimulus to aid in decision making about future behaviors. Satisfaction data can assist the rehabilitation professional in improving services (quality-improvement efforts), in responding to accountability demands (outcome measurements), and in marketing services to future consumers (customer satisfaction). The Quebec User Evaluation of Satisfaction With Assistive Technology (QUEST; see chapter 5) is a consumer- and disability-friendly tool that assesses a user's satisfaction with an assistive device (Demers, Weiss-Lambrou, & Ska, 1996; see Table 2.1). The

QUEST is based on the MPT model (Scherer Associates, 1991) and the subjective and personal nature of attitudes and personal standards. Device users are asked to first attribute a degree of importance to different satisfaction variables that cover the three domains of technology, user, and environment. Next, the AT user is asked to rate his or her level of satisfaction with specific variables across a 5-point scale. A summary of the satisfaction of only those areas of importance allows this tool to be individualized to the specific and personal concerns of the AT user (Demers, Weiss-Lambrou, & Ska, 1997). The QUEST can aid in providing outcomes data for reimbursement issues and in person-centered justification of ATs.

Focus on Specific Populations: Children and Families

The Individuals With Disabilities Education Act Amendments of 1990 (P.L. 101-476) extended the ages of mandatory special education down to the preschool years and included provisions for AT as a separate service for children with disabilities. Per this law, consideration of the need for AT, which is defined in the same manner as in the Technology-Related Assistance of Individuals With Disabilities Act of 1988 (P.L. 100-407), is mandated in each child's individualized education plan or individualized family service plan.

Previous assessment techniques for determining the appropriateness of an AT for a child with a disability have been criticized for their narrow view and for failure to include families in the formula for effective match (Parette & Brotherson, 1996). Family-centered care is a person-focused principle that sees the family as central to the evaluation process and related services for children with disabilities (Shelton, Jepson, & Johnson, 1987). It has been found that children respond best to technology when they have peer support and the technology can act as social support to families by decreasing performance of certain stressful tasks (Parette & VanBiervliet, 1991; VanBiervliet, Parette, & Bradley, 1991).

A comprehensive model of involving families in the process of AT service delivery for children with disabilities incorporates collaboration and individualization (Parette & Brotherson, 1996). This model first calls for an approach to assessment that recognizes the roles of families in all areas (technology, service system, family, and child) and addresses the linkages between these areas. Examining the effects of the AT on the family system, a family systems assessment, is the second area required for comprehensive AT service delivery to children with disabilities and their families. The last area of the model describes providing families with necessary information about ATs to ensure informed decision making. Scherer's MPT model and MATCH assessment process also reflect the growing movement toward ensuring that families are viewed as the constant in the child's life (Scherer, 1997).

For children with disabilities, person-centered variables with a focus on developmental needs and milestones should be considered in all interventions, including the match of a child with an AT (Holder-Brown & Parette, 1992). The appropriateness of an assistive device should relate to any learning or developmental need of the child. Child characteristics can include present level of functioning, cognitive and pre-academic skills, behavior and social skills, and consideration for the child's preferences (Parette, Hourcade, & VanBiervliet, 1993).

Factors that could influence a child's AT use include motor skills; cognitive–developmental readiness; temperament factors, such as motivation, attention, and persistence; and sensorimotor integration (Furumasu, Tefft, & Guerette, 1996). Technology access for children with disabilities should not be limited to certain environments; AT needs to be multifaceted (Holder-Brown & Parette, 1992). The family has a great deal of impact on AT use for children with disabilities, yet they have historically been ignored (Parette & Brotherson, 1996). A comprehensive AT assessment should include an evaluation of family factors, needs, expectations, and systems, allowing for avoidance of unintended negative outcomes. Such family factors can include caregiving practices, routines, economic resources, and physical layout of the home environment. Attention to these is important, because an AT device can affect the quality of life of the family as well as the child. What is seen as a positive effect may often produce an unintended negative effect on the family, such as added stress, change in family roles, and disruption of routines. An AT device for a child may turn out to be problematic when a family has to make a trade-off of the positive aspects and benefits of the AT versus overall family quality-of-life factors (Parette & Brotherson, 1996).

Advocates of AT for children with disabilities emphasize the need for the device to be compatible with the areas with which and the persons with whom it will be associated (Holder-Brown & Parette, 1992; Scherer & Galvin, 1996). It is imperative that the technology results in a desirable and sufficient outcome of increasing skill and independence. The device needs to be compatible within an environment over time, and the AT must meet the available cost, training, and maintenance resources of the environment and the affiliated technology users. Holder-Brown and Parette (1992) considered AT devices for children a means to increasing a child's experiences and a facilitator of behavior change rather than an ends.

Many times AT is limited by what is available or known. A specific technology doesn't necessarily have to be the most recently developed type of its kind; what is important in decision making is that the technology in question is the most accepted in the child's world. Aspects such as convenience, ease of use for adults, and expense should be considerations, but not the only deciding factors, in regard to appropriate technology for young children with disabilities. Thought also should be given to use of assistive devices that draw undue attention to the child's disability. This sort of technology match highlights the child's differences, which might be a pertinent factor for some children or in some environments. AT aspects worthy of further consideration include its goals of use; availability; customization or modification needs; simplicity of operation; initial and ongoing costs, such as installation or replacement expenses; the device's reliability; and its ability to be adaptable to other needs of the child over time.

CASE STUDIES

The following case studies are representative of AT assessment processes. The first scenario includes a typical AT assessment process but one that did not focus on the individual until a retrospective review was done. The second case represents a focus on the individual and family in a work environment that was less formal and nontraditional.

Becky

Becky was 21 years old at the time of her evaluation, which occurred 1 year after her discharge from a pediatric rehabilitation facility with a research AT device that would help Becky with standing. The device was in the research and design phase of development and thus not widely available. This device had been used by others for mobility, exercise, and access to high places in home and social environments. Becky had incurred a spinal cord injury at the low thoracic level following a gunshot wound when she was 18. Becky was attending a technical school full-time at the time of evaluation. She had used the AT to do household chores, such as putting dishes away on high shelves and doing laundry. In the 2 months before the evaluation she had not used her device and had never used it in other, nonhome environments. Becky stated as her reason for abandonment that the device took too much time to put on and take off. No formal person-centered tests that evaluate personality or temperament had been conducted before Becky was given the device. She did, however, go through a comprehensive rehabilitation evaluation that included psychosocial screening by a social worker and physical and strength evaluations by various rehabilitation professionals (such as physical therapists, medical doctors, occupational therapists, and rehabilitation engineers). Becky's training for the device included a lengthy inpatient hospital stay, minor surgical procedures, and strength and endurance training.

A postintervention evaluation of person-centered factors (Brown, 1996) was conducted and included collection of disability-specific data of personal independence using the Personal Independence Profile (Nosek, Fuhrer, & Howland, 1991), degree of societal handicap using the Craig Handicap Reporting Technique (Whiteneck, Charlifue, Gerhart, Overholser, & Richardson, 1992), device match information using the Assistive Technology Device Predisposition Assessment (Scherer Associates, 1991), and developmental information on self-image using the Offer Self-Image Questionnaire (Offer, Ostrov, Howard, & Dolan, 1992). Results showed a young adult with low average self-image and feelings of inability to control her emotions, frequent depressive symptoms and family tension, and a focus on the negative. Becky showed an ability to deal with frustration and felt relatively confident of ultimate success, but she also showed symptoms of being at risk for single-episode depression and suicidal ideation and attempts. Becky showed a relatively high degree of perceived control of her life yet low psychological self-sufficiency and physical autonomy. Her ATD PA match results revealed that the standing device posed a potential problem in the technology–person match. Becky's only reason for not using the standing device was device related, and she did not use the device during the 2 months prior to her evaluation. Becky's use responses and her decision to abandon the AT device reflect the mismatch between her and the standing system. This assistive device mismatch seems to be due to a variety of interrelated factors, including low psychological self-sufficiency, perceived lack of appropriate psychosocial and family support, and symptoms of affective depression. It became clear that Becky had ambiguous feelings about the standing device. Involvement in the process of fitting the device (an extended inpatient hospitalization stay) met her immediate needs of disability peer group socialization, associated boosts in self-esteem, and relief from a problematic family situation as well as a means to work on independence skills. A more comprehensive and formal assessment of person-centered factors conducted before Becky began the AT training program could have added insight into the needs she felt the program would meet for her and helped in developing alternative plans for having those needs met. Specifically, it would have been prudent to incorporate a screening device, such as the ATD PA or PIADS, prior to device implementation. Such information could have identified family support needs, affective state and traits relative to Becky's feelings about herself and disability, and areas needing further assessment. Through tools such as these Becky's primary needs—those of social integration with disabled peers and autonomy from an undesirable family situation—could have been identified and addressed.

George

George was an 18-year-old high school student in a special education program for individuals with developmental disabilities and delays. He had spastic quadriplegic cerebral palsy and had received special education services and related interventions since preschool. George used a power wheelchair for mobility and had visual–spatial and speech difficulties. He wore eyeglasses yet did not use AT for communication. He was at the point where he was preparing for life after high school and had just become involved in a transition program in which he was exposed to a variety of job-related skills and tasks and expected to gain meaningful job experiences.

Evaluation for job skills training would entail job modifications using technology and related accommodation means. George's AT experiences were assessed with the Survey of Technology Use (Scherer Associates, 1991). An informal vocational evaluation of George indicated that he had interests in sports, social activities, and computers. Problem solving to develop appropriate job experiences and technological solutions for ultimate participation included meetings with George, his teacher, a technology and accommodations consultant, his physical therapist, and a work–study coordinator. Initial experiences in janitorial work with the necessary adaptations to his wheelchair were identified. After consultation with George's parents, it was found that this type of work was unacceptable to them because of its stigmatizing nature. Additional team meetings for problem solving involving the parents were conducted, and the alternative job of mail delivery within an office setting was identified. Wheelchair adaptations, floor plan layouts, and job coaching were used to help give George the tools necessary to complete the job functions.

George became quite productive and successful in this position, which met a variety of needs. He was able to socialize with peers and coworkers, his family felt confident that he would not be stereotyped by a stigmatizing job often left for those with disabilities, and he was able to gain important transferable skills and work behaviors that he could apply to a multitude of jobs and environments. By considering the family's needs as well as George's in a problem-solving process, the intervention team was able to identify necessary changes to the initial plan, eliminating the opportunity for abandonment of technology.

CURRENT TRENDS

Measuring the outcomes of ATs has become a driving force behind AT assessment in recent years (DeRuyter, 1995, 1997; RESNA, 1998;

Scherer, 1996; Smith, 1996). All health care professionals have found it necessary to document the effectiveness of their interventions for third-party reimbursement. Monitoring professional abilities through outcomes has become a necessary component of marketing rehabilitation services and ensuring ethical and professional work. The World Health Organization's (WHO's) classification of disablement has been a catalyst in outcomes measurement in health care (WHO, 1980). The *International Classification of Impairments, Disabilities and Handicaps* (*ICIDH*; WHO, 1980) is a model intended to classify diseases into three areas. *Impairment* occurs at the body or organ level and includes losses or abnormality in function; *disability* occurs at the person level and includes limiting conditions; and *handicap* occurs at the societal level and relates to how well a person is able to fulfill society's expectation of appropriate roles (WHO, 1980).

Recently the WHO initiated a campaign to revise the *ICIDH* to incorporate social understandings of disablement. This new model is based on a universal model of human functioning and recognizes not only the medical and societal variants of disabilities but also the impact of the social and human-built environments on the individual (WHO, 2001). The *ICF* (WHO, 2001) includes four dimensions: (a) impairments at the body level, (b) activities at the person level (formerly disability), (c) participation at the social level (formerly handicap), and (d) contextual factors. These contextual factors list physical environment features, such as climate, and social environment factors, such as attitudes, laws, and institutions. Interaction of the environmental factors with the three levels of functioning result in functioning that is either positive or negative. The addition of this new dimension reflects the needed recognition of the unique and personal nature of a disability's impact on a person's life.

This newer classification system can assist AT professionals in standardizing assessment efforts for clinical and research purposes. According to the *ICF* nomenclature, assistive devices and accommodations are seen as interventions for the negative outcomes of activity and participation because of impairments (WHO, 2001). The addition of the emphasis on the interaction of environmental features, both physical and social, adds an important context within which persons with disabilities can be evaluated. Professionals need not see this as an additional area of assessment and thus an added burden to one's responsibilities; rather, this recognition could just be the incentive that compels AT professionals to further consider the person behind the technology, in interaction with all his or her environments, during the match of that person and AT. AT assessments of the future should incorporate contextual interactions and measure these effects on the person with a disability.

Each of the three assessment methods just described—the MPT model instruments, the PIADS, and the QUEST—add a unique aspect to the field of AT service delivery. Much of the scope of AT user needs is addressed in these instruments, from looking at multidimensional screening of the match between a person and an AT to the specific outcome of satisfaction after AT service delivery. All, however, are psychometrically similar in the testing principles of purpose for testing, level of measurement, referencing or comparison methods, reliability and validity, and overall evaluation principles. All have similar purposes: to screen—to discriminate one kind of individual from another or to identify those needing further assessment; to assess—to evaluate specific behaviors in depth, to provide means of monitoring progress, or to determine who gets what; and to provide research data—to further describe a phenomenon, to predict behaviors, or to evaluate outcomes. All use ordinal measurement levels by which the collected data are scored using a logical hierarchy with unequal intervals. All three use criterion referencing, versus norm referencing, for comparison. These tests look at individual performance based on a specified standard rather than comparison with a larger population. The reliability and validity of two of these tools, the MPT model instruments and the PIADS, have been systematically addressed (Day & Jutai, 1996; Scherer, 1993; Scherer & McGhee, 1992). All three tools have easy-to-use administration procedures and scoring criteria, and all incorporate descriptive methods to report the data collected.

What are missing from the available procedures to assess person-centered aspects of ATs, although not necessarily outside the scope of the next generation of these tools, are methods that are more sophisticated psychometrically. These first attempts to provide clinicians and AT specialists with tools to accurately and adequately measure the particular needs of individuals who use AT have provided a necessary missing piece to the puzzle. Yet because of the external pressures to measure outcomes of rehabilitation, there exists a need for measurement techniques that have high levels of reliability and validity, use normative samples for comparison, and use more precise means of measurement. Without imposing too many qualifications on the evaluator, next-generation evaluation tools need to also incorporate test administration strategies and evaluator training procedures that eliminate procedural and scoring error. These challenges are coupled with the practicalities facing the AT professional: those of needing (a) a tool that can be used routinely, (b) within the service delivery system, and (c) with a multitude of assistive devices and disabilities (Jutai, Ladak, Schuller, Naumann, & Wright, 1996).

SUMMARY

Although AT has potential for increasing the quality of life of persons with disabilities, success is not guaranteed. With the high rate of technology abandonment, and the costs and energies seemingly wasted though misuse and abdication of AT devices, it is important that technology becomes integrated into the lives of those who will use it and benefit from it. One of the best ways to ensure this is for AT professionals to look beyond the technology and physical features of the user and focus on the unique characteristics of that user. Through a thorough investigation of areas associated with levels of use (Scherer, 1996) and application of that knowledge to real world events, AT can result in the outcomes intended: skill acquisition and independence in the lives of persons with disabilities. At the same time, unintentional yet synergistic outcomes such as quality-of-life enhancement can be realized.

REFERENCES

Brooks, N. A. (1991). Users' responses to assistive devices for physical disability. *Social Science and Medicine, 32,* 1417–1424.

Brown, D. L. (1996). Personal implications of functional electrical stimulation standing for older adolescents with spinal cord injuries. *Technology and Disability, 5,* 295–311.

Caudrey, D. J., & Seeger, B. R. (1983). Rehabilitation engineering service evaluation: A follow-up survey of device effectiveness and patient acceptance. *Rehabilitation Literature, 44,* 80–85.

Day, H., & Jutai, J. (1996). Measuring the psychosocial impact on assistive devices: The PIADS. *Canadian Journal of Rehabilitation, 9,* 159–168.

Demers, L., Weiss-Lambrou, R., & Ska, B. (1996). Development of the Quebec User Evaluation of Satisfaction With Assistive Technology (QUEST). *Assistive Technology, 8,* 3–13.

Demers, L., Weiss-Lambrou, R., & Ska, B. (1997). Quebec User Evaluation of Satisfaction With Assistive Technology (QUEST): A new outcome measure. In D. Brienza & E. Trefler (Eds.), *Proceedings of the RESNA '97 annual conference* (pp. 94–96). Arlington, VA: RESNA Press.

DeRuyter, F. (1995). Evaluating outcomes in assistive technology: Do we understand the commitment? *Assistive Technology, 7,* 1–8.

DeRuyter, F. (1997). The importance of outcomes measures for assistive technology service delivery systems. *Technology and Disability, 6,* 89–104.

Furumasu, J., Tefft, D., & Guerette, P. (1996, October). Pediatric powered mobility: Readiness to learn. *Team Rehab Report, 29, 32,* 34–36.

Gjøderum, J. (1994). User involvement in assessment and user influence in standardization of consumer products and assistive technology. In M. Binion (Ed.), (1988) *Proceedings of the RESNA '94 annual conference* (pp. 240–242). Arlington, VA: RESNA Press.

Heinemann, A.W., Magiera-Planey, R., Schiro-Geist, C., & Gimines, G. (1987). Mobility for persons with spinal cord injury: An evaluation of two systems. *Archives of Physical Medicine and Rehabilitation, 68,* 90–93.

Holder-Brown, L., & Parette, H. P. (1992). Children with disabilities who use assistive technology: Ethical considerations. *Young Children, 47*(6), 73–77.

Individuals With Disabilities Education Act Amendments, 20 U.S.C § 1401 (1990).

Jutai, J., & Gryfe, P. (1998). Impact of assistive technology on clients with ALS. In S. Springer (Ed.), *Proceedings of the RESNA '98 annual conference* (pp. 54–56). Arlington, VA: RESNA Press.

Jutai, J., Ladak, N., Schuller, R., Naumann, S., & Wright, V. (1996). Outcome measurement of assistive technologies: An institutional case study. *Assistive Technology, 8,* 110–120.

McGrath, P. J., Goodman, J. T., Cunningham, J., MacDonald, B. J., Nichols, T. A., & Unruh, A. (1985). Assistive devices: Utilization by children. *Archives of Physical Medicine and Rehabilitation, 66,* 430–432.

Nosek, M. A., Fuhrer, M. J., & Howland, C. A. (1991). *Measuring the independence in people with disabilities: The Personal Independence Profile.* Houston, TX: ILRU Research and Training Center on Independent Living.

Offer, D., Ostrov, E., Howard, K. I., & Dolan, S. (1992). Offer Self-Image Questionnaire, Revised (OSIQ–R) manual. Los Angeles: Western Psychological Services.

Parette, H. P., & Brotherson, M. J. (1996). Family participation in assistive technology assessment for young children with mental retardation and developmental disabilities. *Education and Training in Mental Retardation, 31,* 29–43.

Parette, H. P., Hourcade, J. J., & VanBiervliet, A. (1993). Selection of appropriate technology for children with disabilities. *Teaching Exceptional Children, 25*(3), 18–22.

Parette, H. P., & VanBiervliet, A. (1991). School-age children with disabilities: Technology implications for counselors. *Elementary School Guidance and Counseling, 25,* 182–193.

Phillips, B., & Zhao, H. (1993). Predictors of assistive technology abandonment. *Assistive Technology, 5,* 36–45.

Rehabilitation Engineering and Assistive Technology Society of North America. (1998). *RESNA resource guide for assistive technology outcomes: Volume II: Assessment instruments, tools and checklists from the field.* Arlington, VA: Author.

Reswick, J. B. (1994). What constitutes valid research? Qualitative vs. quantitative research. *Journal of Rehabilitation Research and Development, 31,* vii–ix.

Scherer Associates. (1991). *The Scherer MPT model: Matching people with technologies.* Webster, NY: Author.

Scherer, M. J. (1988). Assistive device utilization and quality-of-life in adults with spinal cord injuries or cerebral palsy. *Journal of Applied Rehabilitation Counseling, 19*, 21–30.

Scherer, M. J. (1990). Assistive device utilization and quality of life in adults with spinal cord injuries or cerebral palsy two years later. *Journal of Applied Rehabilitation Counseling, 21*, 36–44.

Scherer, M. J. (1993, October). *The Assistive Technology Device Predisposition Assessment: How does it measure up as a measure?* Paper presented at the 70th Annual meeting of the American Congress of Rehabilitation Medicine, Denver, CO.

Scherer, M. J. (1994). *Matching person and technology.* Webster, NY: Author.

Scherer, M. J. (1996). Outcomes of assistive technology use on quality of life. *Disability and Rehabilitation, 18*, 439–448.

Scherer, M. J. (1997). *Matching assistive technology and child.* Webster, NY: Institute for Matching Person and Technology.

Scherer, M. J., & Galvin, J. C. (1996). An outcomes perspective of quality pathways to most appropriate technology. In M. J. Scherer & J. C. Galvin (Eds.), *Evaluating, selecting, and using appropriate assistive technology* (pp. 1–26). Gaithersburg, MD: Aspen.

Scherer, M. J., & McGee, B. G. (1991, April). *The development of two instruments assessing the predispositions people have toward technology use: The value of integrating quantitative and qualitative methods.* Paper presented at the Annual Meeting of the American Educational Research Association, Chicago. (ERIC Document Reproduction Service No. TM 016 608)

Scherer, M. J., & McGee, B. G. (1992, April). *Early validity and reliability data for two instruments assessing the predispositions people have towards technology use: Continued integration of qualitative and quantitative methods.* Paper presented at the Annual Meeting of the American Educational Research Association, San Francisco. (ERIC Document Reproduction Service No. TM 018 385)

Shelton, T. L., Jepson, E. S., & Johnson, B. H. (1987). *Family-centered care for children with special health care needs.* Washington, DC: Association for the Care of Children's Health.

Simon, S. E., & Patrick, A. (1997). Understanding and assessing consumer satisfaction in rehabilitation. *Journal of Rehabilitation Outcome Measures, 1*, 1–14.

Smith, R. O. (1996). Measuring the outcomes of assistive technology: Challenge and innovation. *Assistive Technology, 8*, 71–81.

Technology-Related Assistance of Individuals With Disabilities Act, 29 U.S.C. § 3002 (1988).

VanBiervliet, A., Parette, H. P., & Bradley, R. H. (1991). Infants with disabilities and their families: A conceptual model for technology assessment. In J. Presparin (Ed.), *Proceedings of the 14th annual RESNA conference* (pp. 219–221). Washington, DC: RESNA Press.

Walker, M. L. (1995). Transforming disability research. *ReHab Network, 38*, 12–17.

Whiteneck, G. G., Charlifue, S. W., Gerhart, K. A., Overholser, J. D., & Richardson, G. N. (1992). *Guide for the use of the CHART: Craig Handicap and Reporting Technique*. Englewood, CO: Craig Hospital.

World Health Organization. (1980). *International classification of impairments, disabilities and handicaps: A manual of classification relating to the consequences of disease*. Geneva, Switzerland: Author.

World Health Organization. (2001). *ICF: International classification of functioning, disability and health, final draft* [On-line]. Retrieved from http://www.who.int/icidh/

3

PERSONALITY ASSESSMENT IN MEDICAL REHABILITATION

TIMOTHY R. ELLIOTT, MONICA KURYLO, AND MICHELE N. CARROLL

Many people who are considered for rehabilitative services participate in a psychological assessment. This assessment ideally informs decisions concerning need for services, the expense that accompanies sponsorship, and the provision of assistive equipment that can enhance quality of life. Psychological assessment is of particular importance during this era when many health care delivery systems limit access to care, which in turn can result in higher costs associated with the subsequent treatment of preventable conditions. Unfortunately, many psychologists are not trained to face the issues inherent in the assessment of persons with physical disabilities. These problems exist despite the original mandates of the Rehabilitation Act of 1973 for psychologists to have the rudimentary skills to conduct informed assessments of people with disabilities. In fact, the Rehabilitation Act of 1973 clearly stipulates that assessment may be necessary for the determination of eligibility and "vocational rehabilitation needs" and that the assessment might include the evaluation of "personality, interests, interpersonal skills, intelligence and related functional capacities . . . vocational aptitudes, personal and social adjustments and . . . other pertinent . . . cultural, social, . . . and environmental factors that affect the employment and rehabilitation needs of the individual" (Sec. 504, Rehabilitation Act of 1973).

Generally, assessment of personality and psychological adjustment are included within an informed and comprehensive battery, yet differences in qualifications and training can result in the differential use of these instruments and subsequent interpretation of results. For example, whereas classically trained clinical psychologists are sensitive to displays of psychopathology and aberrant behaviors, neuropsychologists focus intently on

This work was support in part by Grants HI33B30025-96 and HI33N50009-96A from the National Institute on Disability Rehabilitation and Research.

neurological impairment and brain–behavior relations, and those trained in counseling psychology usually are well versed in assessing career development concerns and vocational adjustment. Few psychology training programs adequately prepare doctoral students for the informed use of personality instruments with people who have physical or sensory disabilities (Elliott, 1993).

In this chapter we describe the historical background of personality assessment within medical rehabilitation. We also discuss the appropriate use of personality assessment in medical rehabilitation. Personality assessment ideally can inform consumers, health care workers, and financial providers of the costs and benefits of assistive technology (AT) for individuals from a psychological standpoint. Finally, we discuss ethical issues inherent in personality assessment in a medical rehabilitation setting.

HISTORICAL OVERVIEW

Psychological opinions about behavioral disorders among people with disabilities have historically displayed a lack of congruence. In the developing years of rehabilitation, practicing psychologists were few in number, and mental health specialists from a variety of other disciplines leaned heavily on impressionistic models of adjustment to disability. Many of these convenient and atheoretical models borrowed loosely from neo-Freudian concepts of stagelike dynamics in reaction to acute loss, and these guided many assessment practices. It was erroneously presumed, for example, that any person who acquired a physical disability would become depressed soon after injury onset, and this was considered adaptive and necessary for optimal adjustment (e.g., Nemiah, 1957). It is interesting that there was a separate camp of psychologists who believed that emotional disorders found among psychiatric populations traditionally served by mental health specialists were rare among medical patients (Belar, 1988). From this perspective, depression, anxiety, and characterological problems were often unrecognized and untreated, because clinicians suspected these behaviors were representative of transitory states.

These practices and beliefs have resulted in several unfortunate trends in assessment practices. First, there is a tendency toward use of instruments without regard to the theoretical background of the instrument and its intended use. Atheoretical models ignore individual differences and environmental influences on respondent behavior and their effects on adjustment. Second, psychologists often rely on assessment methods and instrumentation that are ill suited for the rehabilitation setting. The data that result from such methods inadvertently reinforce and perpetuate negative expectations in interpretations of behavior among people with disability.

Third, subjective interview methods are often used as a diagnostic tool (Williams & Mourer, 1990). This is a poor method for assessing enduring personality characteristics (Meehl, 1954), and clinical judgments based on interview methods are highly unreliable and inconsistent, regardless of the clinician's experience and training (Faust et al., 1988; Wedding & Faust, 1989).

Fourth, assessment is typically driven toward the detection of problems and is generally insensitive to the assessment of potential (Wright & Fletcher, 1982). Psychologists are primed to determine areas of concern and deficit and are generally insensitive to the assessment of abilities, resources, and personal and social assets. Psychologists, like others in the helping professions, are often insensitive to the situational and environmental determinants of behavior among people with physical and sensory disabilities. Consequently, many psychologists are apt to attribute the locus of a particular problem within the respondent and ignore contributing environmental and situational factors that frame, precipitate, or define a particular problem experienced by a client.

Finally, many clinicians are guided by the expectations that people with disabilities are preoccupied with the limitations imposed by the condition, and they are less sensitive or attentive to displays of commonplace, nonpathological behavior (Wright, 1983). Clinical observations are thus influenced by the clinicians' expectation that a person with a disability will exhibit advertent behavioral patterns (Wright, 1983). Thus, an overview of the extant research reveals a widespread use of measures of psychopathology and maladjustment in the assessment of people with physical disabilities (e.g., the Minnesota Multiphasic Personality Inventory [MMPI]; Elliott & Umlauf, 1995). Clinicians often infer personality characteristics from measures of distress, yet these measures were designed to assess problems and symptoms rather than routine and stylistic ways of thinking, behaving, and emoting under ordinary circumstances. Appropriate assessment of personality can and should take into account both nonpathological and potentially pathological aspects of the individual to provide a well-rounded and accurate cost–benefit psychological analysis for each individual who may be a potential AT user.

PERSONALITY EVALUATION FOR AT

When evaluating an individual with a disability for the explicit purpose of providing recommendations regarding AT, several concerns arise. What personality assessments are available? How should the results of the assessment be interpreted as they regard physical and sensory disabilities? What can the results of the evaluation tell health care professionals in terms of providing recommendations for AT?

Nonpathological and Pathological Assessment Devices

Nonpathological personality measures typically encompass trait or social–cognitive measures of personality. Trait measures, such as the NEO Personality Inventory and the NEO Five Factor Inventory (Costa & McRae, 1989), emphasize nonpathological assessment of personality in comparison to a normative sample. Social–cognitive measures, such as measures of problem-solving ability and locus of control, attempt to account for the situational context of an individual's character by examining nonpathological social–cognitive factors involved in everyday emotional functioning. In contrast, pathological personality measures typically include the more "traditional" personality measures in psychological assessment, such as the MMPI–2 (Butcher, Dahlstrom, Graham, Tellegen, & Kaemmer, 1989) and the Millon Clinical Multiaxial Inventory–III (MCMI–III; Millon, 1997).

Obvious differences between nonpathological and pathological types of assessments include (a) the manner in which the items are worded and in which the respondents answer, (b) the length of the measures and the time necessary to complete them, and (c) the theoretical and clinical interpretation of the resulting profile. It is important to consider that individuals who are asked to complete these assessment instruments may also notice these more obvious differences when given both types of measures. The manner of development and the theoretical background provide more subtle differences between the two types of measures.

Personality profiles from most psychopathological assessment devices imply that a respondent with a physical disability is preoccupied with physical sensations or ailments in comparison to the normative–nondisabled population (Elliott & Umlauf, 1995). This interpretation reinforces a stereotypic belief that people with acquired disability are preoccupied with limitations imposed by the physical condition (Wright, 1983). Established instruments should be used with caveats kept in mind for considering the influence of physical disability experiences on responses to certain items.

The selection of any assessment device should ideally be intricately connected to a logical intervention program that would enhance rehabilitation efforts for the respondent (Glueckauf, 1993). From this perspective, psychologists should be aware of a variety of assessment methods and the unique strengths and limitations of each. Moreover, these clinicians should know how to integrate assessment data within meaningful theoretical models of behavior so that logically derived intervention efforts may ensue. Psychometric data can provide a basis for a scientific approach to development of well-informed interventions. For example, cognitive–behavioral models of behavior often have clear directives for therapeutic intervention. Certain cognitive–behavioral skills (e.g., problem-solving skills), which would otherwise remain unmeasured and unnoticed by a treatment team that relies on interview methods or measures of psychopathology, have been related to the incidence of secondary complications and long-term adjustment among people with physical disabilities (Elliott & Jackson, 1996). Collectively, empirical data available across several patient populations indicate that psychological characteristics are crucial in patient adjustment, quality of life, and overall health above and beyond features of the chronic condition, etiology, or initial medical procedures (Taylor, 1991). Furthermore, use of nonpathological inventories to assess personality and behavioral functioning can be useful in appreciating the influence of the situation and environment on current behaviors and can aid in the interpretation of behavior within its particular context (Wright, 1983).

Interpreting the Results

There is a tendency for psychologists to administer psychometric instruments to people with disabilities and interpret the scores as if the respondents were not disabled (Myerson, 1957). Psychologists should use appropriate norms for people with disabling conditions. Unfortunately, appropriate norms and comparison groups are often not available. When appropriate norms are collected, personality profiling may reveal more important information than the typical finding of "preoccupation with physical sensations." In addition, appropriate norms may clarify the extent of symptomatology compared to peers who have similar physical limitations. For example, research has provided profile corrections for some populations on certain instruments (i.e., the Premorbid Somatic Complaint Questionnaire; Rodevich & Wanlass, 1995, correction for the MMPI–2 for use with individuals with spinal cord injury). Most important, however, psychologists should use theory-based perspectives in administering, interpreting, or conceptualizing data to develop theory-based interventions (Elliott & Umlauf, 1995).

Making Recommendations for AT

Few published studies to date have examined the association between personality and use or nonuse of ATs (Scherer, 1988, 1990), and no studies have examined personality profiles on pathological measures (e.g., the MMPI or MCMI) and their relation to use or nonuse of ATs. Although it is important that client behavior be understood and interpreted within the perspective of the interaction between person and environment (e.g., the field-theory perspective; Leung, 1984), it is equally as important that the relation between person and technology be understood. The technology must fit the person. For example, personality screening for potential sociopathy is important to complete before individuals are provided with videoteleconferencing equipment at home. There have been cases in which sociopathic individuals were provided with such technology and later pawned the device because the value they placed on the device was different from that of the provider of the technology. In this case, personality assessment conducted prior to the dispensation of the devices would have provided vital information regarding the potential for nonuse or misuse of the technology.

Until published studies examining personality inventories and use–nonuse of ATs are performed, we can provide only hypotheses and clinical anecdotes as a method of illuminating the need for personality evaluation when assessing an individual's suitability for AT. For example, individuals who are open to novel techniques and are emotionally stable (e.g., the Openness and Neuroticism factors on the NEO Five Factor Inventory) are probably more likely to use assistive devices than individuals who are resistant to novelty and who are anxious by nature. The case studies that follow provide powerful examples of the importance of personality testing in relation to provision of AT.

Clinical Anecdotes

Timothy R. Elliott was asked to evaluate a 30-year-old male with a spinal cord injury, Bob, who had been referred by vocational rehabilitation services after it was discovered that he was not using an expensive, specially designed bed purchased for him with vocational rehabilitation services funds. Despite Bob's history of several pressure sores, which initially prompted the suggestion of the purchase of the special bed, he was apparently sleeping on the floor. This in turn resulted in yet another pressure sore. He apparently continued to sleep on the floor after the special bed was provided. Because his demeanor was consistently pleasant, optimistic, and cooperative when he met with his caseworkers, they were confused regarding his nonuse of the technologies provided.

Dr. Elliott decided to assess Bob's personality with the MCMI–2, which provides a profile of personality styles that suggest potential for personality disorders. Bob's responses to the MCMI–2 suggested that he tended to display characteristics often found among people with antisocial and passive–aggressive personality disorders, as defined by the *Diagnostic and Statistical Manual of Mental Disorders* (4th ed.; *DSM–IV*; American Psychiatric Association, 1994) and *DSM–III* (1980). In other words, he was unlikely to conform to behavior that was expected of him, and he tended to be deceitful and irresponsible and lack remorse for his behavior. In addition, his profile suggested that he may also be likely to passively agree with and report compliance with treatment regimens and use of AT while actually being noncompliant when he was not in the caseworkers' presence (at home).

If the psychological assessment had been conducted before the expensive AT was purchased, this information could have been considered before investing considerable financial resources in this case, given that Bob's profile suggested that he would likely be nonadherent to the ATs provided. In addition, behavioral intervention, such as setting up a reward schedule, could have been recommended to boost his compliance with ATs. Specifically, Bob would be offered a reward for consistent use of the ATs provided with the understanding that he would not receive his reward if he could not show consistent use of the technological device.

A second clinical anecdote provides an example of the use of nonpathological devices in assessing personality. Mary, a 16-year-old girl who received a severe head injury in an automobile accident, underwent a neuropsychological evaluation approximately 6 months after her injury. As a part of this evaluation, she was given the Children's Depression Inventory and Revised Children's Manifest Anxiety Scale, and her parents completed the Child Behavior Checklist. In addition, Mary was interviewed individually by the psychologist; her parents also were interviewed. Although the measures given and the interviews were appropriate, the information gained through these methods focused on potential pathological behaviors and did not provide an adequate picture of the more positive, nonpathological aspects of her emotional functioning. Mary and the examiner may have benefited from administration of a measure of commonplace personality characteristics and social–cognitive abilities or attributes (e.g., the Hope Scale, a social–cognitive measure of goal orientation; Snyder et al., 1991). An additional measure of nonpathological personality functioning would have provided the examiner with a more positive orientation toward the aspects of Mary's personality that may have elucidated and informed decisions regarding recommendations for AT use. Mary and her parents ultimately decided, without benefit of the psychologist's input, that use of audiorecordings of classes would assist her learning and would allow her to continue to progress toward her life goals of graduating high school and eventually attending college.

ETHICAL ISSUES

Several ethical issues have accumulated and increased under the prevailing winds of managed care and health care costs. Despite the fact that opportunities for psychologists in rehabilitation have been increasing over the past 10 years (Frank, Buckelew, & Gluck, 1990), adequate training of psychologists for conducting assessments with people who have physical and sensory disabilities is lacking. Clinical assessment is a key component of psychological practice with people who have disabling conditions (Eisenberg & Jansen, 1987). However, inappropriate and insensitive use of psychological instruments with people who have disabling conditions can produce an array of inappropriate and misleading interpretations to the detriment of the client, the clinic, and the profession.

Elliott and Umlauf (1995) noted that psychological assessment with people who have disabling conditions is no longer a function of a simple, well-defined psychologist–client relationship. Psychologists should carefully consider prior to any psychometric assessment "who is the client" in any given assessment (Monahan, 1980). In medical systems, for example, the psychologist may be part of a larger rehabilitation team, and the "client" may be the medical system, the physician, the third-party health care provider, or the rehabilitation team. In fact, in many of these situations it is the system and the team that have requested psychological assessment and consultation in determining how to work best with a given patient. In addition, legal systems may be involved, and psychological data resulting from the assessment may be used to monitor client behavior. Moreover, in the current managed-care environment psychometric data may be used to deny or restrict treatment options for a person with a disability. In business and industrial settings, psychologists representing a given company are obviously required to give informative feedback to the client who is requesting and reimbursing the psychologist for the assessment. Similarly, health maintenance organizations and other health care payors may be well deserving of feedback from the psychologist concerning assessment results.

The degree of confidentiality and a frank explanation of the use of test data must be discussed with the client. Most people who agree to psychological assessment simply have no idea how such information may be used for or against them. It is incumbent on the administering psychologist to discuss these issues with the respondent prior to any formal assessment so that the respondent can make an informed choice regarding his or her degree of cooperation and have an opportunity to make any special requests or inquiries regarding the procedure. It may be difficult at times, then, to please both the consumer and the managed-care organization. Although the consumer may not want the information he or she shares with the psychologist to be released to the managed-care entity, the managed-care organization might desire and expect full disclosure of information deemed important to allocating its resources and services. Similarly, personal information about the client that is somewhat tangential to the overall vocational rehabilitation process (e.g., past experimentation with marijuana, elevated scores on a measure of personality disorders from a client with a stable vocational history, etc.) may be inappropriately used by vocational rehabilitation professionals to deny sponsorship or support for assistive devices.

Within standard rehabilitative practices, the Rehabilitation Act of 1973 stipulates that "applicants and eligible individuals must be active and full partners" in the process, including "assessments to determine eligibility and vocational rehabilitation needs." Unfortunately, in many cases the assessment is used to "screen out" eligible participants, as clinicians focus on problems and characteristics that might pose difficulties to the rehabilitative process, and the degree of actual "partnership" is thus dubious indeed. This lack of partnership is also obvious in the increased pressure on health care systems and rehabilitation programs to provide the most inexpensive and streamlined program for an eligible or potential client, regardless and independent of client opinion. These issues should be openly discussed and presented to a participant prior to the assessment. The clinician should be judicious and thoughtful concerning which assessment tools should be used and how results may be interpreted by the multiple clients involved in the assessment process.

The demand to efficiently manage health care resources now limits input into the rehabilitation program, and it compromises the ability of the client to participate as an equal partner in the rehabilitation program. The perspective of the client is often considered immaterial or it is altogether ignored by the rehabilitation team members who may be compelled to economically provide services. Efficient and thorough assessment involves considerable expertise and time investment; reimbursement should be expected. Minimizing or eliminating psychological assessment data and client opinion in any rehabilitation plan may produce short-term financial gain, but this will be negated when characteristics previously ignored are manifested in subsequent resistance, distress, or secondary complications that require costly rehospitalizations or attendant care.

Other challenges may emanate from societal changes, such as an increase in the incidence of severe physical disability due to acts of violence (Elliott, Richards, DeVivo, Jackson, & Stover, 1994). In addition, other issues are important to address, such as the assessment of children and elderly individuals who have sustained physically disabling conditions (Richards, Elliott, Cotliar, & Stevenson, 1995) and assessment of people from different minority ethnic and cultural backgrounds (Uswatte & Elliott, 1997). Furthermore, psychologists working in emerging health care delivery systems must be adept at providing informed psychological assessment and interpretations at all levels of health care delivery. This involves the strategic use of assessment devices at the individual level of service delivery as well as at the higher echelons where decisions are made concerning resource allocation, formation of health care policy, seamless continuum of service delivery across the life span and across acute care episodes, and overall integration of psychological services into health systems (Elliott & Klapow, 1997; Elliott & Shewchuk, 1996; Elliott & Shewchuk, cited in Johnstone et al., 1995).

SUMMARY

In this chapter we have reviewed both historical and contemporary issues that exist within the profession of psychology to deliver competent and expert personality assessment services to people with debilitating conditions, particularly regarding recommendations for provision of AT. We also have described the appropriate use of personality assessment in medical rehabilitation, including a brief description of the typical measures used to assess personality. Research is still required to address the validity and reliability of many assessment instruments for use with people with physical and sensory disabilities to ensure accurate interpretation and application of assessment data. Moreover, research in the relation between personality and use of AT is critical. In the meantime, psychologists must strive to understand the relation between person and environment, as well as the relation between person and technology, when assessing individuals with severe disability. Personality assessment will soon become the hallmark of a thorough evaluation for assistive technology when a broader understanding of the Person × Technology fit is formed.

REFERENCES

American Psychiatric Association. (1980). *Diagnostic and statistical manual of mental disorders* (3rd ed.). Washington, DC: Author.

American Psychiatric Association. (1994). *Diagnostic and statistical manual of mental disorders* (4th ed.). Washington, DC: Author.

Belar, C. D. (1988). Education in behavioral medicine: Perspectives from psychology. *Annals of Behavioral Medicine, 10,* 11–14.

Butcher, J. N., Dahlstrom, W. G., Graham, J. R., Tellegen, A., & Kaemmer, B. (1989). *Manual for the restandardized Minnesota Multiphasic Personality Inventory: MMPI-2*. Minneapolis, MN: University of Minnesota Press.

Costa, P. T., Jr., & McRae, R. R. (1989). *The NEO personality inventory/NEO five-factor inventory manual supplement*. Odessa, FL: Psychological Assessment Resources.

Eisenberg, M., & Jansen, M. (1987). Rehabilitation psychologists in medical settings: A unique specialty or a redundant one? *Professional Psychology: Research and Practice, 18,* 475–478.

Elliott, T. (1993). Training psychology graduate students in assessment for rehabilitation settings. In R. Glueckauf, L. Sechrest, G. Bond, & E. C. McDonel (Eds.), *Improving the quality of assessment practices in rehabilitation and health* (pp. 196–211). Newbury Park, CA: Sage.

Elliott, T., & Jackson, W. T. (1996). Psychological assessment in spinal cord injury rehabilitation: Benefiting patient, treatment team, and health care delivery system. *Topics in Spinal Cord Injury Rehabilitation, 2*(2), 34–45.

Elliott, T., & Klapow, J. (1997). Training psychologists for a future in evolving health care delivery systems: Building a better Boulder model. *Journal of Clinical Psychology in Medical Settings, 4*, 255–267.

Elliott, T., Richards, J. S., DeVivo, M., Jackson, A., & Stover, S. (1994). Spinal cord injury model systems of care: The legacy and the promise. *NeuroRehabilitation, 4*, 84–90.

Elliott, T., & Shewchuk, R. (1996). Defining health and well being for the future of counseling psychology. *The Counseling Psychologist, 24*, 743–750.

Elliott, T., & Umlauf, R. (1995). Measurement of personality and psychopathology in acquired disability. In L. Cushman & M. Scherer (Eds.), *Psychological assessment in medical rehabilitation settings* (pp. 325–358). Washington, DC: American Psychological Association.

Faust, D., Guilmette, R. J., Hart, K., Arkes, H. R., Fishbume, F. J., & Davey, L. (1988). Neuropsychologists' training, experience and judgment accuracy. *Archives of Clinical Neuropsychology, 3*, 145–163.

Frank, R. G., Buckelew, S., & Gluck, J. (1990). Rehabilitation: Psychology's greatest opportunity? *American Psychologist, 45*, 762–765.

Glueckauf, R. L. (1993). Use and misuse of assessment in rehabilitation: Getting back to the basics. In R. L. Glueckauf, L. B. Sechrest, G. R. Bond, & E. McDonel (Eds.), *Improving assessment in rehabilitation and health* (pp. 135–155). Newbury Park, CA: Sage.

Johnstone, B., Frank, R. G., Belar, C., Berks, S., Bieliaukas, L. A., Bigler, E. D., Caplan, B., Elliott, T., Glueckauf, R., Kaplan, R. M., Kreutzer, J., Mateer, C., Patterson, D., Puente, A., Richards, J. S., Rosenthal, M., Sherer, M., Shewchuk, R., Siegel, L., & Sweet, J. J. (1995). Psychology in health care: Future directions. *Professional Psychology: Research and Practice, 26*, 341–365.

Leung, P. (1984). Training in rehabilitation psychology. In C. Golden (Ed.), *Current topics in rehabilitation psychology* (pp. 17–27). Orlando, FL: Grune & Stratton.

Meehl, P. E. (1954). *Clinical versus statistical prediction: A theoretical analysis and a review of the evidence.* Minneapolis: University of Minnesota Press.

Millon, T. (1997). *Millon clinical multiaxial inventory III manual* (2nd ed.). Minneapolis, MN: National Computer Sysytems.

Monahan, J. (1980). *Who is the client? The ethics of psychological intervention in the criminal justice system.* Washington, DC: American Psychological Association.

Myerson, K. (1957). Special disabilities. *Annual Review of Psychology, 8*, 437–457.

Nemiah, J. C. (1957). The psychiatrist and rehabilitation. *Archives of Physical Medicine and Rehabilitation, 38*, 143–147.

Rehabilitation Act of 1973. September 26, 1973. Pub. L. No. 93-112, 93rd Congress (HR 8070).

Richards, J. S., Elliott, T., Cotliar, R., & Stevenson, V. (1995). Pediatric medical rehabilitation. In M. C. Roberts (Ed.), *Handbook of pediatric psychology* (2nd ed., pp. 703–722). New York: Guilford Press.

Rodevich, M. A., & Wanlass, R. L. (1995). The moderating effects of spinal cord injury on MMPI–2 profiles: A clinically derived *T*-score correction procedure. *Rehabilitation Psychology, 40,* 181–190.

Scherer, M. J. (1988). Assistive device utilization and quality-of-life in adults with spinal cord injuries or cerebral palsy. *Journal of Applied Rehabilitation Counseling, 19,* 21–30.

Scherer, M. J. (1990). Assistive device utilization and quality of life in adults with spinal cord injuries or cerebral palsy two years later. *Journal of Applied Rehabilitation Counseling, 21,* 36–44.

Snyder, C. R., Harris, C., Anderson, J. R., Holleran, S. A., Irving, L. M., Sigmon, S. T., Yoshinobu, L., Gibb, J., Langelle, C., & Harney, P. (1991). The will and the ways: Development and validation of an individual differences measure of hope. *Journal of Personality and Social Psychology, 60,* 570–585.

Taylor, S. E. (1991). *Health psychology* (2nd ed.). New York: McGraw-Hill.

Uswatte, G., & Elliott, T. (1997). Ethnic and minority issues in rehabilitation psychology. *Rehabilitation Psychology, 42,* 61–71.

Wedding, D., & Faust, D. (1989). Clinical judgment and decision making in neuropsychology. *Archives of Clinical Neuropsychology, 4,* 233–265.

Williams, G., & Mourer, S. (1990). Psychological assessment of newly injured SCI patients: Survey results. *SCI Psychosocial Processes, 3*(3), 12–15.

Wright, B. A. (1983). *Physical disability: A psychological approach.* New York: Harper & Row.

Wright, B. A., & Fletcher, B. (1982). Uncovering hidden resources: A challenge in assessment. *Professional Psychology, 12,* 229–235.

4

PAIN AND ITS INFLUENCE ON ASSISTIVE TECHNOLOGY USE

DAVID R. PATTERSON, MARK JENSEN,
AND JOYCE ENGEL-KNOWLES

Pain is a crucial element, and often the cause, of disability. The treatment of pain is a worthy clinical and empirical endeavor, because pain is identified as the primary complaint for more than 10 million office visits annually to U.S. physicians (Knapp & Koch, 1984). Traumatic injuries, cancer, and surgery account for millions of people experiencing moderate to severe pain each year (Turk & Melzack, 1992). Pain is inherent in both new-onset disability as well as chronic conditions. For example, traumatic brain and spinal cord injuries are both a potential source of pain, particularly early after their onset. Chronic disability, such as cystic fibrosis and multiple sclerosis, also have pain as a frequent component. As such, it is valuable to treat pain in people with disabilities as well as in the general population. Unfortunately, this issue has been woefully neglected with respect to disability, both in terms of assessment and treatment.

Successful treatment of both acute and chronic pain is often predicated on accurate assessment of this problem. The International Association for the Study of Pain Task Force on Taxonomy defines *pain* as "an unpleasant sensory and emotional experience associated with actual or potential tissue damage, or described in terms of such damage" (Merskey & Bogduk, 1994, p. 210). This definition acknowledges that pain has both sensory and affective components. It also suggests that actual tissue damage need not be present for an individual to experience pain. Because pain is highly subjective and potentially multilayered, treatment may potentially be far off the mark if the nature of the pain is misunderstood. Similarly, outcome studies on pain must rest on a foundation of accurate assessment.

A model that conceptualizes the multilayered nature of pain can be critical in assessment. In this vein, a model put forth by Loeser and Fordyce

(1983) is extremely useful in conceptualizing this phenomenon. These authors view pain as elements of discomfort in a series of circles, as in a "bull's eye." In this model, *nociception,* the detection of potentially tissue-damaging thermal or mechanical energy by specialized nerve endings, is considered at the heart of pain. Beyond nociception is *pain,* or a perceived noxious input to the nervous system. *Suffering* extends beyond pain and refers to a negative affective response engendered by pain and by such diverse phenomena as depression, isolation, anxiety, and fear. Finally, *pain behaviors*—or any and all outputs of the individual that a reasonable observer would characterize as suggesting pain, such as posture, facial expression, verbalizing, lying down, taking medicines, seeking medical assistance, and receiving compensation—lie at the farthest-out circle. One of the characteristics of this model, which is not readily apparent in one's day-to-day experience of pain, is that these layers are distinct. It is possible to experience or show some elements of this context in the absence of the others. For example, in the case of chronic pain, pain behaviors and suffering often exist in the absence of nociception. Conceptualizing pan through this multilayered model can be useful in assessment as well as treatment. For many people with disability, assistive technology (AT) is essential to generating an accurate assessment of pain. However, the use of AT will only be as good as the principles of assessment that underlie its application. As such, the focus of this chapter is on basic pain assessment, with brief mention of how AT can enhance this for people with disability.

With pain being the complex construct that it is, multiple approaches to assessment are discussed in the literature. Although the brevity of this chapter precludes us from covering all such approaches, we are able to summarize some of the primary ones. The areas of self-report procedures, behavioral assessment, and psychological factors are particularly relevant to disability and are the focus of this chapter. After discussing the valid and reliable instruments on which AT must be predicated, we then touch on their applications to people with disability.

SELF-REPORT SCALES

Self-report measures are certainly the most common type of pain assessment technique available. In keeping with Loeser and Fordyce's (1983) model of pain, it is useful to divide self-report scales as to whether they assess pain *intensity* or pain *affect.* We address each of these areas in turn. This categorization is useful for describing the various self-report measures that have been reported in the literature.

Assessing Pain Intensity

Verbal Rating Scales

Verbal rating scales (VRSs) list a series of adjectives as a means of describing the intensity of pain. Any number of adjectives may be used. The lists typically provide extremes of pain at either end of a continuum. For example, one 5-point scale includes the adjectives *none, mild, moderate, severe,* and *very severe* (Frank, Moll, & Hort, 1982). Patients are instructed to read over the list of adjectives and pick the one that best describes their current, typical pain intensity. A number of such scales have been published, and the number of adjectives provided to patients often differs (Gracely, McGrath, & Dubner, 1978; Joyce, Zutshi, Hrubes, & Mason, 1975). Several weaknesses of VRSs have been identified. The scale uses a rank scoring method, but people may assume that equal intervals exist between adjectives. However, it is likely that the intervals between scales are not equal. Thus, there is no way to account for the magnitude of differences between adjectives. A second problem is that VRSs are treated as if they produce interval-level data (i.e., with equal intervals between points), yet they are in fact ordinal (ranked) scaling data. Cross-modality matching procedures can be used to correct for these measurement problems, but they are time consuming and require an additional step (Jensen & Karoly, 1992). The strengths of VRSs include the ease with which they can be administered and scored (although they should undergo a correction procedure), the compliance rate they elicit, their positive relation to other pain measures, and their ability to be sensitive to treatments. However, Jensen and Karoly (1992) recommended that VRSs be used in conjunction with other measures because, among other reasons, the limited adjectives may not truly capture the patient's experience.

Visual Analogue Scales

Visual analogue scales (VASs) are usually a 10-cm line with descriptors of extremes of pain at each end (e.g., *worst possible pain, no pain at all*). Patients are instructed to make a mark along this line that indicates their level of pain. Some VASs have numbers or adjectives along the line and are referred to as *graphic rating scales*. VASs have two primary weaknesses. First, because scoring involves measuring the difference between the endpoint and the patient's mark, it can be time consuming and more prone to error. Second, some patients have difficulty understanding this measure (Jensen, Karoly, & Braver, 1986). Despite these weaknesses, the VAS has been studied extensively and has several strengths. VAS scales are reported to correlate positively with other measures (Downie et al., 1978); to relate to observed pain behavior (Teske, Daut, & Cleeland, 1983); to be sensitive to treatment effects (Turner, 1982); to be amenable statistically as ratio data (Price & Harkins, 1987); and, with their increased number of response categories, to be more sensitive to change (Jensen & Karoly, 1992). However, the weaknesses make it advisable not to use the VAS as a sole measure.

Behavior Rating Scale

The Behavior Rating Scale (BRS) was developed by Budzynski, Stoyva, Adler, & Mullaney (1973) to provide a behaviorally based means of assessing pain intensity. Patients are provided with a series of behavior descriptors of their pain (e.g., "Pain exists, but can be ignored at times") and asked to pick the one that describes their pain intensity. Although BRSs have demonstrated some correlation with other measures of pain intensity (Jensen et al., 1986), are easy to administer, and have shown sensitivity to treatment effects (Budzynski et al., 1973), they may confound pain intensity with pain interference and should be considered only an indirect measure of subjective experience (Jensen & Karoly, 1992; Jensen, Karoly, O'Riordan, Bland, & Burns, 1989).

Picture Scales

Perhaps one of the best known and frequently used picture scales is The Oucher (Beyer, Denyes, et al., 1992). It presents a number of vertically arranged photographs of a child's face depicting different levels of pain intensity. It is for use with children ages 6–8 years and is available with pictures of children from different ethnic backgrounds. The picture scale (Frank et al., 1982) is a measure on which patients are asked to indicate their level of pain intensity by rank ordering (from 0 to 7) a series of drawn facial expressions according to the degree to which they reflect the patient's experience. This type of scale has not been researched well, and the nature of the facial expressions are such that affective dimensions of pain may be confused with sensory dimensions of pain. However, picture scales may hold promise for patients who lack the ability to complete other pain intensity scales secondary to language, literacy, or cultural reasons. As we discuss later in the chapter, picture scales may be particularly useful for people with some disabilities. The Faces Pain Scale (Bieri, Reeve, Champion, Addicoat, & Ziegler, 1990) is another potentially useful measure of pain intensity. This scale consists of seven drawings of facial expressions of pain in rank order. It has been tested for use in children, adults, and elderly people (Herr, Mobily, Kohout, & Wagenaar, 1998; Hunter, McDowell, Hennessy, & Cassey, 2000; Stuppy, 1998).

Numerical Rating Scales

Numerical rating scales (NRSs) are weighted on either end with descriptors (e.g., *no pain at all*) like VASs. Patients are asked to choose a number from 0 to 10 or from 0 to 100 that best describes their pain. There are a number of strengths to NRSs, including positive correlations with other pain intensity measures (Downie et al., 1978), sensitivity of pain treatments (Seymour, 1982), sensitivity to pain, and ease of administration and scoring. Although there are few weaknesses associated with NRSs, one study (Turner, 1982) indicated that they are less sensitive to treatment effects than are VASs. More research is needed on the sensitivity of NRSs relative to other pain scales, but they hold particular promise for people with disabilities who have limited verbal or motor expression.

Box Scale

The box scale is essentially an 11-point NRS in which the numbers are put into boxes. Patients are instructed to mark the box (containing the numbers 0–10) that best indicates their pain level. The simplicity and ease of administration of this measure leads to high levels of compliance, and it is easy to score. Although not a lot of research has examined the box scale, initial studies of its psychometric properties are promising (Jensen et al., 1986; Jensen et al., 1989).

Descriptor Differential Scale

The Descriptor Differential Scale (Gracely & Kwilosz, 1988) lists a series of adjectives; for each, patients are instructed to rate the degree to which it reflects the intensity of their pain. Twelve adjectives are presented to patients (e.g., *faint, strong, very intense*), and they indicate whether their pain is equal to, less than, or more than each descriptor. The multiple-item nature of this scale allows for more complex assessment of its psychometric validity, and early reports have suggested that it is strong in terms of internal consistency and internal reliability. Although promising, this is a new scale that is in need of additional studies (Jensen & Karoly, 1992).

Brief Pain Inventory

The Brief Pain Inventory (Cleeland & Ryan, 1994) measures both the intensity of pain (sensory dimension) and interference of pain in the patient's life (reactive dimension). It also asks patients to report about pain relief, pain quality, and patient perception of the cause of pain. It has demonstrated reliability and validity across cultures and languages and has been adopted for use in many countries (Caraceni et al., 1996; Ger, Ho,

Sun, Wang, & Cleeland, 1999; Uki, Mendoza, Cleeland, Nakamura, & Takeda, 1998; Radbruch et al., 1999; Saxena, Mendoza, & Cleeland, 1999; Wang, Mendoza, Gao, & Cleeland, 1996).

Assessing Pain Affect

Pain affect refers to the degree to which patients suffer emotionally from pain. It is never an easy task to quantify emotional experience, and assessing the affective component of pain is no exception. The goal of measuring pain affect, rather than simply assessing the strength of nociceptive input, is often to assess how accurately various adjectives reflect the patient's internal experience.

McGill Pain Questionnaire

The McGill Pain Questionnaire (MPQ; Melzack, 1975) was designed to assess more subjective components of pain experience, such as affective pain, and is the most often used and researched measure of this nature to date. The MPQ includes a series of different pain descriptors that fall into four major groups: sensory, affective, evaluative, and miscellaneous. Patients are instructed to go through 20 clusters of adjectives and circle those that best reflect their pain. The questionnaire yields three major indices: the pain rating index, the number of words chosen, and the number–word combination. The pain rating index provides separate scores for the sensory, affective valuative, and miscellaneous subclasses as well as an overall score. The MPQ appears to meet the psychometric qualities of being valid, reliable, and consistent (Chapman et al., 1985; Melzack, 1983). It is a practical measure that has been used in more than 100 studies on pain of various types (Melzack & Katz, 1992), but it can be a bit cumbersome to administer and score. There is a short form of the MPQ that can be useful for this reason. In general, the MPQ can provide an effective means of evaluating a patient's subjective, affective–evaluative experience of pain. Most clinicians and researchers will likely choose to supplement the MPQ with measures of pain intensity, behavior, or both.

Other Measures of Pain Affect

Means to assess pain other than the MPQ have been developed; most of them follow the strategies of measuring pain intensity just described. On VRSs (Gracely et al., 1978; Tursky, Jamner, & Friedman, 1982) patients choose an adjective from a list of descriptors that increase in the degree to which they reflect the unpleasantness of pain. VASs are weighted with affective descriptors rather than indications of intensity; thus, patients who are administered affective VAS scales may mark a line that reads *not bad at all* on one end and *the most unpleasant feeling possible for me* at the other (Price, Harkins, & Baker, 1987). The Descriptor Differential Scale of Pain Affect (Gracely & Kwilosz, 1988) lists 12 adjectives and has an administration and scoring strategy like the DDS for pain intensity described previously (p. 63). The scales differ only in that adjectives for the Pain Affect scale describe qualitative elements of pain (i. e., emotional descriptors), rather than pain intensity. In general, the strengths and weaknesses of these pain measures are almost identical to those described for the corresponding measures of pain intensity just described. Finally, the Pain Discomfort Scale (Jensen, Karoly, & Harris, 1991) provides patients with 10 items affirming or denying an affective component of pain (e.g., "I am scared about the pain I feel"). Patients are asked to indicate on a 5-point Likert scale the degree to which they agree with each statement. Although this measure has initially yielded promising factors reflecting multidimensional components of pain, it is early in its development and requires substantially more research (Jensen & Karoly, 1992).

Assessing Pain Behaviors

There are several dimensions to the experience of pain, and assessment may fall short if only sensory and affective components are examined. Assessment and treatment should consider the contributions of *pain behaviors*, the means through which people communicate that they are in pain. Such behaviors may include grimacing, limping, saying "ouch," or withdrawing and becoming silent. They can also include more subtle communication of pain, such as taking analgesic medications, pursuing a more sedentary lifestyle, or seeking disability payments. Effective treatment of chronic pain often relies on accurately determining the presence of such behaviors.

There are two components that are useful to consider when assessing pain behavior. The first has to do with describing pain behavior as an isolated phenomenon. In preverbal children or cognitively impaired adults, for example, the only means available to assess their pain may be observation of their behavior. As we discuss, this is often also the case with people with severe disabilities. The second component involves functional analysis (Ferster, 1965), or observing pain behaviors in the context of the stimuli that cause them or the response that they create. With regard to stimuli, simply asking a person how he or she feels may result in a change from that person displaying content and happy behavior to grimacing or even tearfulness. In the case of consequences, rewards such as solicitous behavior from a spouse may serve to increase pain behavior. Functional analysis can determine the degree to which pain behavior changes as a result of social and environmental variables. In assessing and sampling pain behavior, Keefe and Williams (1992) described five options that are available: continuous observation, duration measure, frequency counts, time sampling, and interval recording.

Continuous Observation

Continuous observation typically occurs in a patient's home or workplace. This form of sampling behavior involves continuously noting any changes in behavior over a relatively long duration of time. Continuous observation at the workplace, for example, may involve watching a patient for a period of time at his or her workstation and noting changes in posture and potential operants. Because behavior is complex and occurs in a ongoing stream, continuous observation is useful as it recognizes this quality and makes some attempt to conceptualize and measure it. However, continuous observation is time consuming and yields a plethora of data that are not easily analyzed (Keefe & Williams, 1992).

Duration Measures

Duration measures involve recording how long it takes a patient to complete a particular behavior. For the sake of accuracy, such measures can be completed by an observer, although more convenient (but less accurate) duration measures can be completed by the patient. Fordyce (1976) emphasized collecting duration measures on activities that are incompatible with pain, such as ambulation or working. Other examples or duration measures might be the length of time it takes a person to complete physical therapy or the length of time he or she wears a splint. Duration measures form the basis for pain diaries, which are one of the more frequently used techniques to assess chronic pain. Patients are instructed to use such diaries to keep track of the amount of time spent performing various behaviors, usually "well" behaviors, such as walking or exercising.

Frequency Counts

Frequency accounts simply involve recording the number of times a behavior occurs. Examples might include the number of physician visits, analgesics taken, or exercises performed. The major limitation to both frequency counts and duration measures is that long periods of time may be necessary to reliably record infrequently occurring behavior (Keefe & Williams, 1992).

Time Sampling

Time sampling involves taking counts of behavior at prespecified intervals of time. For example, patients in an inpatient pain setting may be observed for 20-minute intervals during each nursing shift (Keefe, Crisson,

& Trainor, 1987). Like the aforementioned approaches, time sampling is also more difficult to use when assessing low-frequency behavior.

Interval Recording

In interval recording a period of observation is broken into equal-length intervals. The frequency with which a target behavior occurs over those intervals is then recorded. Interval recording works particularly well when a sample of behavior is videotaped. This approach can be useful for reliably recording behaviors that occur over several hours.

Fordyce (1976) championed the importance of assessing behavior in the treatment of chronic pain, and his book still provides one of the best resources for defining and measuring pain behaviors.

PSYCHOLOGICAL ASSESSMENT

As has been repeatedly emphasized in the literature, pain, particularly that of a chronic nature, is a multidimensional construct. Because pain is influenced by myriad cultural, psychological, and environmental variables even evaluations that consider sensory, affective, and behavioral components of pain may be inadequate in addressing the patient's complete picture. For example, 33% of patients with chronic pain experience depression (Romano & Turner, 1985), and the incidence of generalized anxiety and somatization are higher in this patient group than in the general population. Determining the causal relation between psychological factors and chronic pain is a vexing challenge; dispositional factors in humans can predispose them to experience pain differently, and situational factors can exacerbate or alleviate this experience. As such, effective psychological assessment considers both long-term personality factors as well as more transient influences on a patient's emotional status. A number of other psychological factors, such as the manner in which the patient's pain affects his or her functioning and the manner in which the patient copes with pain, also should be considered.

Personality and Emotional Status

There are a number of self-report measures that are useful for measuring psychological status as it might relate to chronic pain. The Minnesota Multiphasic Personality (MMPI; Graham, 1977) and the MMPI–2 (Graham, 1990) have been used with several studies of chronic pain. The more typical application of this instrument has been to investigate personality type as it may relate to chronic pain (Costello, Hulsey, Schoenfield, & Ramamurthy, 1987; McGill, Lawlis, Selby, Mooney, & McCoy, 1983). The revised Symptom Checklist–90 (SCL–90–R; Derogatis, 1983) is another instrument developed for general psychiatric assessment that is used with chronic pain (Jamison, Rock, & Parris, 1988); it is preferred by many clinicians and patients because of its shorter length. Similarly, the Millon Behavioral Health Inventory (Bradley, McDonald-Haile, & Jaworski, 1992) can provide valuable information about personality characteristics of patients with chronic pain and is short and more practical than most other measures. The Illness Behavior Questionnaire (Pilowsky, Bassett, Barrett, Petrovic, & Minniti, 1983) focuses more specifically on whether the patient has a tendency to somaticize. Bradley et al. (1992) recommended the MMPI and Millon Behavioral Health Inventory for assessment of chronic pain, although they warned that the length of these measures can be problematic.

Situational Stressors

Patients with almost any medical condition, as well as chronic pain, can have their condition exacerbated by situational stressors, so it is reasonable that assessment of such factors be considered. As such, instruments that investigate the impact of major life stressors, such as the Life Experiences Survey (Sarason, Johnson, & Siegel, 1978), or day-to-day problems, such as the Hassles Scale (Kanner, Coyne, Schaefer, & Lazarus, 1981), can be valuable components of an assessment battery.

Coping

The manner in which patients cope with their pain at baseline and the degree to which cognitive–behavioral strategies can alter such ways of coping are of obvious interest to clinicians and researchers who study chronic pain. The Ways of Coping Questionnaire (Folkman & Lazarus, 1980) was designed to assess coping with general life stressors but has been found to also be useful in research with patients who have chronic pain (Felton & Revenson, 1984). Two other measures that might be useful with this population include the Coping Strategies Questionnaire (Rosenstiel & Keefe, 1983) and the Chronic Pain Coping Inventory (Jensen, Turner, Romano, & Strom, 1995). The Waldron/Varni Pediatric Pain Coping Inventory might be considered for use for children (Varni et al., 1996).

Health Quality of Life

A frequent area of interest is how chronic pain affects the quality of a person's life. The Medical Outcomes Survey Symptom–Function Checklist (SF–36; Ware, Snow, Kosinski, & Gandek, 1993) is a short measure that is valuable because it has been applied to numerous medical populations and allows comparisons of health quality of life. The Sickness Impact Profile

(Bergner, Bobbitt, Carter, & Gibson, 1981) has been applied more specifically to individuals with chronic pain (Jensen, Turner, & Romano, 1991) but is a much more cumbersome measure to administer and score. As such, more efficient alternatives, such as the Chronic Illness Problem Inventory (Kames, Naliboff, Heinrich, & Schag, 1984), have been considered.

Other Psychological Assessment Approaches

Some psychological approaches are expansive enough that they address several of the psychological variables discussed in this section. Structured interviews might serve this purpose. The Psychosocial Pain Inventory (Getto, Heaton, & Lehman, 1983) gathers information about 25 psychosocial aspects of chronic pain. The interview can take as long as 2 hours to administer, but the authors reported good reliability data on this instrument. Bradley et al. (1992) discussed semistructured behavioral interviews at length, indicating that their objectives are to obtain a pain history, identify factors that serve as stimuli and reinforcers for pain, evaluate patients' daily activities, determine the family history of chronic pain, and assess patients for affective disturbances.

A final approach to assessing psychological factors in chronic pain that deserves mention is the West Haven–Yale Multidimensional Pain Inventory (Kerns, Turk, & Rudy, 1985). This measure includes several items that assess the impact of pain both on a person and on his or her family. In contrast to the structured interviews, the West Haven–Yale Multidimensional Pain Inventory is a self-report inventory, but it does assess multiple dimensions of pain.

PAIN ASSESSMENT AND DISABILITY

Little has been written on the subject of assessing pain in people with disability, and this subject has in fact been largely neglected in general. Pain can be an ongoing problem with genetically based disabilities, such as cystic fibrosis. It can be a transient challenge (e.g., burn injuries), or it can be an ongoing component of acquired disabilities (such as amputations or spinal cord injuries). In many such disabilities the measurement of pain can follow the types of approaches outlined thus far in this chapter. The degree to which pain has sensory, affective, and behavioral components will likely not differ on the basis of whether a person has a disability; however, many of the approaches we have discussed will present challenges to people with disabilities when they are limited in terms of speech, motor, cognitive functioning, or some combination of these.

The interaction between pain and AT is certainly worth mentioning. Although the focus of this chapter is measuring pain and how AT may facilitate such assessment, one should also consider the prevalence of pain associated with AT use. As an example, prolonged wheelchair use might result in rotator cuff pain, or keyboard use might cause pain from carpal tunnel syndrome. Such types of pain are likely frequently underdiagnosed, and differentiating between whether pain is caused by the initial disability or by resulting AT use can be a vexing task. From this perspective it is important to understand that pain can have a modifying effect on the degree to which AT contributes to quality of life. At times, the improvements in function that result through AT use will have to be weighed against the pain that such devices might create.

AT providers can adapt several of the available pain measurement approaches for people limited by disability. For people with speech deficits, the augmentative communication devices used facilitate communication of pain complaints. Many of the self-report scales discussed (VASs, NRSs, the MPQ) can be used as assistive devices in themselves. For patients who cannot speak, the clinician can present these scales in their present form, with instructions that patients respond by pointing, or even with eyeblinks. For patients with motor and visual limitations, the scales may be enlarged to facilitate pointing and readability. The clinician can determine reliability of the patient's response by stating aloud what he or she believed the response to be.

For young children and elderly people, faces scales have proved to be useful when verbal communication is a challenge (Beyer et al., 1992, Frank et al., 1982). Patients are presented with a series of photographs or drawings ranging from happy (pain free) faces to ones representing individuals in substantial pain (as discussed, this is a means of assessing pain intensity through the use of picture scales). The pictures on a faces scale often make the concept of pain measurement more comprehensible to patients with limitations in their cognitive capacity. As such, a faces scale not only represents a good option for people with disabilities, but it also can be particularly useful for those with mild cognitive limitations.

For patients with motor function deficits that preclude writing or marking answers, many of the pain scales reviewed can be administered orally. In such cases NRSs (which require choosing a number rather than making a mark) will be preferable to VASs, for obvious reasons. Descriptor differential scales and the MPQ will be useful because the patient can respond verbally to the items and will allow the assessment of affective components of pain.

People with both motor and speech deficits will certainly be the ones most in need of AT to express their pain. Adaptive devices, such as pencil grips and computers with touch screens, can potentially facilitate motor responses. Augmentative communication devices, such as boards fit with pictoral and numerical scales, or computerized voice systems, may be essential to elicit verbal responses. Eyeblinks may be an important resource in patients without motor or speech responses, such as those with locked-in syndrome. In such patients an NRS for pain can be administered with instructions that the patient is to blink when the number that describes his or her pain is reached. It is important to obtain some type of estimate of the reliability of eyeblink communications before this approach is used to assess pain. It is also important for clinicians not to anticipate a patient's responses and allow him or her sufficient time to respond.

Some disabilities will be of a nature that precludes a person with a disability from communicating his or her pain verbally or motorically, even with the use of AT. In such cases the use of behavioral observations may be the only available means of assessing pain. This is also the case with infants and many elderly people; in such individuals, cognitive limitations preclude the use of virtually any technique other than behavior observations. The methods for recording pain behaviors discussed earlier can be useful with people who have such disabilities; however, the challenges can be greater, because contractures, spasticity, and decreased active movement can be mistakenly attributed to pain.

Physiological measures may be the only other means of assessing pain in people whose disabilities rule out all other assessment techniques. Indicators such as heart rate, blood pressure, or breathing rate may provide useful indexes of pain with patients who are unable to provide their subjective opinions. A combination of behavioral and physiological measures may be used as cross-references for a noncommunicative patient. For instance, elevated physiological parameters can be used to determine whether grimacing is an indication of pain or is some type of other involuntary response.

SUMMARY

The concepts behind pain assessment in general are appropriate for people with disabilities, independent of whether they require assistive devices. Even when AT is used in assessing pain, however, it will likely be necessary for it to be superimposed on a basic understanding of what is known about the theory and practice of pain measurement. Consequently, we have reviewed evaluations of sensory, affective, and pain behavior components of pain and have paid particular attention to self-report measures. AT can play a critical role in enabling patients to communicate the pain they experience on the measures that are available. Once it is established whether a person's disability influences a person's verbal communication, motor communication, or both, AT can be combined with known, psychometrically sound pain assessment instruments to provide the most accurate picture of pain possible.

REFERENCES

Bergner, M., Bobbitt, R. A., Carter, W. B., & Gibson, B. S. (1981). The Sickness Impact Profile: Development and final revision of a health status measure. *Medical Care, 19,* 787–805.

Beyer, J. E., Denyes, M. J., et al. (1992). The creation, validation, and continuing development of the Oucher: A measure of pain intensity in children. *Journal Pediatric Nursing, 7*(5), 335–345.

Bieri, D., Reeve, R. A., Champion, G. D., Addicoat, L., & Ziegler, J. B. (1990). The Faces Pain Scale for the self-assessment of the severity of pain experienced by children: Development, initial validation, and preliminary investigation for ratio scale properties. *Pain, 41,* 139–150.

Bradley, L. A., McDonald-Haile, J., & Jaworski, T. M. (1992). Assessment of psychological status using interviews and self-report instruments. In D. C. Turk & R. Melzack (Eds.), *Handbook of pain assessment* (pp. 193–213). New York: Guilford Press.

Budzynski, T. H., Stoyva, J. M., Adler, C. S., & Mullaney, D. J. (1973). EMG biofeedback and tension headache: A controlled outcome study. *Psychosomatic Medicine, 35,* 484–496.

Caraceni, A., Mendoza, T. R., Mencaglia, E., Baratella, C., Edwards, K., Forjaz, M. J., Martini, C., Serlin, R. C., de Conno, F., & Cleeland, C. S. (1996). A validation study of an Italian version of the Brief Pain Inventory (*Breve Questionario per la Valutazione del Dolore*). *Pain, 65,* 87–92.

Chapman, C. R., Casey, K. L., Dubner, R., Foley, K. M., Gracely, R. H., & Reading, A. E. (1985). Pain measurement: An overview. *Pain, 22,* 1–31.

Cleeland, C. S., & Ryan, K. M. (1994). Pain assessment: Global use of the Brief Pain Inventory. *Annals of the Academy of Medicine, Singapore, 23,* 129–138.

Costello, R. M., Hulsey, T. L., Schoenfield, L. S., & Ramamurthy, S. (1987). P-A-I-N: A four-cluster MMPI typology for chronic pain. *Pain, 30,* 199–209.

Derogatis, L. (1983). *The SCL–90R manual–II: Administration, scoring and procedures.* Baltimore: Clinical Psychometric Research.

Downie, W. W., Leatham, P. A., Rhind, V. M., Wright, V., Branco, J. A., & Anderson, J. A. (1978). Studies with pain rating scales. *Annals of the Rheumatic Diseases, 37,* 378–381.

Felton, B. J., & Revenson, T. A. (1984). Coping with chronic illness: A study of illness controllability and the influence of coping strategies on psychological adjustment. *Journal of Consulting and Clinical Psychology, 52,* 343–353.

Ferster, C. B. (1965). Classification of behavioral pathology. In L. Krasner & L. P. Ullman (Eds.), *Research in behavior modification* (pp. 6–26). New York: Holt, Rinehart & Winston.

Folkman, S., & Lazarus, R. S. (1980). An analysis of coping in a middle-aged community sample. *Journal of Health and Social Behavior, 21*, 219–239.

Fordyce, W. E. (1976). *Behavioral methods for chronic pain and illness*. St. Louis: Mosby YearBook.

Frank, A. J. M., Moll, J. M. H., & Hort, J. F. (1982). A comparison of three ways of measuring pain. *Rheumatology and Rehabilitation, 21*, 211–217.

Ger, L. P., Ho, S. T., Sun, W. Z., Wang, M. S., & Cleeland, C. S. (1999). Validation of the Brief Pain Inventory in a Taiwanese population. *Journal of Pain Symptom Management, 18*, 316–322.

Getto, C. J., Heaton, R. K., & Lehman, R. A. (1983). PSPI: A standardized approach to the evaluation of psychosocial factors in chronic pain. *Advances in Pain Research and Therapy, 5*, 885–889.

Gracely, R. H., & Kwilosz, D. M. (1988). The Descriptor Differential Scale: Applying psychophysical principles to clinical pain assessment. *Pain, 35*, 279–288.

Gracely, R. H., McGrath, P., & Dubner, R. (1978). Ratio scales of sensory and affective verbal pain descriptors. *Pain, 5*, 5–18.

Graham, J. R. (1977). *The MMPI: A practical guide*. New York: Oxford.

Graham, J. R. (1990). *MMPI-2: Assessing personality and psychopathology*. New York; Oxford University Press.

Herr, K. A., Mobily, P. R., Kohout, F. J., & Wagenaar, D. (1998). Evaluation of the Faces Pain Scale for use with the elderly. *Clinical Journal of Pain, 14*, 29–38.

Hunter, M., McDowell, L., Hennessy, R., & Cassey, J. (2000). An evaluation of the Faces Pain Scale with young children. *Journal of Pain and Symptom Management, 20*, 122–129.

Jamison, R. N., Rock, D. L., & Parris, W. C. V. (1988). Empirically derived Symptom Checklist 90 subgroups of chronic pain patients: A cluster analysis. *Journal of Behavioral Medicine, 11*, 147–158.

Jensen, M. P., & Karoly, P. (1992). Self-report scales and procedures for assessing pain in adults. In D. C. Turk & R. Melzack (Eds.), *Handbook of pain assessment* (pp. 135–168). New York: Guilford Press.

Jensen, M. P., Karoly, P., & Braver, S. (1986). The measurement of clinical pain intensity: A comparison of six methods. *Pain, 27*, 117–126.

Jensen, M. P., Karoly, P., & Harris, P. (1991). Assessing the affective component of chronic pain: Development of the Pain Discomfort Scale. *Journal of Psychosomatic Research, 35*, 149–154.

Jensen, M. P., Karoly, P., O'Riordan, E. F., Bland, F. J., & Burns, R. S. (1989). The subjective experience of acute pain: An assessment of the utility of 10 indices. *Clinical Journal of Pain, 5*, 153–159.

Jensen, M. P., Turner, J. A., & Romano, J. M. (1991). Self-efficacy and outcome expectancies: Relationship to chronic pain coping strategies and adjustment. *Pain, 44*, 263–269.

Jensen, M. P., Turner, J. A., Romano, J. M., & Strom, S. E. (1995). The Chronic Pain Coping Inventory: Development and preliminary validation. *Pain, 60,* 203–216.

Joyce, C. R. B., Zutshi, D. W., Hrubes, V., & Mason, R. M. (1975). Comparison of fixed interval and visual analogue scales for rating chronic pain. *European Journal of Clinical Pharmacology, 8,* 415–420.

Kames, L. D., Naliboff, B. D., Heinrich, R. L., & Schag, C. C. (1984). The Chronic Illness Problem Inventory: Problem-oriented psychosocial assessment of patients with chronic illness. *International Journal of Psychiatry in Medicine, 14,* 65–75.

Kanner, A. D., Coyne, J. C., Schaefer, C., & Lazarus, R. S. (1981). Comparison of two modes of stress measurement: Daily hassles and uplifts versus major life events. *Journal of Behavioral Medicine, 4,* 1–39.

Keefe, F. J., Crisson, J. E., & Trainor, M. (1987). Observational methods for assessing pain: A practical guide. In J. A. Blumenthal & D. C. McKee (Eds.), *Applications in behavioral medicine and health psychology: A clinician's source book* (pp. 67–94). Sarasota, FL: Professional Resource Exchange.

Keefe, F. J., & Williams, D. A. (1992). Assessment of pain behaviors. In D. C. Turk & R. Melzack (Eds.), *Handbook of pain assessment* (pp. 277–292). New York: Guilford Press.

Kerns, R. D., Turk, D. C., & Rudy, T. E. (1985). The West Haven–Yale Multidimensional Pain Inventory (WHYMPI). *Pain, 23,* 345–356.

Knapp, D. A., & Koch, H. (1984). *The management of new pain in office-based ambulatory care. National ambulatory medical care survey, Advance data from vital and health statistics* (DHHS Publication No. PHS 84-1250, Vol. 97). Hyattsville, MD: Public Health Service.

Loeser, J. D., & Fordyce, W. E. (1983). Chronic pain. In J. E. Carr & H. A. Dengerink (Eds.), *Behavioral science in the practice of medicine* (pp. 331–345). New York: Elsevier.

McGill, J., Lawlis, F., Selby, D., Mooney, V., & McCoy, C. E. (1983). The relationship of Minnesota Multiphasic Personality Inventory (MMPI) profile clusters to pain behaviors. *Journal of Behavioral Medicine, 6,* 677–692.

Melzack, R. (Ed.). (1983). *Pain measurement and assessment.* New York: Raven Press.

Melzack, R. (1975). The McGill Pain Questionnaire: Major properties and scoring methods. *Pain, 1,* 277–299.

Melzack, R., & Katz, J. (1992). The McGill Pain Questionnaire: Appraisal and current status. In D. C. Turk & R. Melzack (Eds.), *Handbook of pain assessment* (pp. 152–168). New York: Guilford Press.

Merskey, H., & Bogduk, N. (Eds.). (1994). Classification of chronic pain: Descriptions of chronic pain syndromes and definitions of pain terms (2nd ed.). Seattle: IASP Press.

Pilowsky, I., Bassett, D., Barrett, R., Petrovic, L., & Minniti, R. (1983). The Illness Behavior Assessment Schedule: Reliability and validity. *International Journal of Psychiatry in Medicine, 13,* 11–28.

Price, D. D., & Harkins, S. W. (1987). Combined use of experimental pain and visual analogue scales in providing standardized measurement of clinical pain. *Clinical Journal of Pain, 3*, 1–8.

Price, D. D., Harkins, S. W., & Baker, C. (1987). Sensory–affective relationships among different types of clinical and experimental pain. *Pain, 28*, 297–307.

Radbruch, L., Loick, G., Kiencke, P., Lindena, G., Sabatowski, R., Grond, S., Lehmann, K. A., & Cleeland, C. S. (1999). Validation of the German version of the Brief Pain Inventory. *Journal of Pain Symptom Management, 18*, 180–187.

Romano, J. M., & Turner, J. A. (1985). Chronic pain and depression: Does the evidence support a relationship? *Psychological Bulletin, 97*, 18–34.

Rosenstiel, A. K., & Keefe, F. J. (1983). The use of coping strategies in low-back pain patients: Relationship to patient characteristics and current adjustment. *Pain, 17*, 33–40.

Sarason, I. G., Johnson, J. H., & Siegel, J. M. (1978). Assessing the impact of life changes: Development of the Life Experiences Survey. *Journal of Consulting and Clinical Psychology, 46*, 932–946.

Saxena, A., Mendoza, T., & Cleeland, C. S. (1999). The assessment of cancer pain in north India: The validation of the Hindi Brief Pain Inventory—BPI-H. *Journal of Pain Symptom Management, 17*, 27–41.

Seymour, R. A. (1982). The use of pain scales in assessing the efficacy of analgesics in post-operative dental pain. *European Journal of Clinical Pharmacology, 23*, 441–444.

Stuppy, D. J. (1998). The Faces Pain Scale: Reliability and validity with mature adults. *Applied Nursing Research, 11*, 84–89.

Teske, K., Daut, R. L., & Cleeland, C. S. (1983). Relationships between nurses' observations and patients' self-reports of pain. *Pain, 16*, 289–296.

Turk, D. C., & Melzack, R. (1992). The measurement of pain and the assessment of people experiencing pain. In D. C. Turk & R. Melzack (Eds.), *Handbook of pain assessment* (pp. 3–12). New York: Guilford Press.

Turner, J. A. (1982). Comparison of group progressive-relaxation training and cognitive–behavioral group therapy for chronic low back pain. *Journal of Consulting and Clinical Psychology, 50*, 757–765.

Tursky, B., Jamner, L. D., & Friedman, R. (1982). The Pain Perception Profile: A psychophysical approach to the assessment of pain report. *Behavior Therapy, 13*, 376–394.

Uki, J., Mendoza, T., Cleeland, C. S., Nakamura, Y., & Takeda, F. (1998). A brief cancer pain assessment tool in Japanese: The utility of the Japanese Brief Pain Inventory—BPI-J. *Journal of Pain Symptom Management, 16*, 364–373.

Varni, J. W., Waldron, S. A., Gragg, R. A., Rapoff, M. A., Bernstein, B. H., Lindsley, C. B., & Newcomb, M. D. (1996). Development of the Waldron/Varni Pediatric Pain Coping Inventory. *Pain, 67*, 141–150.

Wang, X. S., Mendoza, T. R., Gao, S. Z., & Cleeland, C. S. (1996). The Chinese version of the Brief Pain Inventory (BPI–C): Its development and use in a study of cancer pain [see comments]. *Pain, 67,* 407–416.

Ware, J., Snow, K., Kosinski, M., & Gandek, B. (1993). *SF–36 Health Survey: Manual and interpretation guide.* Boston: Nimrod Press.

5

SATISFACTION AND COMFORT

RHODA WEISS-LAMBROU

Over the past 20 years the field of assistive technology (AT) has developed and grown into a well-grounded and recognized body of knowledge, practice, and research. Consumer satisfaction and comfort are among the current key issues in AT assessment that need to be considered by rehabilitation practitioners and researchers.

AT research began to grow dramatically in the early 1990s. Several conceptual frameworks for interfacing people with AT underscored the relation among person, technology, and environment. Of particular significance is the matching person and technology (MPT) model that emerged from Scherer's (1993, 1996) research on technology use and quality of life. The MPT model was the first theoretical model that placed the focus on involving the consumer in the AT service delivery process. Two other conceptual models followed that also played a significant role: the human activity assistive technology model (Cook & Hussey, 1995) and the human–environment/technology model (Smith, 1991). These three conceptual models provided a framework for organizing the many factors that needed to be considered when evaluating, selecting, and using appropriate technology. From an educational perspective these paradigms became an integral part of university curricula in most of the undergraduate rehabilitation programs, thereby providing a more universal and common framework for studying AT.

AT consumers have participated in studies that have used various methodologies, including self-report questionnaires, interviews, and focus groups. Batavia and Hammer (1990) were the first to address the issue of developing consumer-based criteria for the evaluation of assistive devices. For this purpose, consumers participated in a focus group and generated the criteria that should be used in evaluating technology. Scherer's (1993) participatory-action research is another example of consumers being involved in AT research. *Living in the State of Stuck* (Scherer, 1993, 1996, 2000) was the first textbook to chronicle the perspectives and experiences of AT consumers and to explain how technology affects their lives.

Whereas the consumer-centered approach provided an important foundation for identifying consumer needs together with reasons for device use, nonuse, and abandonment, AT specialists, researchers, and third-party payers have increasingly recognized the need for outcomes-based research. The demand for outcomes data and outcomes measurement instruments emerged as the topic of foremost importance because it concerns all stakeholders (Scherer & Vitaliti, 1997; Trachtman, 1994). In his comprehensive review article Smith (1996) addressed numerous measurement issues and explained the meaning and importance of outcomes research in today's changing health care climate. The domains of AT outcomes measurement most typically documented to date are clinical results, functional status, quality of life, cost, and satisfaction (DeRuyter, 1995). These five dimensions play a pivotal role in providing qualitative and quantitative data on the comprehensiveness and effectiveness of AT.

It is in this outcomes-measurement context that recent studies have found that failure to consider user opinions and preferences is often associated with abandonment and rejection of AT (Phillips & Zhao, 1993; Scherer, 1996) and that *user satisfaction* needs to be defined and measured (Demers, Weiss-Lambrou, & Ska, 1996). In a new study on consumer satisfaction, sources of user satisfaction and dissatisfaction with wheelchair seating aids were reported, and the results brought to light that although consumers considered comfort to be the most important factor, it was also the least satisfying one (Weiss-Lambrou, Tremblay, LeBlanc, Lacoste, & Dansereau, 1999). Just like satisfaction, comfort is a desirable and important AT outcome, and it needs to be considered together with the other domains of AT outcomes. Providing comfort and satisfying consumers are among the principal goals of technology, so why are these goals not always met? The answer to this question lies in a better understanding of the meaning and importance of satisfaction and comfort and in the development of assessment tools that measure these concepts.

SATISFACTION

Meaning and Importance of Satisfaction

Etymologically, the word *satisfy* means "make enough." It comes by means of the Old French *satisfier* and from the Latin *satisfacere*, meaning "content." Satisfaction is a complicated multidimensional concept, and to date there has been little agreement about the factor structure of satisfaction measures. Although satisfaction can mean different things to different people, there is a general consensus that satisfaction is an attitude about a service, a product, a service provider, or an individual's health status.

From a psychological perspective, satisfaction is a state of pleasantness, well-being, or gratification (Chaplin, 1985). According to Linder-Pelz (1982), satisfaction is a positive attitude, an affect that results from social-psychological determinants, including perceptions, evaluations, and comparisons. On the basis of the theory and research underlying satisfaction, Simon and Patrick (1997) defined *consumer satisfaction* as a level of pleasantness, well-being, or gratification felt in reaction to a total specified experience or to its components.

In his comprehensive review article on patient satisfaction and rehabilitation services, Keith (1998) explained that satisfaction comprises affective components that reflect positive or negative feelings as well as cognitive components that are concerned with what is important and how it is evaluated. He maintained that if the factors that influence a patient's opinion cannot be identified, then the satisfaction measures have limited value. Keith also contended that unless there is some uniformity in satisfaction questionnaires and instruments, comparison of levels of satisfaction across settings and programs will not be possible.

Consumer Satisfaction

Measuring consumer satisfaction with AT has become regarded as a key means of obtaining AT outcomes data. It indicates how consumers perceive the quality of the services or the product (DeRuyter, 1995), and it is based on the real-life experience of the users. The measurement of user satisfaction with AT has been encouraged and driven by the consumer movement in health care.

Measuring consumer satisfaction is important to all stakeholders, because it provides information on AT specialists' success at meeting consumers' needs and expectations. If AT specialists want to be accountable for their actions and decisions, then they must be willing to ask consumers whether they are satisfied with the AT services and products they receive. Measurement of satisfaction is also necessary for showing that the technology is being used and that it makes a difference to the person with a disability; the consumer becomes empowered when he or she is asked to give a meaningful judgment of the device's value and impact. Data showing that the person is using the device and is satisfied with it provide the AT specialist with proof that the technology selected was the best match for that person. Identifying the sources of user satisfaction and dissatisfaction are indispensable in explaining the reasons for use, nonuse, or abandonment of an assistive device.

Measurement of satisfaction is also essential for tracking how the consumer's use of the device evolves over time. This kind of information is needed for conducting follow-up evaluations of AT use and performance as well as for establishing consumer profiles congruent with the changes in the person's condition, needs, and desires. From the perspective of third-party payers and manufacturers of the technologies, consumer satisfaction demonstrates the benefits of the AT device in terms of cost. Finally, consumer satisfaction is important because it enables rehabilitation professionals to monitor and evaluate the effectiveness of the AT programs and interventions as well as to improve the quality of the products and services provided.

Recent studies have reported a growing and widespread interest in consumer satisfaction, and they have underscored the need for a valid and reliable measure of satisfaction (Demers et al., 1996; Nochajski, Tomita, & Mann, 1996; Philipps & Zhao, 1993; Weiss-Lambrou et al., 1999). A *valid* assessment instrument is one that measures what is intended to be measured, whereas a *reliable* assessment instrument is one that produces the same result each time it is used, given that the phenomenon addressed is unchanged (Sheikh, 1986). To be useful as a standard of user opinion such a satisfaction measure should also be appropriate for use with a wide range of assistive devices as well as sufficiently sensitive to differentiate among consumers in terms of their degree of satisfaction. In the context of instrument development, such a tool needs to evolve over time and improve itself through field testing and controlled studies. Finally, rather than providing only a global score of satisfaction, it must encompass all the factors that influence user satisfaction.

Assessing Satisfaction

Some research has been directed toward developing consumer-based criteria that can be used for decisions in designing, manufacturing, and selecting assistive devices as well as for assessing consumer satisfaction. In Batavia and Hammer's (1990) study 17 general factors for 11 types of ATs were ranked in order of their perceived importance by a group of 13 consumers. The results revealed that, on average, the four most important factors for all the technologies assessed were the effectiveness, affordability, operability, and dependability of the device. The rankings of the other factors depended largely on the specific type of technology assessed. At the Rehabilitation Engineering Research Center on Technology Transfer at the University at Buffalo, State University of New York, Lane, Usiak, and Moffatt (1996) developed a subset of Batavia and Hammer's 17 criteria by combining variables that were considered by consumers to be redundant. The result was a list of 11 consumer-based criteria, with the four most important ones being effectiveness, affordability, reliability, and portability. The consumer-based criteria generated in both studies represent factors that are important to consumers when selecting their assistive devices.

To assess a consumer's satisfaction with his or her device, the dimensions of user satisfaction need to be identified. For this purpose, the development of an outcomes measurement tool of user satisfaction with assistive devices was the goal of Demers et al. (1996), the authors of the Quebec User Evaluation of Satisfaction With Assistive Technology (QUEST). QUEST is an outcomes-measurement instrument designed to evaluate a person's satisfaction with his or her AT device. Although some general satisfaction questionnaires and checklists have been developed (Rehabilitation Engineering and Assistive Technology Society of North America, 1998), QUEST is the first and only standardized satisfaction assessment tool that was designed specifically for AT devices. Data from several sources contributed to item generation for the instrument, including Batavia and Hammer's (1990) evaluation criteria. Scherer's (1996) MPT model served as the theoretical foundation for the instrument. Since the first publication of QUEST (Demers et al., 1996), the instrument has undergone pilot and field testing at research centers in Canada, the United States, and the Netherlands (Wessels, de Witte, Weiss-Lambrou, Demers, & Wijlhuizen, 1998). This testing resulted in a reduction of the number of items from 27 to 12 (see Exhibit 5.1) together with important changes to the measuring scales and assessment materials. I next present a brief description of the instrument and then discuss some of the latest findings of QUEST validity and reliability studies. Two examples of how and why QUEST can be applied in a research outcomes context conclude this section.

Quest

The concept of satisfaction as defined in the original QUEST was based on a person's critical evaluation of several aspects of the technology. The person's expectations, perceptions, attitudes, and personal values affect this assessment. This definition is consistent with current satisfaction theoretical bases (Keith, 1998; Simon & Patrick, 1997) and was originally inspired by Linder-Pelz's (1982) theoretical work on satisfaction. The 27 items that constituted the original QUEST were the criteria considered to most likely influence consumer satisfaction (Demers et al., 1996).

The original QUEST was divided into three parts. Part 1 consisted of 18 closed-ended questions aimed at describing the context in which the user's satisfaction or dissatisfaction with the assistive device developed. In Part 2 the person was asked to rate the degree of importance he or she attributes to 27 items associated with specific characteristics of the person, the device, and the environment. Using a 5-point scale, the respondent rated the degree of importance of each item, on a scale that ranged from 1 (*of no importance*) to 5 (*very important*). Inasmuch as QUEST was designed

EXHIBIT 5.1
Comparison of Consumer-Based Criteria for Evaluating Assistive Devices

Batavia & Hammer (1990)	Lane, Usiak, & Moffatt (1996)	Demers, Weiss-Lambrou, & Ska (1996)	Demers, Weiss-Lambrou, & Ska (2000)
1. Effectiveness	1. Effectiveness	1. Usefulness	1. Comfort
2. Affordability	2. Affordability	2. Repairs/servicing	2. Dimensions
3. Operability	3. Reliability	3. Adjustments	3. Simplicity of use
4. Dependability	4. Portability	4. Training	4. Effectiveness
5. Portability	5. Durability	5. Support from family/peers/employer	5. Durability
6. Durability	6. Securability	6. Durability	6. Adjustments
7. Compatibility	7. Physical security/safety	7. Accommodation by others	7. Safety
8. Flexibility	8. Learnability	8. Safety	8. Weight
9. Ease of maintenance	9. Physical comfort/ acceptance	9. Comfort	9. Professional service
10. Securability	10. Ease of maintenance/ reparability	10. Dimensions	10. Follow-up services
11. Learnability	11. Operability	11. Simplicity of use	11. Repairs/servicing
12. Personal acceptance		12. Follow-up services	12. Service delivery
13. Physical comfort		13. Professional assistance	
14. Supplier repair		14. Appearance	
15. Physical security		15. Compatibility	
16. Consumer repair		16. Effort	
17. Ease of assembly		17. Maintenance	
		18. Reaction of others	
		19. Weight	
		20. Functional performance	
		21. Transportability	
		22. Flexibility	
		23. Service delivery	
		24. Personal acceptance	
		25. Cost	
		26. Installation	
		27. Effectiveness	

to assess a wide range of AT devices, not all items were applicable to every user and every situation; consequently the respondent was allowed to score an item as nonapplicable. In Part 3 of QUEST the user was asked to rate his or her satisfaction with the variables using a 5-point satisfaction scale that ranged from 1(*not satisfied at all*) to 5 (*very satisfied*). For each item that was scored 3 (*more or less satisfied*), 2 (*not very satisfied*), or 1 (*not satisfied at all*) the user was asked to comment on or explain the source(s) of dissatisfaction. Finally, the user was asked to rate his or her overall satisfaction with the AT device. The QUEST took approximately 45 min to administer, and it was administered in a face-to-face interview context. QUEST was developed simultaneously in French and English, and a Dutch version translation was later constructed (Wessels et al., 1998).

Three studies were conducted concurrently to establish the psychometric properties of QUEST. The purpose of the first study was an international content validation of QUEST (Demers, Wessels, Weiss-Lambrou, Ska, & de Witte, 1999). For this purpose, a questionnaire was developed to assess the value of the QUEST items and to critique the administration and scoring procedures. The questionnaire was completed by an international group of 12 content experts from the United States, the Netherlands, and Canada, who were given several months to apply and test the instrument in a clinical or research context. At the test level the findings revealed that QUEST had been adequately sampled in terms of embracing all the important facets of satisfaction with AT.

The aim of the second study was to determine, at the item level, the test–retest stability and the interrater reproducibility of QUEST (Demers, Ska, Giroux, & Weiss-Lambrou, 1999). On the basis of the results of this study the Satisfaction scale was deemed reliable in terms of stability and reproducibility; however, the Importance scale did not prove to be reliable for discriminating between and among users of AT. From a validity perspective these results confirmed that QUEST had adequate content coverage, because it contained those aspects of satisfaction that were considered important to the users. However, in terms of reliability the obtained coefficients did not support the usefulness of rating the importance of each QUEST item. The task of scoring the importance of the items was dropped in the subsequent revision of QUEST.

The third study was an item analysis of 24 items comprising QUEST (Demers, Weiss-Lambrou, & Ska, 2000). To assess the psychometric properties of these items, and to select a subset of items that demonstrate optimal measurement performance, several criteria were used: general acceptability, content validity, criterion validity, contribution to internal consistency, test–retest stability, and sensitivity. The items that ranked best in terms of these measurement properties were then submitted to factorial analysis. The results of the factor analysis revealed that the underlying structure of satisfaction with AT consists of two dimensions related to the AT device (8 items) and services (4 items). This finding was cross-validated in a Dutch sample of 375 device users, and an identical structure was obtained, thereby strongly supporting the stability of the QUEST satisfaction model. The final 12 items constituting QUEST are presented in Exhibit 5.1.

At the same time as these psychometric studies were being conducted, a QUEST-based approach was being used in two investigations (Vachon, Weiss-Lambrou, Lacoste, & Dansereau, 1999; Weiss-Lambrou et al., 1999). In a study of consumer satisfaction with wheelchair seating aids (n = 24), comfort was found to be the most important variable, while at the same time it was the least satisfying variable (Weiss-Lambrou et al., 1999). The findings also revealed that there tended to be a difference in satisfaction scores between male and female respondents as well as between respondents who lived at home and those who lived in an institution. The results of Weiss-Lambrou et al.'s (1999) study clearly underscore the meaning and usefulness of satisfaction data for better understanding the consumer's needs, expectations, and preferences as well as for improving wheelchair products and services. In a second study, Vachon et al. (1999) examined the satisfaction of elderly nursing home residents (n = 32) who use a manual or powered wheelchair. The authors used a QUEST-based approach, and the results showed that the variables rated as being the most satisfying were simplicity of use, effectiveness, professional services, and safety of the wheelchair. On the other hand, respondents were most dissatisfied with their wheelchair's comfort, adjustments, and weight, as well as with the follow-up services provided. Differences in the satisfaction scores between manual and powered wheelchair users were also found, and respondents offered several reasons for their dissatisfaction. These results disclosed the sources of wheelchair satisfaction and dissatisfaction from an elderly person's viewpoint. The QUEST-based approach used in both Weiss-Lambrou et al.'s (1999) and Vachon et al.'s studies confirms the importance of assessing consumer satisfaction in a systematic and ecologically valid manner and illustrates how and why QUEST can be applied in a research outcomes context.

The current version of QUEST (paper-and-pencil format) consists of 12 satisfaction items that can be either self-administered or completed by the practitioner–evaluator. As a clinical tool, QUEST provides AT practitioners with a means of collecting satisfaction data that can be used to document the real-life benefits of AT devices and to justify the need for these devices. As a research tool, QUEST allows researchers to compare satisfaction data with other outcome measures, such as clinical results, quality of life, functional status, cost factors, and comfort. It can also serve to compare satisfaction results obtained with different user groups, in different service settings, and in different countries. Finally, because the new QUEST is easier and shorter to complete than its original version, it can be used for types of research (such as mail surveys) that require rapid acquisition of satisfaction data.

COMFORT

Meaning and Importance of Comfort

Etymologically, the word *comfort* means "make someone stronger," and its original English sense was "encourage, support." It comes by means of the Old French *conforter* and from the Latin *confortare*, meaning to strengthen greatly. Semantically speaking, comfort can be a verb, a noun, or an adjective, and it can refer to a process or an outcome. Like satisfaction, the construct of comfort is complex because it embraces a multidimensional, personal experience with differing degrees of intensity (Kolcaba, 1992).

In the context of AT, the consumer's comfort is not always considered to be an important criterion. If rehabilitation professionals are to ensure the best possible match of technology and user, it is imperative that they consider the person's psychological and physical comfort with the technology. Unlike the widespread interest in consumer satisfaction, the meaning and importance of comfort from the AT user's perspective have been to date relatively unexplored. It is important that AT practitioners and researchers interested in consumer comfort understand the varied perspectives from which the definitions of comfort have evolved. Both the nursing discipline and the field of ergonomics have long been interested in comfort.

From a nursing perspective, comfort is reported to be a desirable and important outcome for patient care (Kolcaba & Kolcaba, 1991). It is considered to be both physical and mental, and the concept of comfort is generally qualified as being pleasant and positive. In the nursing literature, Paterson and Zderad (1988, p. 112) defined *comfort* as "a state in which the person is free to be and become, controlling and planning his own destiny in accordance with his potential at a particular time in a particular situation." Nursing researchers strongly advocate that interventions must be based on the comfort needs of patients and that instruments for measuring the outcome of comfort must be developed (Kolcaba, 1992). In two qualitative nursing studies, Hamilton (1985, 1989) has inquired into the meaning of comfort from the patient's perspective. Patients were asked what comfort meant to them and what factors contributed to and detracted from their personal comfort. Although the results did not lead to an operational definition of comfort, Hamilton (1989) concluded that comfort is multidimensional, meaning different things to different people.

Researchers in the field of ergonomics also have investigated the multi-dimensional nature of comfort and discomfort. Of particular interest is the recent questionnaire survey study of Zhang, Helander, and Drury (1996), in which office workers were asked to identify factors associated with sitting comfort and discomfort and to rate their degree of importance. Forty-three of the descriptors of comfort and discomfort generated were retained and classified into groups using factor analysis, cluster analysis, and multidimensional scaling. Two main factors emerged that were identified as Comfort and Discomfort. On the basis of these findings Zhang et al. proposed a hypothetical model in which sitting comfort and discomfort are considered as different yet complementary entities. In this model, discomfort is associated with fatigue and biomechanical factors (e.g., joint angles, muscle contractions, and pressure distribution), whereas comfort is associated with feelings of relaxation and well-being. Zhang et al. (1996) explained that although good biomechanics will not necessarily increase the level of sitting comfort, it is likely that poor biomechanics will result in discomfort. Furthermore, if discomfort is increased (such as with increased time on a task), comfort will decrease; however, reducing discomfort does not necessarily result in increasing the level of comfort.

Consumer comfort with AT, just like satisfaction, is important to all stakeholders. Providing comfort is one of the primary goals of technology, and knowing whether the consumer is comfortable provides information as to whether his or her comfort needs and expectations have been met. It can be assumed that the importance of comfort will vary with the type of AT being evaluated and, consequently, the meaning of comfort will most likely vary with distinct AT user groups. Unlike consumer satisfaction, however, the importance of developing a valid and reliable outcome measure of consumer comfort has not yet been underscored in the literature.

The measurement of comfort is essential for studying how the consumer's comfort or discomfort differs with the type of activity being performed and how it changes with increased time and effort. This kind of information is important for conducting follow-up evaluations of AT use and performance, to confirm that the technology selected was the best match for that person and for improving the design and quality of devices. From the perspective of AT designers and manufacturers, consumer comfort is therefore essential for attracting new customers and for satisfying their comfort needs. Knowing the sources of user comfort and the reasons for any discomfort can help explain the reasons for use, nonuse, or abandonment of the AT. Finally, AT specialists must evaluate the effectiveness of interventions aimed at providing comfort, and they need to reidentify their mission as providers of comfort.

Assessment of Sitting Comfort

The assessment of AT consumer comfort is central to the role of AT, yet little research has been conducted to define comfort from the AT user's perspective and to develop a valid and reliable measure of this construct. Experts in ergonomics research on sitting comfort have developed both objective and subjective assessment measures for evaluating chair comfort of office workers (Christiansen, 1997; Drury & Coury, 1982; Shackel, Chidsey, & Shipley, 1969). According to Christiansen (1997), objective assessment methods of sitting comfort often use sophisticated techniques such as x-rays; electromyography investigations of muscle action potentials and observations of body position, movement, and posture; and observation of task performance. Although these objective techniques provide quantitative and objective measurements of the variables they can influence participants' health (e.g., x-ray studies), are usually very time consuming, and generally are restricted to the research laboratory. Christiansen (1997) further argued that although subjective assessments of sitting comfort may be somewhat less reliable than objective methods, they are very useful. In a series of studies aimed at exploring various testing methods for assessing chair comfort, Shackel et al. (1969) used four subjective measurement methods: (a) general comfort rating, (b) body area comfort rating, (c) chair feature checklist, and (d) direct ranking of different chairs. To date, there is no general agreement as to which of these techniques is the most valid and reliable; however, it is important that they be examined in terms of how they might be applied or adapted to the context of assessing wheelchair sitting comfort.

In an ergonomic study aimed at developing a multidimensional scale for assessment of chair comfort and discomfort, Helander and Zhang (1997) developed a checklist, the Chair Evaluation Checklist, which has 14 items describing comfort and discomfort. Each descriptor is a short statement suggestive or indicative of a degree of sitting comfort or discomfort. The Chair Evaluation Checklist consists of 12 descriptors of comfort and 12 descriptors of discomfort together with 3 overall ratings of comfort and discomfort (see Exhibit 5.2). To assess the intensity of each descriptor, a 9-point Likert scale is used. The checklist was field tested with 37 nondisabled office workers, and the results of the factor analysis confirmed the factor structure of Comfort and Discomfort. Helander and Zhang's (1997) findings are of conceptual and methodological significance in that they can serve as basis for defining comfort and discomfort from the viewpoint of AT consumers.

As a first step in the construction of an outcomes tool for measuring wheelchair sitting comfort and discomfort, Monette, Weiss-Lambrou, and

Dansereau (1999) identified the factors associated with sitting comfort and discomfort from the viewpoint of wheelchair users. For this purpose, they conducted two focus groups to define the multidimensional nature of wheelchair sitting comfort and discomfort and to generate a list of descriptors that represent the factors most likely to be associated with comfort and discomfort. Helander and Zhang's (1997) conceptual model served as the theoretical foundation for the instrument's design, and the methodologies used by Shackel et al. (1969) and Melzack (1975) inspired and guided Monette et al. The focus groups were composed of wheelchair users with a range of disabilities and occupational therapists who specialized in the area of wheelchair seating (Monette, 1999; Monette et al., 1999).

A total of 31 descriptors emerged from Monette et al.'s (1999) study: 14 of comfort, 15 of discomfort, and 2 overall ratings of comfort and discomfort. In Exhibit 5.2 the comfort–discomfort descriptors from the wheelchair users' perspective are compared with the descriptors of the nondisabled office worker group. Both groups associated feelings of well-being with sitting comfort. Unlike the nondisabled group, however, the study participants did not identify the aesthetics of the wheelchair as being an important factor associated with sitting comfort; rather, they described their feelings of comfort in terms of their ability to perform specific functional activities. The discomfort descriptors for both groups were closely related to biomechanical factors and fatigue. Unlike the nondisabled group, though, the AT participants identified particular wheelchair components and physical constraints as factors associated with sitting discomfort.

The descriptors generated by Monette et al.'s (1999) study participants confirm the multidimensional nature of sitting comfort–discomfort and constitute the first step in the development of the Wheelchair Sitting Comfort/Discomfort (CD) outcomes measure. These descriptors are used with a 5-point scale on which the wheelchair user rates the degree to which each descriptor is *always false* (1) or *always true* (5). Other components of the CD tool include an intensity scale, for assessing the degree of discomfort; a body diagram, on which the person is asked to locate the body area of his or her discomfort; and a diagram of a wheelchair, on which the person is asked to locate the technology component associated with discomfort. The CD tool needs to be field tested and its psychometric properties established. Until the time that future studies determine the instrument's relative strengths and weaknesses, the work described here can serve as an example of how research methods used in other disciplines can be linked and applied in AT outcomes research.

EXHIBIT 5.2
Comparison of Descriptors of Comfort and Discomfort

Comfort		Discomfort	
Nondisabled office workers (Helander & Zhang, 1997)	Wheelchair users (Monette, Weiss-Lambrou, & Dansereau, 1999)	Nondisabled office workers (Helander & Zhang, 1997)	Wheelchair users (Monette, Weiss-Lambrou, & Dansereau, 1999)
1. I feel relaxed.	1. I feel good.	1. I have sore muscles.	1. I have pain.
2. The chair feels soft.	2. I feel supported in the right spots.	2. I feel stiff.	2. I need to move.
3. The chair looks nice.	3. I feel little pressure under my buttocks.	3. I feel tired.	3. The wheelchair's surface is too hard.
4. I feel refreshed.	4. My wheelchair and I are one.	4. I feel restless.	4. The wheelchair limits my activities.
5. The chair is spacious.	5. I can perform my activities.	5. I have heavy legs.	5. I feel unstable.
6. I like the chair.	6. I feel stable.	6. I feel uneven pressure from the seat/back.	6. I need a better seat or backrest support.
7. I feel comfortable.	7. The dimensions of my wheelchair are adequate.	7. I feel uncomfortable.	7. I am preoccupied by my seated position.
	8. I can easily change positions in my wheelchair.		8. The wheelchair hinders my movements.
	9. I have a good endurance level in my wheelchair.		9. I feel physically tired.
	10. I can move effortlessly.		10. I have to make an extra effort in order to maintain my position.
	11. I can easily adjust the wheelchair components.		11. I need to radically change position.
	12. I feel satisfied.		12. I feel a burning sensation.
	13. I can maneuver my wheelchair.		13. I lose my balance.
	14. I feel relaxed.		14. I feel stiff.
	15. I feel comfortable.		15. I slide in my wheelchair.
			16. I feel uncomfortable.

To prepare for the future direction in which technology for people with disabilities might lead it is important to reflect on how the issues addressed in this chapter can serve to develop a more comprehensive and unifying framework for AT practice and research. The assistive technology outcomes measurement (ATOM) model (see Figure 5.1) proposed here is presented as a future framework for studying and evaluating the outcomes of AT on people with disabilities.

The ATOM model was designed to link theory and practice and define areas of concern for AT outcomes-based practice and research. The model was formulated using concepts mainly from DeRuyter's (1995) domains of AT outcomes, Scherer's (1996) MPT model, and the newly revised version of the *International Classification of Functioning, Disability and Health*, also known as *ICF* (World Health Organization, 2001). The *ICF* is a multipurpose classification providing a common framework for understanding and communicating different dimensions of disablement and health. The new version was prompted by the need to measure the consequences or outcomes of health conditions, and it will be finalized after the results of field trials are interpreted. In the *ICF* disablement is seen as an interaction between one's health condition and contextual factors (i.e., environmental and personal factors). In the context of "consequences of health conditions" the classification includes three distinct but parallel dimensions: Impairment (a loss or abnormality of body structure or of a physiological or psychological function), Activity (personal phenomena influencing the nature and extent

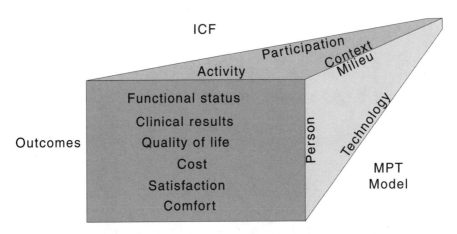

Figure 5.1. Assistive technology outcomes model (ATOM). AT outcomes: domains of AT outcomes (DeRuyter, 1995). MPT model = matching person and technology model (Scherer, 1993, 1996); *ICF* = *International Classification of Functioning, Disability and Health* (World Health Organization, 2001).

of a person's activities associated with everyday life), and Participation (societal phenomena affecting the nature and extent of a person's involvement in life situations). Although the dimensions of Activity and Participation have been defined, instruments to measure them have yet to be determined. As the classification and terminology of the ICF evolves, so will the terms and components of the ATOM model.

Currently, the ATOM model consists of three main components: the domains of outcomes, the MPT model, and the ICF (see Figure 5.1). These components are arranged in a cubic form to illustrate their dynamic interaction as well as their complex relation with contextual factors. The component outcomes consists of six principal domains: clinical results, functional status, quality of life, cost, satisfaction, and comfort. The three components of the MPT model (characteristics of the milieu, the person, and the technology) constitute the second determinant of the ATOM model and underscore the principle that the consumer's experience and opinion must serve as the foundation for assessing AT outcomes (Scherer, 1996). The third component of the ATOM model integrates two of the dimensions of the ICF—Activity and Participation—and emphasizes the importance of considering contextual factors.

The ATOM model is flexible in that it can interface with other perspectives, theories, and practices. It is this adaptability that offers a practical tool to AT specialists practicing in many different roles and settings. The model was conceptualized to facilitate communication within and outside the AT field, and the terminology can be communicated in various languages and cultures. Although it is only in its early stage of development, the ATOM model has the potential for successfully engaging AT specialists and collaborators from other disciplines in a systematic approach to assessing AT outcomes. It is most likely that AT research in the next millennium will lead to further development and refinement of this conceptual model.

REFERENCES

Batavia, A. J., & Hammer, G. S. (1990). Predictors of assistive technology abandonment. *Assistive Technology, 5,* 36–45.

Chaplin, J. P. (1985). *Dictionary of psychology.* New York: Dell.

Christiansen, K. (1997). Subjective assessment of sitting comfort. *Collegium Antropologicum, 21,* 387–395.

Cook, A. M., & Hussey, S. M. (1995). *Assistive technologies: Principles and practice.* St. Louis, MO: Mosby.

Demers, L., Ska, B., Giroux, F., & Weiss-Lambrou, R. (1999). Stability and reproducibility of the Quebec User Evaluation of Satisfaction With Assistive Technology (QUEST). *Journal of Rehabilitation Outcomes Measurement, 3*(4), 42–52.

Demers, L., Weiss-Lambrou, R., & Ska, B. (1996). Development of the Quebec User Evaluation of Satisfaction With Assistive Technology (QUEST). *Assistive Technology, 8,* 3–13.

Demers, L., Weiss-Lambrou, R., & Ska, B. (2000). Item analysis of the Quebec User Evaluation of Satisfaction With Assistive Technology (QUEST). *Assistive Technology, 12,* 96–105.

Demers, L., Wessels, R. D., Weiss-Lambrou, R., Ska, B., & de Witte, L. P. (1999). An international content validation of the Quebec User Evaluation of Satisfaction With Assistive Technology (QUEST). *Occupational Therapy International, 6,* 159–175.

DeRuyter, F. (1995). Evaluating outcomes in assistive technology: Do we understand the commitment? *Assistive Technology, 7,* 3–16.

Drury, C. G., & Coury, B. G. (1982). A methodology for chair evaluation. *Applied Ergonomics, 13,* 195–202.

Hamilton, J. (1985). *Comfort on a palliative care unit: The client's perception.* Unpublished master's thesis, School of Nursing, McGill University, Montreal, Quebec, Canada.

Hamilton, J. (1989). Comfort and the hospitalized chronically ill. *Journal of Gerontology Nursing, 15*(14), 28–33.

Helander, M.G., & Zhang, L. (1997). Field studies of comfort and discomfort in sitting. *Ergonomics, 40,* 895–915.

Keith, R. L. (1998). Patient satisfaction and rehabilitation services. *Archives of Physical Medicine and Rehabilitation, 79,* 1122–1128.

Kolcaba, K. (1992). Holistic comfort: Operationalizing the construct as a nurse-sensitive outcome. *Advances in Nursing Science, 15,* 1–10.

Kolcaba, K., & Kolcaba, R. (1991). An analysis of the concept of comfort. *Journal of Advanced Nursing, 16,* 1301–1310.

Lane, J. P., Usiak, D. J., & Moffatt, A. (1996). Consumer criteria for assistive devices: Operationalizing generic criteria for specific ABLEDATA categories. In *Proceedings of the 19th Annual Conference on Rehabilitation Technology* (pp. 146–148). Arlington, VA: RESNA Press.

Linder-Pelz, S. (1982). Toward a theory of patient satisfaction. *Social Science and Medicine, 16,* 577–582.

Melzack, R. (1975). The McGill Pain Questionnaire: Major properties and scoring methods. *Pain, 1,* 277–299.

Monette, M. (1999). *Le développement d'un instrument de mesure du confort et de l'inconfort de la position assise des usagers d'aides techniques à la mobilité et à la posture* [*The development of an assessment tool to measure wheelchair sitting comfort and discomfort*]. Unpublished master's thesis, University of Montreal, Montreal, Quebec, Canada.

Monette, M., Weiss-Lambrou, R., & Dansereau, J. (1999). In search of a better understanding of wheelchair sitting comfort and discomfort. In *Proceedings of the RESNA '99 Annual Conference* (pp. 218–220). Arlington, VA: RESNA Press.

Nochajski, S. M., Tomita, M. R., & Mann, W. C. (1996). The use and satisfaction with assistive devices by older persons with cognitive impairments: A pilot intervention study. *Topics in Geriatric Rehabilitation, 12*(2), 40–53.

Paterson, J., & Zderad, L. (1988). *Humanistic nursing* (2nd ed.). New York: National League for Nursing.

Phillips, B., & Zhao, H. (1993). Predictors of assistive technology abandonment. *Assistive Technology, 5,* 36–45.

Rehabilitation Engineering and Assistive Technology Society of North America (1998). *RESNA resource guide for assistive technology outcomes. Volume II: Assessment instruments, tools, and checklist from the field.* Arlington, VA: RESNA Press.

Scherer, M. J. (1993). *Living in the state of stuck: How technology impacts the lives of people with disabilities.* Cambridge, MA: Brookline Books.

Scherer, M. J. (1996). *Living in the state of stuck: How technology impacts the lives of people with disabilities* (2nd ed.). Cambridge, MA: Brookline Books.

Scherer, M. J. (2000). *Living in the state of stuck: How technology impacts the lives of people with disabilities* (3rd ed.). Cambridge, MA: Brookline Books.

Scherer, M. J., & Vitaliti, L. T. (1997). A functional approach to technological factors and their assessment in rehabilitation. In S. S. Dittmar & G. E. Gresham (Eds.), *Functional assessment and outcome measures for the rehabilitation health professional* (pp. 69–80). Gaithersburg, MD: Aspen.

Shackel, B., Chidsey, K. D., & Shipley, P. (1969). The assessment of chair comfort. *Ergonomics, 12,* 269–306.

Sheikh, K. (1986). Disability scales: Assessment of reliability. *Archives of Physical Medicine and Rehabilitation, 67,* 245–249.

Simon, S. E., & Patrick, A. (1997). Understanding and assessing consumer satisfaction in rehabilitation. *Journal of Rehabilitation Outcomes Measurements, 1*(5), 1–14.

Smith, R. (1991). Technological approaches to performances enhancement. In C. Christiansen & C. Baum (Eds.), *Occupational therapy: Overcoming human performance deficits* (pp. 747–788). Thorofare, NJ: Slack.

Smith, R. O. (1996). Measuring the outcomes of assistive technology: Challenge and innovation. *Assistive Technology, 8,* 71–81.

Trachtman, L. (1994). Outcome measures: Are we ready to answer the tough questions? *Assistive Technology, 6,* 91–92.

Vachon, B., Weiss-Lambrou, R., Lacoste, M., & Dansereau, J. (1999). Elderly nursing home residents' satisfaction with manual and powered wheelchairs. In *Proceedings of the RESNA '99 Annual Conference* (pp. 221–223). Arlington, VA: RESNA Press.

Weiss-Lambrou, R., Tremblay, C., LeBlanc, R., Lacoste, M., & Dansereau, J. (1999). Wheelchair seating aids: How satisfied are consumers? *Assistive Technology, 11,* 43–53.

Wessels, R. D., de Witte, L. P., Weiss-Lambrou, R., Demers, L., & Wijlhuizen, G. (1998). A Dutch version of QUEST (D-QUEST) applied as a routine follow-up within the service delivery process. In E. Placencia & E. Ballabio (Eds.), *Improving the quality of life for the European citizen* (pp. 420–424). Washington, DC: IOS Press.

World Health Organization. (2001). *ICF: International classification of functioning, disability and health: Final draft* (English full version) [On-line]. Retrieved from http://www.who.int/icidh/

Zhang, L., Helander, M. G., & Drury, C. G. (1996). Identifying factors of comfort and discomfort in sitting. *Human Factors and Ergonomics Society, 38,* 377–389.

6

GENDER AND ETHNORACIAL DIFFERENCES IN THE OWNERSHIP AND USE OF ASSISTIVE TECHNOLOGY

DIANA H. RINTALA

In this chapter I describe and evaluate the sparse literature on gender and ethnoracial differences regarding ownership and use of assistive technology (AT). The implications of the findings are discussed, particularly for members of the rehabilitation team who help people make appropriate selections.

Gender differences in health, health care use, and health behaviors have been documented (Verbrugge, 1985). These differences may stem from a number of factors, such as biological differences, diverse lifestyles, and different socialization patterns in childhood. Gender differences may result in various attitudes toward disability and use of AT.

Ethnoracial labels such as *African American* and *Hispanic* have sometimes been associated with certain cultural characteristics (i.e., values, attitudes, and beliefs) thought to be typical of particular groups (Rojewski, 1997). However, it is recognized that there is more variation within these groups than between them (e.g., Phinney, 1996). Thus, simply assigning an ethnoracial label to an individual does not help us to know what values,

This work was supported in part by the Center of Excellence on Healthy Aging With Disabilities, Rehabilitation Research and Development Service, Veterans Health Administration, Department of Veterans Affairs. This work was also supported in part by the Rehabilitation Research and Training Center in Community Integration for Individuals with Spinal Cord Injury, funded by Grant H133B40011-95 from the National Institute on Disability and Rehabilitation Research. The opinions contained in this chapter are those of the author and do not necessarily reflect those of the Department of Veterans Affairs or the U.S. Department of Education.

attitudes, and beliefs the person may have regarding AT. Nevertheless, it is important for rehabilitation professionals to be aware that culture can vary along a number of dimensions that may be relevant to issues of AT. These include independence versus interdependence, degree of family affiliation, degree of assimilation into a dominant culture, degree of shame or punishment associated with disability, direct versus indirect communication style, and internal versus external locus of control. Unfortunately, the studies in the literature regarding the relation of race and ethnicity with AT simply categorize the participants according to broad ethnoracial labels. For the most part, they do not directly address values, beliefs, and attitudes but primarily focus on ownership and use of AT.

It is important for professionals who are consulted regarding AT to be aware of where the service recipient "fits" along the dimensions just noted. Each person brings to an interaction his or her own cultural bias that tends to filter or screen one's perceptions of a situation (Barney, 1991; Krefting & Krefting, 1991). If one is ignorant of customs, beliefs, and practices other than one's own, a very poor understanding of the needs and desires of the client may result. Furthermore, if the service provider believes that his or her views are the only "right" views, the perspective of the client and family may be ignored. Thus, it is important to work with cultural differences rather than against them (Smart & Smart, 1997). Ignoring the influence of culture can lead to less effective service (Aminzadeh & Edwards, 1998). Gitlin, Luborsky, and Schemm (1998) asserted that devices are not value-neutral tools. It is important to be aware that the social meaning of device use is not static: It varies, not only across cultures but also across time periods. For example, canes were considered fashionable during the 19th century but are now often viewed as being used only by frail or elderly people (Aminzadeh & Edwards, 1998; Krefting & Krefting, 1991). Relatively few studies have focused on gender or ethnoracial differences in attitudes and behaviors regarding AT. These studies have varied widely with respect to characteristics of the samples (e.g., ages, cultures, and countries) and types of technology studied (e.g., general, cognitive, mobility, and home modifications). I sought appropriate references through searches of the PubMed and PsycINFO databases. I obtained additional references through citations in already-identified publications. Keywords used in the searches included terms such as *assistive, technology, equipment, aids,* and *devices,* combined with terms such as *gender, racial, ethnic, culture, African-American, Hispanic, Latino, Native American, Asian, Chinese, Japanese, Vietnamese,* and *Korean.* I found no publications that investigated the relation of Native Americans or any Asian groups to AT, and only three that involved Hispanic groups.

Fifteen studies have investigated gender differences in ownership or use of AT. Seven of the studies found that women were more likely to own or use various devices, three found mixed results for gender differences depending on age of respondent or type of device, and five found no gender differences. Macken (1986) analyzed data obtained from the 1982 Long-Term Care Survey conducted by the U.S. Bureau of the Census. Approximately 5,000 Medicare enrollees ages 65 or older (64% female) were interviewed. They were identified from a screening sample of 36,000 as having problems performing basic activities of daily living (ADLs; e.g., bathing, dressings, toileting, and eating) and instrumental activities of daily living (IADLs; e.g., doing housework, preparing meals, doing laundry, shopping for groceries, and managing money). Women were more likely than were men (32% vs. 25%) to have at least one "special feature" in their home and were more likely to have extra handrails or grab bars (23% vs. 19%) and raised toilet seats (7% vs. 4%). Other special features studied included ramps (used by 4%), elevators or stair lifts (3%), extra-wide doors or hallways (4%), and push bars on doors (1%). Women were also more likely than were men (38% vs. 27%) to identify at least one special feature they did not have that they believed would facilitate performance of ADLs or IADLs. Extra handrails or grab bars were the most desired features (21% desired them).

Penning and Strain (1994) analyzed survey data obtained from 749 noninstitutionalized adults ages 65 or older (65% female) living in the province of Manitoba, Canada, who reported difficulty with one or more ADLs. The sample was drawn from the Manitoba Health Services Commission database, which includes nearly all residents of the province. Men were more likely than were women (54% vs. 44%) to neither receive personal assistance nor use AT to perform specified ADLs. Women were more likely than were men to both receive personal assistance and to use AT. For both genders, most people who received personal assistance were also likely to use AT; however, a minority used only one or the other exclusively. Items reportedly used included mobility aids, rails and grab bars, and raised toilet seats.

Sonn and Grimby (1994) interviewed 595 people in Sweden who were age 76 (55% female). Respondents were asked about assistive devices they owned and used. These included devices for hygiene, mobility, beds and chairs (e.g., raising cushions, electric bed), grip and reach, and other (e.g., magnifying glasses, bicycle ergometer). Women were more likely than were men (52% vs. 37%) to have assistive devices.

Watts, Erickson, Houde, Wilson, and Maynard (1996) analyzed a subsample of data from the U.S. National Health Interview Survey: Assistive

Devices Supplement, conducted in 1990. Their analyses included only the 3,297 respondents (58% female) who were ages 65 or older and had at least one assistive device. Women were more likely than were men (36% vs. 27%) to report using more than one assistive device.

In a study of 498 single people (82% female) ages 75 or older living independently in the Netherlands, de Klerk, Huijsman, and McDonnell (1997) differentiated between aids for ADLs (buttonhook, stocking aid, raised bed, grab bar, and shower stool) and mobility aids (cane, walker, and wheelchair). For each of the two types of equipment (ADL or mobility), women were more likely than were men to use at least one device (γ: ADL aids = $-.43$, mobility aids = $-.25$). However, for those people who used at least one device, there was no relation between gender and the number of each type of device used.

Carrasquillo, Lantigua, and Shea (2000) analyzed a subset of data from the Medical Expenditure Panel Survey in 1996. Their sample included the 2,590 adults ages 65 or older who were White (58% female), African American (60% female), or Hispanic (56% female). One question concerned the use of assistive devices such as a walker, grab bars in the bathtub, or any other special equipment for personal care or everyday activities. Women were more likely than were men (22% vs. 14%) to use at least one device.

Tabbarah, Silverstein, and Seeman (2000) analyzed data from 6,551 respondents (61% female) to the U.S. Survey of Asset and Health Dynamics of the Oldest Old (AHEAD; 1993–1994). Their sample included people ages 70 and older who resided in the general community rather than in age-segregated communities and housing. Respondents were asked about the presence of grab bars and shower seats, special railings, ramp access to the street, and wheelchair access within the home. A separate, hierarchical logistic regression analysis was performed for each of the four categories of technology, first entering as predictors sociodemographic characteristics, followed by health conditions/events, and then types of disability. Twenty-three percent of the total sample had grab bars, a shower seat, or both; 8% had special railings; 5% had ramp access to the street; and 9% had wheelchair access within the home. Women were more likely than were men to have grab bars or shower seats (odds ratio in full model = 1.19) and special railings (odds ratio in full model = 1.34). There were no gender differences in the full models for the presence of ramp access to the street and wheelchair access within the home.

Black (1980) analyzed data from the U.S. National Health Interview Survey obtained in 1977 from approximately 41,000 households that included 111,000 people. She reported that among people younger than age 65, men were more likely to use special aids than were women (2.1% vs. 1.8%). However, among people ages 65 or older, women were more likely than were men (13.9% vs. 12.6%) to use special aids. In general, men were more likely than were women (0.24% vs. 0.14%) to use leg or foot braces and crutches, and women were more likely than were men (0.44% vs. 0.20%) to use walkers. There were no gender differences found for the use of canes, special shoes, or wheelchairs.

Forbes, Hayward, and Agwani (1993) reported on data obtained from the Canadian Health and Activity Limitation Survey. Among people ages 55 and older who reported a mobility, vision, or hearing impairment, women tended to use devices to aid hearing and vision more often than did men, whereas men tended to use mobility aids more often than did women. However, the differences were small and varied by age group.

Edwards and Jones (1998) conducted interviews with 500 people in Wales who were randomly selected from three Family Health Service Authority registries. All participants were at least age 65, and 60% were female. A significantly greater proportion of women than men (77% vs. 70%) owned at least one assistive device. Women were more likely than were men to have a walking frame (5% vs. 1%), a wheelchair (5% vs. 2%), a commode chair (10% vs. 6%), and bathroom rails (26% vs. 20%). Men were more likely than were women to have a walking stick (35% vs. 27%). In terms of use of devices, women were more likely than were men to use walking frames (4% vs. 1%) and bathroom rails (24% vs. 16%). No gender differences were found for ownership or use of crutches, raised lavatory seats, nonslip bath mats, bath seats, bath boards, stair rails, or bed hoists.

Geiger (1990) interviewed 40 people (62% female) ranging in age from ages 16 to 95 who had received occupational therapy services at one acute hospital rehabilitation unit in a U.S. city. Each had received more than one of the following devices: reacher, long-handled sponge, long-handled shoehorn, dressing stick, and sock aid. The interviews were conducted 4–6 weeks following discharge. There were no gender differences found in the percentage of items (45%) that were still in use at the time of the interview.

Brooks (1991) investigated the types of assistive devices used in particular social settings (public, employment, educational, friendship, family, and alone). The sample consisted of a group of 595 scientists and engineers (22% female) ranging in age from ages 19 to 88 (M = 47 years) who had disabilities and were members of the American Association for the Advancement of Science (AAAS). The sample constituted 47% of the 1,254 members to whom surveys were mailed. No gender differences were found with regard to types of devices used overall or used in particular social settings. Types of devices included those used for personal care and hygiene (e.g., grooming devices, eating devices), employment (e.g., computers, stand aids), transportation (e.g., vehicle lifts, hand controls), homemaking (e.g., cooking devices, cleaning devices), child care (e.g., bathing devices, monitors), communication (e.g., hearing aids, electronic larynxes), education (e.g., page turners, talking calculators), and mobility (e.g., wheelchairs, canes).

Mann, Karuza, Hurren, and Tomita (1992) analyzed a subset of the data from the Consumer Assessments Study conducted by the University at Buffalo Rehabilitation Engineering Center on Aging. The subsample consisted of 31 noninstitutionalized people (55% female) who were identified as having a cognitive impairment (81% with Alzheimer's disease, 19% with "other"). All were ages 65 or older. In multiple regression analyses gender was not among the variables that were predictive for number of assistive devices of any type used or number of cognitive devices used.

Gitlin, Schemm, Landsberg, and Burgh (1996) interviewed 86 of 250 eligible people who were ages 55 or older (69% female) 5 days prior to discharge to home and 1, 2, and 3 months following discharge from either of two rehabilitation hospitals in Pennsylvania. The remaining respondents participated at some, but not all, data collection points. The primary diagnosis for each person was cerebrovascular accident, orthopedic deficit, or lower limb amputation. Each was discharged with one or more assistive devices for mobility, dressing, bathing, toileting, feeding, or seating for use at home. There were no gender differences in use of the devices at any of the three follow-up contacts, neither were there gender differences in consistency of use across time (*consistent* users used at all three contacts, *delayed* users did not use at first contact but did use by third contact, *temporary* users used at first contact but did not use by third contact, and *nonusers* rarely or never used).

Ostchega, Harris, Hirsch, Parsons, and Kington (2000) analyzed a subset of the data from the National Health and Nutrition Examination Survey (NHANES III). Their sample consisted of the 6,866 people (53% female) ages 60 and older who were interviewed in their home between 1988 and 1994. The results of one question on the use of aids for walking (i.e., cane, wheelchair, crutches, or walker) were included in the report. No significant gender difference in regard to device use was found.

In addition to these 15 studies of device ownership and use, Gitlin et al. (1998) analyzed 131 spontaneous qualitative comments made by 52 participants (50% female) ages 55 or older who had been hospitalized with a primary diagnosis of a cerebrovascular accident. The comments were made while responding to a structured interview regarding AT. Men were more likely than women (63% vs. 41%) to make a spontaneous comment. The qualitative comments were categorized as positive, negative, or mixed. No gender differences were found in the proportion of comments in each category.

The quality of the studies just described varies enormously. Of the studies that found that women were more likely to own or use assistive devices, all had large samples (*Ns* = 498–6,551), and the studies were conducted in a variety of industrialized countries. These characteristics suggest that the findings are generalizable. However, all of those seven samples were of people ages 65 or older, thus limiting generalizability to the elderly population. The studies varied in terms of the specific types of equipment assessed and the outcome measures reported (e.g., number of devices owned or used, ownership or use of either specific devices or groups of devices [e.g., mobility]). They also varied with respect to inclusion criteria, with some including only people known to have a problem with daily activities or to have at least one assistive device. In terms of the studies that found no differences, three of the five had small sample sizes (Ns = 31–86), and four had unique inclusion criteria (e.g., membership in AAAS and disabled, cognitively impaired). Some pertinent details were difficult to find in some of the articles, such as the one by Black (1980), who did not clearly report the percentage of the sample that was female, the age range of the sample, and the inclusion criteria. In general, there is stronger evidence supporting the finding that, among elderly people, women are more likely than men to own and use assistive equipment than supporting the finding of no gender differences.

ETHNORACIAL DIFFERENCES

Nine studies have examined the relation between race–ethnicity (African American, White, and Hispanic) and ownership and use of assistive equipment. Six contrasted only White Americans versus African Americans, whereas three also included Hispanics. Four found that African American respondents owned or used fewer assistive devices than did White respondents, one found that Hispanic respondents were less likely to have one type of device than were White respondents, and five found no differences based on race–ethnicity. In addition, two studies evaluated satisfaction with owned devices. In one, African American respondents were less satisfied than were White respondents, and in the other there was no difference in satisfaction based on race or ethnicity.

Macken (1986), using the data from the long-term care study described earlier (86% White, 14% African American), found that African American participants were less likely than White participants (25% vs. 31%) to have at least one of the special features under study. The only technology that African Americans were more likely to have than White Americans (26% vs. 4%) was ramps. On the other hand, African Americans were more likely than White Americans (41% vs. 28%) to name at least one special feature they did not have that they believed would facilitate their daily activities.

Tomita, Mann, Fraas, and Burns (1997) interviewed 505 frail elders (87% White, 13% African American) ages 60 years or older living in western

New York State. All had difficulty with at least one ADL. Ownership and use of four types of devices (physical, hearing, vision, and cognitive) were assessed. African American elders owned and used fewer vision and hearing devices than White elders, and the African American participants were less satisfied with both their vision and hearing devices than were the White participants. After statistically controlling for age, income, and education, racial differences in number of vision devices owned and used remained statistically significant, but there were no longer racial differences for number of hearing devices owned and used.

In Ostchega et al.'s (2000) study, described earlier, in which a subset of the data from the NHANES III was analyzed, the authors compared results for White Americans (60%), African Americans (19%), and Mexican Americans (18%). For both men and women, African Americans were more likely than White Americans to use a walking aid (men: 17% vs. 11%; women: 22% vs. 12%). Mexican American men and women did not differ significantly from either of the other two ethnoracial groups on this question.

In the analyses of the AHEAD study data (85% White, 11% African American, 4% Hispanic) by Tabbarah et al. (2000), described earlier, African Americans were less likely than White Americans to have grab bars or shower seats (odds ratio for full model = 0.61). Hispanics were less likely than White Americans to have special railings (odds ratio for full model = 0.50). No ethnoracial differences were found for ramp access to the street or wheelchair access within the home. Comparisons between the two minority groups were not reported.

In Mann et al.'s (1992) study, described earlier, of 31 noninstitutionalized people (87% White, 13% African American) who were identified as having a cognitive impairment, race was not among the variables that were predictive for number of assistive devices of any type used or number of cognitive devices used. In the analysis of data from the U.S. National Health Interview Survey by Watts et al. (1996), described earlier, 87% of the sample was White, 12% was African American, and 1% were of "other" ethnicity. There was no relation between race and number of assistive devices used.

Gitlin et al. (1996), in the study described earlier in which respondents (63% White, 37% African American) were contacted each month for 3 months after discharge, no differences were found based on race in patterns of use of assistive devices at any contact point or across time. In Gitlin et al.'s (1998) study, described earlier (65% White, 35% African American), White Americans were more likely than African Americans (61% vs. 38%) to comment spontaneously on AT, but no differences were found based on race in the proportion of comments regarding AT categorized as positive, negative, or mixed.

In the study by Carrasquillo et al. (2000), described earlier, which analyzed a subset of the Medical Expenditure Panel Survey (79% White,

11% African American, 10% Hispanic), there were no significant differences based on race–ethnicity in the proportion (36%) of people who used at least one assistive device.

As with the studies involving gender, the four studies that found ethnoracial differences had large sample sizes (Ns = 505–6,866), whereas three of the five studies that did not find differences had relatively small samples (Ns = 31–86). Furthermore, three of the studies that found differences were national studies. Results of larger national samples are more likely to generalize to similar populations. All of the studies involved U.S. samples, and all involved people ages 55 years or older, thus limiting generalizability to older U.S. residents. Only two of the nine samples attempted to elicit attitudes toward assistive devices as opposed to ownership or use. On balance, there appears to be evidence that African Americans with physical impairments are less likely than White Americans to own and use AT devices. As with gender differences, reasons for this finding are unclear. Explanatory factors may include differences in attitudes, economic status, functional status, or some combination of these. More studies are needed with regard to other ethnoracial groups.

CONCLUSION

Although, to date, scientific evidence on gender and ethnoracial differences regarding AT is relatively meager, and the results are mixed, members of the rehabilitation team, including rehabilitation psychologists, should expect diverse perspectives among their clients and the clients' family members. Thus, it is important to be aware of various potential points of view and respect the fact that more than one perspective is legitimate. When working with a client regarding AT, there are several key points to consider: the client's and family's degree of acculturation, their racial–ethnic identity, the views of their own culture and of the dominant culture, and their level of formal education (Rojewski, 1997). LaPlante, Hendershot, and Moss (1992) found that economic status was related to ownership of devices, who paid for the devices (self or third-party payer), and unmet need for devices. Barney (1991) emphasized that speaking another language is a major barrier to understanding the client's point of view. Furthermore, the impact of AT on self-image and self-esteem must be considered (Kohn, Enders, Preston, & Motloch, 1983; Rojewski, 1997). Other possible consequences of receiving a device should also be taken into account, such as whether the residence is large enough to accommodate the device and whether other devices or modifications are necessary (and attainable) to facilitate use of the device, such as needing a ramp and a van with a lift to effectively use a power wheelchair or scooter, or widening a doorway to allow entry into the bath-room to use bathing and toileting aids (Kohn et al., 1983).

Barney (1991), Cook and Hussey (1995), Kohn et al. (1983), O'Day and Corcoran (1994), and Parrette and Marr (1997) have stressed the importance of understanding both the client's and the family members' points of view regarding AT. In some cases, inclusion of extended family members, in addition to immediate family, may be helpful. The service provider needs to be aware of who in the family makes the health care decisions. Compromises among differing perspectives may need to be consid-ered. If a consensus is not reached, the provider may not get all of the necessary information; there will be poor follow-through by the client, the family members, or both; and distrust of the provider may result (Cook & Hussey, 1995).

Cohen, Tate, and Forchheimer (1994) found that simply receiving more resources (e.g., AT) did not relate to better outcomes. However, congruence between a felt need for a resource and receipt of that resource was related to better long-term outcomes. Scherer and Galvin (1996) empha-sized the importance of matching people with appropriate ATs. They urged professionals to remember to "ask, listen, and respond" (p. 8). They also stressed the importance of providing training on device use and evaluating outcomes of AT ownership and use. In following these suggestions, gender, racial, ethnic, and cultural perspectives must be kept in mind.

Although it is important to be aware of cultural differences regarding AT, it also is important not to stereotype a client's viewpoint based on gender, race, or ethnicity. Rehabilitation psychologists may be able to help other team members to be open to varied points of view and encourage them to listen carefully to what the client and family members say. Being aware of nonverbal cues may also be important. Clients may feel intimidated by the expertise of the provider and therefore may be uncomfortable stating their true feelings about a particular AT item. If the provider is very unfamil-iar with the culture of a particular client, especially if the provider and client speak different languages, it may be helpful to have a person who serves as a culture broker between the client and the provider. A *culture broker*, a term coined by Wolf (1956), is more than a translator of language. Such a person understands the rules and expectations of each of the two cultures and operates successfully in both. Spencer (1991) described the role of such a person as helping people with disabilities living in group housing learn to initiate and manage outside activities. This strategy is likely to be effective in other rehabilitation situations, such as in the selection of AT.

Because of the relative scarcity of scientific evidence of the effects of gender, race, ethnicity, and culture on attitudes toward AT and AT owner-ship and use, further research is needed. Such research should identify subpopulations within racial and ethnic groups that may differ with respect to AT issues. These subpopulations may represent country of origin (e.g., Mexican American, Puerto Rican American, Cuban American), educational level, or economic status. Other grouping variables that may be important are the type and degree of functional limitation people have and the specific types and characteristics of the technology being assessed. Studies that combine qualitative and quantitative methods are likely to yield the most informative results. Rehabilitation professionals must help clients make the best decisions possible regarding AT. To do this they need to understand how decisions are made about acquiring and using such aids.

REFERENCES

Aminzadeh, F., & Edwards, N. (1998). Exploring seniors' views on the use of assistive devices in fall prevention. *Public Health Nursing, 15*, 297–304.

Barney, K. F. (1991). From Ellis Island to assisted living: Meeting the needs of older adults from diverse cultures. *American Journal of Occupational Therapy, 45*, 586–593.

Black, E. R. (1980). Use of special aids: United States—1977. *Vital Health Statistics, 10*, 1–40.

Brooks, N. A. (1991). Users' responses to assistive devices for physical disability. *Social Science and Medicine, 32*, 1417–1424.

Carrasquillo, O., Lantigua, R. A., & Shea, S. (2000). Differences in functional status of Hispanic versus non-Hispanic White elders: Data from the Medical Expenditure Panel Survey. *Journal of Aging and Health, 12*, 342–361.

Cohen, E., Tate, D., & Forchheimer, M. (1994). SCI resources and outcomes: Perceptions of resources needed and received following SCI and long term psychological and functional outcomes: A pilot study. *SCI Psychosocial Process, 7*(2), 47–54.

Cook, A. M., & Hussey, S. M. (1995). *Assistive technologies: Principles and practice.* St. Louis, MO: Mosby.

de Klerk, M. M. Y., Huijsman, R., & McDonnell, J. (1997). The use of technical aids by elderly persons in the Netherlands: An application of the Andersen and Newman model. *The Gerontologist, 37*, 365–373.

Edwards, N. I., & Jones, D. A. (1998). Ownership and use of assistive devices amongst older people in the community. *Age and Ageing, 27*, 463–468.

Forbes, W. F., Hayward, L. M., & Agwani, N. (1993). Factors associated with self-reported use and non-use of assistive devices among impaired elderly residing in the community. *Canadian Journal of Public Health, 84*, 53–57.

Geiger, C. M. (1990). The utilization of assistive devices by patients discharged from an acute rehabilitation setting. *Physical and Occupational Therapy in Geriatrics, 9*, 3–25.

Gitlin, L. N., Luborsky, M. L., & Schemm, R. L. (1998). Emerging concerns of older stroke patients about assistive device use. *The Gerontologist, 38*, 169–180.

Gitlin, L. N., Schemm, R. L., Landsberg, L., & Burgh, D. (1996). Factors predicting assistive device use in the home by older people following rehabilitation. *Journal of Aging and Health, 8*, 554–575.

Kohn, J., Enders, S., Preston, J., & Motloch, W. (1983). Provision of assistive equipment for handicapped persons. *Archives of Physical Medicine and Rehabilitation, 64*, 378–381.

Krefting, L. H., & Krefting, D. V. (1991). Cultural influences on performance. In C. Christian & C. Baum (Eds.), *Occupational therapy: Overcoming human performance deficits* (pp. 101–122). Thorofare, NJ: Slack.

LaPlante, M. P., Hendershot, G. E., & Moss, A. J. (1992, September 16). Assistive technology devices and home accessibility features: Prevalence, payment, need and trends. *Advance Data, 217*, 1–11.

Macken, C. L. (1986). A profile of functionally impaired elderly persons living in the community. *Health Care Financing Review, 7*(4), 33–49.

Mann, W. C., Karuza, J., Hurren, D., & Tomita, M. (1992). Assistive devices for home-based elderly persons with cognitive impairments. *Topics in Geriatric Rehabilitation, 8*, 35–52.

O'Day, B. L., & Corcoran, P. J. (1994). Assistive technology: Problems and policy alternatives. *Archives of Physical Medicine and Rehabilitation, 75*, 1165–1169.

Ostchega, Y., Harris, T. B., Hirsch, R., Parsons, V. L., & Kington, R. (2000). The prevalence of functional limitations and disability in older persons in the US: Data from the National Health and Nutrition Examination Survey III. *Journal of the American Geriatric Society, 48*, 1132–1135.

Parette, H. P., & Marr, D. D. (1997). Assisting children and families who use augmentative and alternative communication (AAC) devices: Best practices for school psychologists. *Psychology in the Schools, 34*, 337–346.

Penning, M. J., & Strain, L. A. (1994). Gender differences in disability, assistance, and subjective well-being in later life. *Journal of Gerontology, 49*, S202–S208.

Phinney, J. S. (1996). When we talk about American ethnic groups, what do we mean? *American Psychologist, 51*, 918–930.

Rojewski, J. W. (1997). Cultural diversity and its impact on career counseling. In *The Hatherleigh guide to vocational and career counseling* (pp. 177–208). New York: Hatherleigh Press.

Scherer, M. J., & Galvin, J. C. (1996). An outcomes perspective of quality pathways to most appropriate technology. In J. C. Galvin & M. J. Scherer (Eds,), *Evaluating, selecting, and using appropriate assistive technology* (pp. 1–26). Gaithersburg, MD: Aspen.

Smart, J. F., & Smart, D. W. (1997). Vocational evaluation of Hispanic clients with disabilities. In *The Hatherleigh guide to vocational and career counseling* (pp. 209–231). New York: Hatherleigh Press.

Sonn, U., & Grimby, G. (1994). Assistive devices in an elderly population studied at 70 and 76 years of age. *Disability and Rehabilitation, 16*, 85–92.

Spencer, J. C. (1991). An ethnographic study of independent living alternatives. *American Journal of Occupational Therapy, 45*, 243–251.

Tabbarah, M., Silverstein, M., & Seeman, T. (2000). A health and demographic profile of noninstitutionalized older Americans residing in environments with home modifications. *Journal of Aging and Health, 12*, 204–228.

Tomita, M., Mann, W. C., Fraas, L. F., & Burns, L. L. (1997). Racial differences of frail elders in assistive technology. *Assistive Technology, 9*, 140–151.

Verbrugge, L. M. (1985). Gender and health: An update on hypotheses and evidence. *Journal of Health and Social Behavior, 26*, 156–182.

Watts, J. H., Erickson, A. E., Houde, L., Wilson, E., & Maynard, M. (1996). Assistive device use among the elderly: A national data-based study. *Physical and Occupational Therapy in Geriatrics, 14*, 1–18.

Wolf, E. R. (1956). Aspects of group relations in a complex society: Mexico. *American Anthropologist, 58*, 1065–1078.

7

ASSISTIVE TECHNOLOGY IN THE HOME AND COMMUNITY FOR OLDER PEOPLE: PSYCHOLOGICAL AND SOCIAL CONSIDERATIONS

LAURA N. GITLIN

Mr. M, a 72-year-old retiree who moved from Puerto Rico to the United States 30 years ago, returned to his two-story row home following a double knee amputation. His wife, of same age, was recently hospitalized for heart disease. Mr. M is unable to ascend or descend his exterior and interior stairs to leave his home or sleep upstairs with his wife. Mrs. M is permitted to ascend stairs only once daily. Mr. M feels trapped and depressed. Mrs. M is upset and fatigued from frequent stair climbing to care for her husband, who must stay on the first floor.

Mrs. T, age 65 and White, takes care of her husband, who has moderate-stage dementia. She must contend with numerous troublesome behaviors, such as his wandering and getting lost in the neighborhood, extreme agitation, and violent outbursts. Mrs. T is unsure how to manage these behaviors. She must watch Mr. T throughout the day and has no time off for herself or to carry out everyday tasks. She is very tired, upset, and anxious.

Mrs. P, age 75 and African American, lives alone. After hospitalization for a hip fracture she is unable to ascend her steep and slippery stairs safely or to transfer in and out of her bed and bath. Her entrance does not have rails, and she has difficulty leaving and entering her home. She feels increasingly socially isolated and depressed and somewhat hopeless about her ability to recover and continue to live alone.

These three real-life scenarios disclose the physical, psychological, social, and environmental challenges older people and their families contend with

This chapter is based on research supported in part by funding from the National Institute on Aging, Grant RO1-AG10947. The opinions contained in this chapter are those of the author and do not necessarily reflect those of the granting agency.

in coping with the onset of functional dependency (Gitlin 1998a). These cases demonstrate that as people age and experience either age-related changes or functional limitations from chronic health conditions they must learn new ways of interacting within their physical environments to successfully carry out daily life activities. Although the personal competencies of the individuals described in these vignettes have declined, their home and community environments remain invariant. Their once easily navigable and comforting settings have become hostile places that pose barriers to safe and independent living. In each of the above scenarios the mismatch between person capabilities and home environmental features resulted in negative psychological and social consequences. Chief among these consequences were feelings of anxiety, depression, social isolation, loss of personal control, and a diminished quality of life.

ROLE OF ASSISTIVE TECHNOLOGY

Assistive technology (AT) is a relatively new strategy that has the potential to break the cycle of functional limitation, poor person–environment fit, and maladaptive psychological consequences and support the efforts of older people and family caregivers in their attempts to successfully age in place at home. In this chapter I describe the role of AT in the lives of older people living at home and the psychological and social considerations in AT use. The snapshots of the lives of Mr. and Mrs. M, Mr. and Mrs. T, and Mrs. P provide the background for the discussion.

What Is AT?

AT has been variably defined in the research literature and refers to widely diverse equipment and devices that range in complexity and cost. These strategies are typically used in combination with other changes that have been categorized as structural alterations, special equipment, assistive devices, material adjustments, and behavioral changes (Pynoos, Cohen, Davis, & Bernhardt, 1987). *Structural alterations* refer to changes made to the original structure of a house and its components, such as widening doors, lowering cabinets, or removing walls. *Special equipment* includes attachments to the original structure of the home, such as handrails, grab bars, or stair glides. *Assistive devices* have been defined as "any item, piece of equipment, or product system, whether acquired commercially off the shelf, modified or customized, that is used to increase, maintain, or improve functional capabilities of individuals with disabilities" (P.L. 100-407, Technology-Related Assistance for Individuals With Disabilities Act of 1988). The term *assistive device* can also refer to an item that is applied to or directly manipulated by a person, such as a wheelchair, walker, cane, or reacher. *Material adjustments* include alterations to the nonpermanent features of a home, such as clearing pathways, removing throw rugs, tacking down carpets, adjusting lighting, rearranging furniture, and color coding and labeling objects. Finally, an *environmentally based behavioral modification* targets the person's interaction with the physical dimensions of the environment. Such strategies may include changing footwear; using task breakdown techniques; modifying task performance through the practice of energy conservation; or changing the function of living areas, such as converting a living room to a bedroom. One could argue that AT should refer only to special equipment and devices; however, because issuing equipment often necessitates instruction in types of modifications in addition to those just described, the discussion that follows includes environmental and home modifications and uses the term *AT* in its broadest sense.

All of the strategies just categorized can be conceptualized as those that either modify physical features of the environment (e.g., a structural renovation, such as widening a doorway to increase accessibility) or those that modify people themselves (e.g., a mobility aid, such as using a walker to improve ambulation). Little is known as to whether there are differential psychological and social impacts when the target of the intervention is the person or the environment. There is some evidence to suggest that older people accept AT that involves modifications to physical features that are hidden from public view, such as a bathroom grab bar, whereas an AT strategy that changes a person's appearance, such as a walker, may be more difficult for a person to accept because it makes the disability publicly visible.

A unifying characteristic of any AT and home modification strategy is that its purpose is to modify the way an individual interacts with his or her immediate environment to afford or maximize that person's capability in performing daily life functions. A combination of strategies is often necessary to address an area of difficulty. For example, Mr. and Mrs. M would have both benefited significantly from a combination of strategies involving structural changes, such as the installation of an exterior ramp and a first-floor powder room; special equipment, such as a stair glide; using behavioral techniques, such as energy conservation; or some combination of these.

Use of AT to Improve Everyday Competencies

A medical model perspective traditionally has prevailed in understanding the role and importance of AT. This model views AT primarily as a compensatory strategy to enhance functional performance in people with physical limitations. However, its potential role is more far-reaching and can be conceptualized as improving everyday competencies and life quality of older people in a number of important life domains (see Table 7.1). AT may be useful to address physical and cognitive limitations as well as improve personal feelings of safety and comfort for older people who as a heterogeneous group reflect a continuum of competency from high to low.

AT for Prevention, Rehabilitation, and Long-Term Care

There are three pivotal points in the aging process for which AT may be effective (Gitlin, 1998c). The first point represents the period prior to the onset of functional decline in which AT may have a preventive role. As a preventive strategy, AT can be introduced to older people to prepare for a future in which they may experience a functional limitation, to avoid disability from an injury, or both. For example, installing a handrail on a steep set of stairs or a grab bar in the bathroom may enhance safety and promote continued stair and safe bathroom use over time prior to the onset of a functional limitation or injury as a result of a fall.

AT also has a preventive function among older people with progressive conditions. In the case of Mrs. T, a number of AT strategies may have helped prevent some of the troublesome behaviors manifested by her husband. For example, the installation and use of deadbolt locks on the doors would have prevented her husband from leaving the house. Mrs. T in turn would have been able to carry out housework without constant vigilance over Mr. T's whereabouts. Also, creating a low-stimulus room by removing unnecessary

TABLE 7.1
Examples of Assistive Technology (AT) Interventions
for Seven Life Domains

Domain	Examples of types of AT interventions	Specific examples
Performance of self-care	Special equipment	Mobility aids, communication devices
Safety	Environmental simplification Special equipment	Grab bars, handrails; removal of throw rugs
Accessibility	Structural renovation	Widen doors, lower cabinets
Orientation and awareness	Material adjustments, simplification of environment, visual cues, adaptive equipment	Removal of clutter; color contrasted objects, large face clock
Physical and emotional comfort	Material adjustments	Quiet, private room; objects of symbolic meaning; photos
Engagement	Special equipment, material adjustments	Leisure aids; control or command center
Caregiving	Behavioral and material adjustments	Energy conservation, task breakdown techniques

items and dimming lights may have provided a comforting, quiet rest place for Mr. T to use periodically throughout the day. This may help to prevent the escalation of feelings of frustration and agitation.

The second point at which AT may be effective is the period following an acute onset of a potentially disabling condition, such as a hip fracture or stroke, in which partial or full recovery may occur over time. In this case, AT is primarily rehabilitative for the purposes of restoring and maintaining function, and its use may be temporary. For example, Mrs. P would have benefited from learning transfer techniques and using a reacher to avoid bending as short-term rehabilitative strategies.

The third point in the aging process for which an AT intervention may be beneficial is long-term care. In long-term care, older people may experience a combination of physical and cognitive impairments that are progressive. The purpose of AT as a long-term care strategy is to maintain social, psychological, and physical function and cognitive awareness and orientation. For example, implementing structural modifications and equipment, such as building a first-floor powder room or installing a stair glide, may prevent nursing home placement or relocation from one's home. Mr. and Mrs. M both clearly have long-term care needs that may be addressed by AT.

In its preventive role AT serves mostly as a safety gap measure. In its rehabilitative and long-term care roles AT improves and maintains physical, cognitive, and emotional well-being. Research has shown that the primary users of AT are older people with physical impairments (Mann, Hurren, Tomita, & Charvat, 1995). AT strategies tend to be used less as a preventive mechanism. One reason for this may be that there are very few opportunities in which older people can develop AT solutions for their future. Also, older people with cognitive impairment tend to use AT solutions with less frequency (Mann, Krauza, Hurren, & Tomita, 1992). This may be due to a diminished capacity to learn how to use new objects with the onset of dementia.

PRINCIPLES THAT GUIDE AT USE

As older people move from high to low levels of physical and mental competencies with age, the onset of multiple chronic health conditions, or both, they will experience a range of AT needs. The model in Figure 7.1 provides a structure for understanding the range of AT needs for older adults at different levels of competencies and different care needs (prevention, rehabilitation, and long-term care; Gitlin, 1998c). The x-axis in Figure 7.1 presents four fundamental interrelated environmental needs that can be conceptualized along a hierarchy (Teresi, Lawton, Ory, & Holmes, 1994).

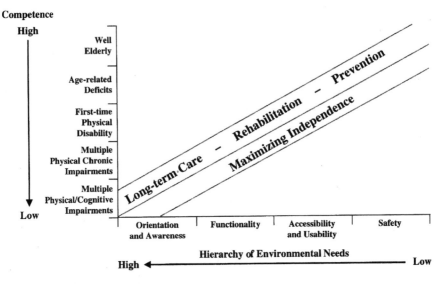

Figure 7.1. A functional–environmental need model for the design of home modification interventions.

This hierarchy reflects the most elemental or basic need for an environment to (a) offer safety and security, (b) be accessible and usable, (c) support functional capacity, and (d) support cognitive awareness and orientation. These represent a progression of environmental needs that are interrelated and not mutually exclusive. Each need cuts across the other in a progressive fashion. For example, safety is the most basic requirement of any living arrangement on which all other environmental needs (accessibility, functionality, orientation, and awareness) build. An environment must first offer safety, and then it can offer accessibility. Likewise, a safe and accessible environment underlies one that enhances functionality (environmental supports to maintain self-care and instrumental activities) and orientation and awareness. A limitation of Figure 7.1 is that it does not show the importance of supporting higher level environmental needs, such as personal comfort, engagement, and continuance of personhood or self-identity. These higher level needs afforded by environments are important at each level of competency (from high to low) and can be conceptualized as underlying the four basic needs shown in the figure.

The y-axis in Figure 7.1 represents different levels of competencies of older people, ordered from high to low. The diagonal suggests that AT intervention can occur at three stages or junctures of aging: (a) prevention, targeting the well elderly population; (b) rehabilitation, targeting older people with a functional limitation; and (c) long-term care, targeting older people with multiple chronic conditions and limitations. Also shown along the diagonal is the overall purpose of an AT intervention at these stages or junctures, that is, to maximize the fit between the person and his or her environment to promote independence, comfort, and positive psychosocial well-being. Thus, this figure provides a basis for identifying the specific environmental needs of older people at different levels of competencies. For example, well elderly people have low environmental needs; their primary need for AT or environmental redesign is to maintain safety, and AT has a preventive role. Therefore, intervention for this group might have as its goal maintaining a safe home environment for prevention of falls. In contrast, elderly people with multiple physical or cognitive impairments have multiple AT needs. Intervention for this group might have as its goal strategies that address all four primary environmental needs as part of long-term care services.

The model in Figure 7.1 suggests several principles to guide AT instruction and use with older people. First, it suggests that AT needs differ among older people on the basis of their level of competency. For example, healthy older people may require AT strategies that address only safety issues in the environment and focus on prevention. An elderly person experiencing disability for the first time, however, may require AT strategies that address safety, accessibility–usability, and function in the environment for the purposes of both rehabilitation and prevention.

A second principle implicit in the model and critical to the use of AT is the concept of universal design. *Universal design* refers to the development of products and environments that account for the broadest possible range of physical and cognitive differences among all people. More products are now being developed and distributed in local stores that fit the criteria of universal design. For example, a can opener with large, easy-to-grip handles is a design that accommodates people with varying degrees of grasping ability and arm strength.

Another principle that guides AT use among the elderly population is the concept of *progressive simplification* of the environment—that is, changes to the home environment are most acceptable to older people and most effective when they occur slowly and over time to address highly specific person–environment transactions that pose difficulty. The environment must fit the emotional, cognitive, and physical needs of a person. Its simplification must match the competencies of the person. The low-stimulus and simplified environment that is appropriate for Mr. T may be isolating, boring, and uncomfortable in the case of Mrs. P. This suggests that a greater number of environmental concerns needs to be addressed as competencies decline. The need for a combination of AT strategies and continual progressive simplification of the environment increases as competencies of older people decline. Implicit in this principle is the need for a service delivery model that permits opportunities for continual re-evaluation of person–

environment transactions from which to identify new AT needs as competencies decline.

PERSONAL-CONTROL THEORY AND AT USE

Previous research has consistently shown that older people are users of a range of AT devices and report the need for more special equipment to optimize their quality of life at home. Nevertheless, the research literature has also shown that older people are selective about the type of AT devices they are willing to use and that people with higher levels of disability are more likely to use special equipment. To date, the psychological and social mechanisms underlying the decision to use or not to use AT to cope with loss of capacity are poorly understood. Early studies of AT use showed that some patients might choose not to use special equipment, even when it is life enhancing, because of the social consequences of being visibly different and disabled (Locker & Kaufert, 1988). Other studies have shown that older people accept and use AT only as it relates to accomplishing the specific goals they personally identify as important (Gitlin, 1998a; Gitlin, Luborsky, & Schemm, 1998). Still, the specific factors that influence elderly people's decisions to use or not to use an AT strategy remain unclear.

Why are people motivated to use AT? A recent advance in personal-control theory and its application to physical disability provides an important theoretical framework from which to understand AT use by older people. Personal-control theory contends that all individuals are motivated to maintain control over difficult situations (Schulz, Heckhausen, & O'Brien, 1994; Williamson & Schulz, 1992). This perspective is based on the premise that control is a human imperative. To maintain control, individuals use various strategies, referred to as *primary* and *secondary mechanisms*. *Primary mechanisms* are attempts people make to change their immediate environment (e.g., people, objects) or actively manipulate external forces to retain control and have a positive effect. *Secondary mechanisms* are attempts to change internal cognitions or emotions and support or enable the use of primary or active behavioral strategies.

Critical to the concept of personal control is the emphasis on the individual's engagement with his or her immediate environment to afford positive outcomes and buffer threats or actual losses to personal abilities to control important outcomes in life. Within this framework, AT use can be understood as an adaptive primary strategy that enables older people to actively control important outcomes in their life. An important outcome of exerting control is enhanced self-efficacy. To the extent that an AT strategy is successful in helping older people sustain control and feel efficacious, negative affective responses to disability, such as anxiety or depression, are minimized. There is some support for this hypothesis. Recent research shows that people with high levels of disability who use AT as the primary source of assistance show enhanced self-efficacy (Verbrugge, Rennert, & Madans, 1997). Also, family caregivers of people with dementia show improved self-efficacy by using principles of progressive simplification and material adjustments (Gitlin, Corcoran, Winter, Boyce, & Hauck, 2001). Most important, previous research suggests that having a sense of control is positively linked to both physical and psychological health. The use of AT, then, might have an important impact beyond that of functional improvement. Its use might influence well-being by enhancing feelings of self-efficacy.

BENEFITS AND BIOGRAPHICAL CONSEQUENCES OF AT USE

Relatively little research has systematically documented the range of benefits afforded to older people who use AT. It seems logical to suggest that AT use may result in the delay of nursing home placement and improve daily quality of life of older people, but again, there is little empirical verification of these major outcomes. One recent study showed that AT use lowers the cost of long-term care at home and postpones relocation (Mann, Ottenbacher, Fraas, Tomita, & Granger, 1999).

A typology of likely benefits of AT use might range from factors that reflect an immediate impact on person–environment transactions (e.g., improved home safety); benefits that reflect a proximal gain in the domain of behavioral competence (e.g., increased independence in functional health or self-care) and psychological well-being (e.g., improved mastery); to benefits that reflect a distal outcome, such as improvement in perceived quality of life (e.g., satisfaction with staying in place, delayed relocation to residential care).

The most compelling evidence of the benefits of AT is derived from qualitative research in which elderly people and their families report the impact of AT use in their daily lives (Gitlin, 1998a; Gitlin, Luborsky, & Schemm, 1998). Chief among the benefits described by AT users is a sense of a return to normalcy, the "way things used to be." For example, installing a stair glide enables a person with a mobility impairment to ascend stairs and conduct "normal" bathing, sleeping, and dressing routines, in contrast to having to convert a living room into a bedroom, use a commode on the first floor, and so on. Other life enhancements that result from AT use have been reported by older people to include increased engagement in valued leisure activities (e.g., use of adaptive playing cards or game boards), maintenance of social contact (e.g., use of door adapter, outside elevator, or handrails to facilitate egress), and reserved energy (e.g., stair glide) to carry out activities of choice.

Despite its important benefits, there may also be negative consequences to AT use. Foremost is the symbolic meaning of AT as a visible reminder of a change in a person's role status from able bodied to being disabled. An environmental adjustment, especially one that is public (e.g., mobility aid, ramp), may heighten feelings of loss and serve as a reminder that life is not like before.

Also, objects in homes may represent hidden meanings and values such that their rearrangement or removal disrupts a person's sense of normalcy and continuity of personal integrity. Consider the case of Mrs. T, who cares for her husband with dementia. Although Mrs. T had a double-bolt lock on the front door that successfully blocked Mr. T's elopement attempts from that location, he was still able to leave the home from a door in the kitchen that led to an open yard. In examining different strategies with an occupational therapist to control his wandering behavior, Mrs. T initially agreed to the installation of a deadbolt lock on the back door. However, once the lock was installed, she was unable to actually use it. She expressed that she felt "locked in" and overwhelmed by its use. Shortly after the installation of the lock, a wandering episode occurred in which Mr. T left their home by that door without Mrs. T's knowledge. Mr. T became lost and was found by a neighbor 4 hours later. He had become extremely agitated, verbally and physically abusive, and had an incontinence incident. Mrs. T in turn was profoundly distressed and overwhelmed. She immediately placed her husband in a nursing home. The lock for Mrs. T symbolized the subjective burden she felt caring for her husband, and she was unable to successfully use that strategy (Gitlin, 2000).

The home and community serve as important sources for maintaining biographical integrity, or a sense of personal continuity in self-definition. Accordingly, alteration of either one may be a source of personal disruption or upset. An individual's difficulty in removing a potential falls hazard, such as a throw rug, may reflect the potential biographical disruption caused by an environmental adjustment. This seemingly simple action influencing the environment may in fact challenge a person's ego integrity and self-definition. The throw rug may reflect a long-standing environmental arrangement with meanings that transcend or are more important than its hazardous placement. Compliance with an environmental change, such as removing the rug, may be low unless the person perceives that he or she is at personal risk (Hindmarsch & Estes, 1989) or that making the environmental change will fit his or her personal goals for self-care (Gitlin, 1998a, 1998b).

The drive for environmental continuity, to keep the home "as it always has been," is a qualitative observation that has been discussed in a number of studies. It is illustrated by the case of an 85-year-old woman caring for her 90-year-old husband, who was at the moderate stage of dementia. The caregiver maintained the home as it had always been and enforced a daily routine that reflected the premorbid activities and behaviors of her husband. Of central importance to this caregiver was maintaining a sense of normalcy and biographical integrity of her husband and how she chose to remember him. Therefore, objects for care, such as a commode, medications, and mobility aids, were concealed and brought out only at the immediate time of need. A number of home modifications were offered by an occupational therapist to offset the objective burden of care. Modifications included a stair glide for safety, adapted utensils to facilitate eating, and bathroom equipment. None, however, were acceptable to the caregiver, because they fundamentally altered her perspective of normalcy that guided her care practices and use of objects in the home (Gitlin, Corcoran, & Leinmiller-Eckhardt, 1995). Modifications that were acceptable to this caregiver were those that were environmentally imperceptible (e.g., cutting up food into smaller portions, serving one item of food, using tactile cueing in descending stairs) and fit into the physical structure and daily routines that she had established.

A fundamental aspect of using AT may be the need to engage in a process of biographical management (Gitlin et al., 1998). This process entails weighing or evaluating the relative gains and importance of accomplishing an activity using AT in view of its sociocultural implications of stigma and feelings of loss that its use often imputes. Accordingly, AT enables older people to continue performing lifelong and valued personal routines but may simultaneously create feelings of personal disruption and a sense of discontinuity of self. Older people must contend with this duality and reconcile feelings of loss with the gains obtained by using AT.

SPECIAL CONSIDERATIONS IN AT INSTRUCTION WITH OLDER PEOPLE

There are a number of special considerations in providing AT solutions to older people and their family members that concern both how service delivery is organized as well as how one-on-one instruction is provided. First, adult learning theory provides a framework from which to understand best practices in providing AT strategies to older people. Research on adult learners has shown that older people learn new skills most effectively within the context or situation in which the skill is actually used. Contextualized learning is therefore very important when introducing AT. Simulation of an activity or real-time in-home instruction provides the optimal learning condition. In the case of Mrs. P, she was instructed in a left-to-right bed transfer technique during hospitalization. However, this type of transfer did not reflect her sleeping arrangement at home. At home, she was unable to translate the transfer technique to match her situation. She thus experienced great difficulty and pain each time she had to rise from her bed. When she received in-home instruction, she was able to master the proper transfer that fit her environmental situation.

Second, adult learning theory also suggests that older people need repeated practice opportunities to absorb new skills. Mrs P was able to practice the transfer technique and receive feedback from a health professional over several home visits. This reinforced her knowledge and ability to use this strategy appropriately. Therefore, in providing instruction at home, visits may need to be spaced over time to allow older people repeated exposure to and practices with an AT solution.

Third, older people and their family members must be considered part of the team in making decisions about the best AT solutions. As discussed earlier, research has shown that older people are users of AT devices that fit their own personal and self-identified goals. AT recommendations by health professionals must match not only environmental setups but also the values and beliefs of the people who use the AT solutions.

With regard to service delivery, assessment for AT solutions and instructional process may require a multidisciplinary team, whose members might include an occupational therapist, case manager, physical therapist, nurse, architect, construction crew, or some combination of these. Each of these professionals brings a particular expertise to the design of an AT solution and its implementation in the home. Occupational therapists are particularly critical to the assessment process given their specialized knowledge of person–environment fit issues. Also, it is important to recognize that as competencies change, older people need to be re-evaluated with new AT solutions offered to fit specific emerging areas of difficulty. Many older people learn about AT in the hospital or rehabilitation setting or receive a one-time home modification service. Consequently, older people have limited access to AT services as they age over time. Therefore, rehabilitation professionals must strive to develop a long-term care delivery system that allows opportunities for re-evaluation and the introduction of new AT solutions as needs develop with time.

CONCLUSION

A persistent finding in research is the strong preference of older people to remain at home as they age. Family members involved in the care of frail older people share this goal. With the dramatic aging of American society, it becomes increasingly important to fully understand the role of AT in maximizing human potential and the manifold consequences, negative and positive, in using AT strategies. In this chapter I have explored the role of AT with older people and showed that its use supports seven important life domains (see Table 7.1), from physical functioning to higher order competencies, such as social and leisure engagement and continuation of a sense of personhood. As a preventive, rehabilitative, or long-term care strategy AT use may provide multiple benefits, including postponement of relocation or nursing home placement, ability to access cabinets and rooms, and a return to a sense of normalcy and personal comfort. There are a number of special considerations in providing AT solutions to older people and their family members. Chief among these is the need to involve the potential user in the assessment process and derive AT solutions that support the particular areas of difficulty identified by the potential AT users themselves. Foremost among the changes necessary to service delivery is provision of repeated opportunities for accessing AT solutions as people age and experience changes in their level of competency.

REFERENCES

Gitlin L. N. (1998a). From hospital to home: Individual variation in the experience with assistive devices among the elderly. In D. Gray, L. A. Quatrano, & M. L. Lieberman (Eds.), Designing and using assistive technology: The human perspective (pp. 117–136). Baltimore, MD: Brookes Press.

Gitlin, L. N. (1998b). The role of social science research in understanding technology use among older adults. In M. G. Ory & G. DeFriese (Eds.), Self-care in late life (pp. 162–169). New York: Springer.

Gitlin, L. N. (1998c). Testing home modification interventions: Issues of theory, measurement, design, and implementation. In R. Schulz, M. P. Lawton, & G. Maddox (Eds.), Annual review of gerontology and geriatrics: Intervention research with older adults (pp. 190–246). New York: Springer.

Gitlin, L. N. (2000). Adjusting "person–environment systems": Helping older people live the "good life" at home. In M. Moss & R. Rubenstein (Eds.), The many faces of aging: Essays in honor of M. P. Lawton (pp. 41–54). New York: Springer.

Gitlin, L. N., Corcoran, M., & Leinmiller-Eckhardt, S. (1995). Understanding the family perspective: An ethnographic framework for providing occupational therapy in the home. American Journal of Occupational Therapy, 49, 802–809.

Gitlin, L. N., Corcoran, M., Winter, L., Boyce, A., & Hauck, W. (2001). A randomized, controlled trial of a home environmental intervention: Effect on efficacy and upset in caregivers and on daily function of persons with dementia. The Gerontologist, 41, 4–14.

Gitlin, L. N., Luborsky, M., & Schemm, R. L. (1998). Emerging concerns of older stroke patients about assistance device use. The Gerontologist, 38, 169–180.

Hindmarsch, J. J., & Estes, H. (1989). Falls in older persons: Causes and interventions. *Archives of Internal Medicine, 149*, 2217–2222.

Locker, D., & Kaufert, J. (1988). The breadth of life: Medical technology and the careers of people with post-respiratory poliomyelitis. *Sociology of Health and Illness, 10*, 23–40.

Mann, W. C., Hurren, D., Tomita, M., & Charvat, B. (1995). The relationship of functional independence to assistive device use of elderly persons living at home. *Journal of Applied Gerontology, 14*, 225–247.

Mann, W. C., Krauza, J., Hurren, D., & Tomita, M. (1992). Assistive devices for home-based elderly persons with cognitive impairments. *Topics in Geriatric Rehabilitation, 8*, 35–52.

Mann, W. C., Ottenbacher, K. J., Fraas, L., Tomita, M., & Granger, C. V. (1999). Effectiveness of assistive technology and environmental interventions in maintaining independence and reducing home care costs for the frail elderly. *Archives of Family Medicine, 8*, 210–217.

Pynoos, J., Cohen, E., Davis, L., & Bernhardt, S. (1987). Home modifications: Improvements that extend independence. In V. Regnier & J. Pynoos (Eds.), *Housing the aged: Design directives, policy considerations* (pp. 277–304). New York: Elsevier Science.

Schulz, R., Heckhausen, J., & O'Brien, A. T. (1994). Control and the disablement process in the elderly. *Journal of Social Behavior and Personality, 9*, 139–152.

Technology-Related Assistance of Individuals With Disability Act, 29 U.S.C. § 3002 (1988).

Teresi, J., Lawton, M. P., Ory, M. G., & Holmes, D. (1994). Measurement issues in chronic care populations: Dementia special care. *Alzheimer Disease and Associated Disorders, 8* (Suppl. 1), 144–183.

Verbrugge, L. M., Rennert, C., & Madans, J. H. (1997). The great efficacy of personal and equipment assistance in reducing disability. *American Journal of Public Health, 87*, 384–392.

Williamson, G. M., & Schulz, R. (1992). Physical illness and symptoms of depression among elderly outpatients. *Psychology and Aging, 7*, 343–351.

8

COPING AND ADJUSTMENT

ALLEN W. HEINEMANN AND THERESA LOUISE-BENDER PAPE

Impairment and illness can result in functional limitations, and these limitations can curtail participation in home and community activities. A reduction in activity participation diminishes one's quality of life. Assistive technology (AT), however, provides a means of circumventing the environmental barriers that limit activity participation. In turn, increased participation provides the basis to cope and adapt to environmental barriers and can favorably influence quality of life. How people appraise their physical, communicative, and cognitive capacity and the technology that maximizes their skills is critically important. Some people are willing to embrace technology, whereas others are reluctant to do so. In this chapter we review AT use and nonuse by (a) older adults, (b) people with acquired and congenital disabilities, and (c) people with functional limitations due to progressive diseases. Three case vignettes are included to illustrate successful integration of AT into people's lives. In the final section we illustrate the sociocultural and psychosocial issues that influence individual appraisals of AT and the extent to which individuals integrate AT into their daily routines.

LITERATURE REVIEW

Aging

AT research has focused on the elderly population, because a large proportion of elderly people own assistive devices. Changes are related to

This chapter was funded in part by the Quality Enhancement Research Initiative Spinal Cord Injury, Grant SCI 98-000, Health Services Research and Development, U.S. Department of Veterans Affairs. The Advanced Rehabilitation Research Training program funding was provided to Theresa Louise-Bender Pape from the National Institute on Disability and Rehabilitation Research. We are indebted to Mike, Joe, and Ken for allowing us the opportunity to interview them and for providing us with feedback that enabled us to accurately portray their charismatic personalities and enriched lives.

the aging process and the desire by elderly people to remain in their homes contribute to the high rate of device ownership (Mann, Hurren, Tomita, & Charvat, 1996). AT reduces the effect that physiological and cognitive changes have on activities of daily living (ADLs) and maximize independence, allowing older people to continue residing in their homes.

The large proportion of older people who own AT devices is well documented in the literature. Hartke, Prohaska, and Furner (1998), for example, in their analysis of the 1990 National Health Interview Survey (NHIS) data, found that 25% of people ages 65 years and older own an assistive device, and approximately one third of these people own multiple devices. Watts, Erickson, Houde, Wilson, & Maynard (1996) analyzed the same NHIS device supplement data and reported a similar proportion (23%) of device ownership.

Early studies reported that older adults own 8–14 assistive devices and use 44%–80% of them. The variability in use rates reflects a number of factors, including type of impairment (Mann, Hurren, & Tomita, 1993). Declining vision, for example, is a common physiological change that occurs with the aging process, but macular degeneration is a chronic and progressive eye disease that affects central vision and often renders a person legally blind (Moore, 1999; Singer, 1999). Mann, Hurren, Tomita, and Charvat (1997) studied the effects that severe visual impairments, such as macular degeneration, have on ADLs and found that these impairments significantly contribute to diminished capacity. They explored changes in device use occurring with changes in vision over a 2-year period in a sample of 38 adults with severe visual impairments. They found that device ownership increased from an average of 19 devices to an average of 29 devices and that this increase was directly related to declining vision. This sample also had a very high use rate (90%) at 2 years; Mann et al. (1997) interpreted this as evidence of the effectiveness of the devices in maximizing independence. They concluded that assistive devices for people with severe visual impairments enhance successful coping.

The effectiveness of devices used by people with cognitive impairments, such as orientation calendars and medication organizers, has been explored. Nochajski, Tomita, and Mann (1996), for example, found that AT use rate by people with cognitive impairments was lower than the rate for people with physical impairments. Although use effectively diminishes the consequences of cognitive impairments, the devices are not as readily accepted as are devices that ameliorate physical limitations. Paradoxically, users of devices intended for cognitive impairments were more satisfied with devices than were users of devices intended for physical limitations. Device use and device satisfaction were not correlated with life satisfaction in Nochajski's sample.

Degree of impairment, as well as impairment type, is another factor that contributes to use rates. Mann et al. (1996) proposed, for example, a prescription model for bathing devices based on the degree of physical impairment: A higher level bathing device is best matched with a greater degree of physical impairment. Hartke et al. (1998) also observed that poorer health is associated with greater AT use and multiple device use.

Personal care attendants were more often employed in the past by older adults to assist with ADLs in their homes. Manton, Corter, and Stallard (1993) reported that recent advances in AT have led to increased used of assistive devices with a concomitant decrease in employment of attendants. A desire for independence, increased control, and cost savings are believed to be responsible for the preference of AT ownership over employing personal care attendants.

In summary, older adults use AT to diminish the effects of physiological and cognitive changes that occur with aging. AT device use reflects the type and degree of impairment, device type, and the time since onset of disability. The rate of use is higher if the device promotes successful coping; however, satisfaction with a particular device does not guarantee that it will be valued and used (Nochajski et al., 1996).

Acquired Disabilities

AT is prescribed during rehabilitation following an acquired disability, such as spinal cord injury (SCI), cerebral vascular accident (CVA; e.g., stroke), or amputation. The goal is to maximize independence; AT is used to achieve this goal (Dittuno, Stover, & Freed, 1992).

Phillips and Zhao (1993) surveyed 227 people with acquired disabilities and reported a nonuse rate of 30%. The strongest influences on device abandonment included nonparticipation in device selection; functional improvements that obviated the need for the device; and poor device performance, reliability, durability, comfort, and ease of use. Cushman and Scherer (1996) evaluated AT use by 47 people with a variety of conditions, including SCI (23%), CVA (36%), and amputation (19%). The 33% nonuse rate 3 months after hospital discharge is similar to findings from other studies. Grooming aids were abandoned by 59% of the sample because functional gains obviated the need. Cushman and Scherer reported that functional gains were the reason for nonuse of other devices for half of their sample.

AT users report many reasons for nonuse, including being less inclined to use a quad cane in public and with friends even though the cane enhances ambulation. Another reason for nonuse is that a daily activity must be completed within an individually defined time period before it is considered "functional." People with SCIs reported the greatest rates of abandonment of devices for dressing (Weingarden & Martin, 1989) because, even with the device, the activity requires too much time. Despite the fact that dressing aids allow independent dressing, survey respondents often delegated this activity to an attendant. Weingarden et al.'s (1989) report illustrates that device abandonment is likely if an activity is not completed within a "functional" time frame. High energy consumption is another reason for device nonuse. Heinemann, Magiera-Planey, Schiro-Geist, and Grimes (1987) surveyed 92 people with paraplegia an average of 15 years after SCI. They found that a majority of the sample (67%) had been prescribed knee–ankle–foot orthoses, but only 26% were still using them occasionally, and only 4% were using them as their sole means of mobility. Wheelchairs were reported to be of greater value by the respondents than leg braces because they permitted a greater level of activity with less energy consumption.

Gauthier-Gagnon, Grise, and Potvin (1998) studied 396 people with amputations and found that adaptation to amputation was the best predictor of prosthetic use. Gauthier-Gagnon, Grise, and Potvin (1994) used the Prosthetic Profile of the Amputee questionnaire to evaluate the factors related to use and nonuse. Adaptation to amputation was measured by responses to the question "How adapted do you feel to the amputation and prosthesis?" The respondents rated their adaptation on a scale that ranged from 1 (not at all adapted) through 5 (completely adapted). One third of the respondents (35%) who did not use their prostheses reported that they were not adapted to their amputation, whereas 69% of the prosthetic users reported that they were well or completely adapted.

People with acquired disabilities use AT to diminish the limiting effects of the environment on their performance of ADLs. Device use rates are greater when (a) users participate in device selection, (b) the device is easy to use and aesthetically pleasing, (c) the time required for activity completion is perceived as being reasonable, (d) the person has achieved a sufficient level of adaptation to the disability, and (e) the device use promotes participation in activities.

THE CASE OF MIKE, AN ASPIRING ATTORNEY WITH AN ACQUIRED SPINAL CORD INJURY (SCI)

Mike, age 29 and unmarried, has C_4 quadriplegia; he was injured in 1988 at age 18. He began attending law school full-time in 1996. After his first semester he switched to a part-time status. He has seven more classes to take; he expects to graduate in the year 2001. He works full-time in the summer as a law clerk and part-time during school. Mike uses a sip-and-puff-controlled wheelchair and a Relax unit that operates a television, video recorder, lights, fan, and radio. Mike replaced his UNIDIALER with the

Relax unit because "It's better than the UNIDIALER. Why ride in a Chevette when you can ride in a Mercedes?"

Mike uses a PC at home with speech recognition software; he has a nearly identical setup at work. He uses a mouth stick with an eraser, a bookboard to elevate books, and a page turner that is connected to his mouth stick. He uses a commercially available telephone and headset, which he prefers over a speakerphone. He lived alone when we spoke with him but was interviewing roommates and planned to choose one soon. He employs an attendant about 90 minutes in the morning and 90 minutes in the evening. Although he does not drive, he owns a minivan equipped with a wheelchair ramp; friends drive his van to social and leisure activities. He also uses public transportation to go to work.

Mike said that many activities have been enhanced with AT. He described living without AT as

> kind of being paralyzed all over again, just totally, completely dependent on others. A feeling that you'll need someone to do everything in your life that you've done before—minus sleeping, breathing, and chewing. That's what being paralyzed is—needing assistance from someone forever and obviously not being able to move. With AT [devices], I don't need someone as much as I would without AT. AT allows me to have independence, which I really miss, and control over my life—the way it was before I was hurt.

Mike said that work and school activities are enhanced by AT. He said that about 90% of his school and work assignments require writing. A PC with speech recognition software allows

> me to be who I was before [my] injury—independent and in control. Along with my wheelchair, [AT devices] get me to work . . . [and allow] me to do the work. My mind has not been affected. During college I wanted to be a psychologist to help people cope with SCI. After a few years, however, I saw that many of my classmates were also disabled and doing just fine. As a result, I figured I could help people like myself on a greater scale working as a lawyer and being a role model.

AT helps Mike minimize the effects of physical limitations. AT

> helps me be more independent. I know I need these devices. They serve their purpose. I appreciate them; I know I'm lucky to have them. They're expensive, not everyone has them. They allow me to live a life thousands of other paralyzed people won't live because they don't have them. They don't help me cure the paralysis. I don't think about them helping me cope with my paralysis; I expect that they'll be there and function. I hope for some breakthrough that will allow me to have use of one or two arms. I'd still be a happy person without such a breakthrough. I like to think positive.

Mike did not identify specific ways in which AT devices have helped his psychological adjustment. He described himself by saying "I don't think of myself as the guy in the wheelchair." He said he tries to do his best in school and work roles. He wishes that voice-activated software were faster. AT devices "help me out, but not exactly like I want to be." When he becomes frustrated with AT devices, he reminds himself that "it's only a machine; it doesn't have feelings."

PEOPLE WITH CONGENITAL IMPAIRMENTS

People born with a disability are likely to perceive AT differently and hold different expectations regarding device performance (Scherer, 1988, 1990). These perceptions and expectations explain why people with congenital disabilities are more likely to use AT than are people with other types of disabilities. Scherer reported that five women with cerebral palsy (CP), for example, viewed AT as a means to perform tasks that they were not able to perform otherwise. In contrast, Scherer also reported that adults with SCIs viewed AT as a poor substitute for their own skills; they said the substitutions serve to remind them of their lost skills.

People with congenital disabilities commonly employ personal care attendants and own multiple assistive devices. People with CP, for example, are likely to use motorized wheelchairs, which can be controlled with a variety of switches, such as joysticks and foot pedals (Stewart, Noble, & Seeger, 1992). People with CP also typically use augmentative and alternative communication (AAC) systems: external communication systems, such as picture boards or computers with synthesized speech, that can serve either as an individual's sole means of communication or as an adjunct to verbal and nonverbal modes. In fact, 35% of the adults with CP surveyed by Balandin and Morgan (1997) owned some form of AAC device. AAC systems can also be controlled through a variety of switches, including head pointers and infrared pointers.

Research regarding AT use by people with congenital disabilities has focused on people with CP and is more limited in size and scope than research conducted with older adults and people with acquired disabilities. A search of three databases (PyscINFO, Cumulative Index to Nursing and Allied Health [CINAHL], and Medline) yielded more than 70,000 articles, of which only 8 addressed congenital disabilities and AT and all of which focused on people with CP.

McCall, Markova, Murphy, Moodie, and Collins (1997) studied 89 adolescents with CP, who used AAC systems, regarding availability and use of vocabulary, use rates for a single communication mode versus a combination of modes, and communication breakdowns. McCall also studied the perspectives of adults with CP and their communication partners regarding communication strategies (as defined by Light, 1988) to (a) express needs and wants, (b) convey information, (c) express social closeness, and (d) convey social etiquette. McCall reported that 74% of the adolescents had a vocabulary that included "ask for a drink," and 89% used this vocabulary. When providing information about a holiday, however, only 48% had vocabulary available, and 90% of these adolescents used this vocabulary to describe a holiday. In contrast, 43% of the AAC users had the vocabulary to "open a conversation," but only 77% actually used this vocabulary to start conversations. Twenty-eight (32%) of the AAC users had the vocabulary required to "close a conversation," and 79% effectively used their vocabulary. Half of the AAC users reported that they used AAC with another mode to "request a drink," and 32% reported that they used a non-AAC mode to describe a holiday. Most (68%) of the AAC users indicated that they used a non-AAC mode exclusively to open and close conversations. The advantage of AAC that was most frequently cited by the communication partners was the effect on the quality of the user's life. Nonuse of available vocabulary and nonuse of AAC for higher level language transactions were attributed by the adult AAC users to frequent communication breakdowns with their partners and consequent frustration. The partners, however, did not perceive communication breakdowns as often. Two main concerns regarding AAC use include (a) technological and maintenance requirements and (b) changes in the communication message as a direct result of the AAC system.

Wanting to feel part of a group is natural for all people, but for people with CP a feeling of belonging can be a significant achievement. People with CP want to fit in social contexts, but feeling left out is likely when communication breaks down. Frustration and anger arise because of communication breakdowns (McCall et al., 1997), and these feelings can contribute to a desire to reduce the number or duration of interactions (Buzolich & Lunger, 1995). Schaller and Garza (1999) reported that social withdrawal is often a symptom of frustration and anger. Communication breakdowns remind the person with CP that he or she is different from others.

Buzolich and Lunger (1995) described Vivian, a 12-year-old girl with CP who used an AAC system in conjunction with verbal and nonverbal communication modes. Vivian used her AAC device primarily when more than a yes–no response was needed and when the setting was not constrained by time limits. After an intervention that taught her how to control conversations, Vivian used her AAC device more frequently. After the intervention, Vivian's topic initiation, during 10-minute conversations with her peers, increased from 20% to 35%, turn taking improved, and communication breakdowns decreased; this illustrates how empowering a person with skills increases AAC use rate.

Older adults with CP are more likely than are children with CP to employ a personal care attendant (Manton et al., 1993; Thyen, Kuhlthau, & Perrin, 1999); this observation reflects that fact that children are more likely to rely on their parents for assistance. Reliance on attendants often results from communication breakdowns with unfamiliar communication partners. Balandin and Morgan (1997) reported that older adults with CP who are able to communicate verbally without difficulty with familiar listeners needed assistance to communicate with their physicians during annual exams. Seventy-six of the 279 (27%) adult respondents reported, however, that they did not require assistance with self-care tasks. Balandin and Morgan also reported that life expectancy and the life expectations were different for these respondents compared to people with other types of disabilities. Only 22% of respondents had made retirement plans, even though a large proportion were employed and 42% had a will.

People with congenital impairments typically have higher AT use rates than do people with other impairments, because they have different physical and communication needs, different expectations regarding device performance, and do not typically experience a single period of disablement that resolves with time. A definable period of identity confusion is not typical, in contrast to people with acquired disabilities, because people with congenital impairments have a lifetime to incorporate a stable physical condition as part of their identity. People with congenital impairments therefore view AT as conferring benefits and few limitations. Nonuse of AT by people with congenital impairments is attributable to (a) frequent communication breakdowns that cause frustration and anger, (b) changes in the message due to the AAC system, (c) wanting to belong to a peer group, and (d) limited skills to control a conversation.

THE CASE OF JOE, WHO USES TECHNOLOGY TO MAKE LIFE BETTER

Joe, age 28, lives with his parents. During the interview, which took place on a warm summer day, he was wearing a t-shirt emblazoned with an NBA logo and shorts; his hair was worn in a crew cut. He graduated from high school at age 20 and received special education services while in school. He has spastic cerebral palsy. He uses a powered wheelchair, which he controls with a foot switch, and an AAC system with an active color matrix LCD, touch screen activation, and speech output. He controls the device with a head pointer and creates speech through a series of keyboard-actuated menus. He uses a keyboard to control Web TV and a PC at work.

Activities at home that are enhanced with AT include communication with family and friends. Joe said he can communicate faster and more accurately with the AAC device. He explained that often people will not wait for him to communicate at his unassisted speed. Joe controls lights, television, and a stereo with an environmental control unit. He acknowledged the ways in which others' assistance is helpful—for example, changing tapes in his stereo.

AT also helps Joe function more independently in his community. Joe works at a United CP program, and his current job is to press public transit labels onto booklets. He expressed appreciation for the opportunity to earn an income. He leaves home for work 5 days per week, weather permitting, using a public transit service for people with disabilities.

Joe prepared a speech for a dinner during the past year in which he discussed his views of AT.

> I used to use my eyes to talk. That worked sometimes, but I always felt that my choices were limited. It was scary to have to depend on other people to guess what I wanted to say. My grandfather did help me to talk. He went to church and gave money because he wanted to see me talk. He had faith it would happen one day. I feel good that I can say what I want to. I have been able to make more friends. AT has helped me to become more independent. I now have my own job responsibilities that I take care of at my vocational program, and I hope to get a job in the community one day. When something goes wrong with my head pointer or my AAC system, I can't communicate. Technology sometimes breaks down, but I hang in there. It's my life.

Joe said that he has used all technology offered to him and has adopted upgrades as they became available. He keeps an older AAC system in his home and still uses it occasionally. Joe summarized his view of AT by saying "It is cool."

PEOPLE WITH PROGRESSIVE DISORDERS

Chronic illnesses have progressive trajectories that diminish a person's ability to perform ADLs (Peace, 1995). Parkinson's disease, Alzheimer's disease, cancer, postpoliomyelitis syndrome, diabetes, and motor neuron disease (e.g., amytrophic lateral sclerosis [ALS]) are chronic, progressive diseases. Each disease introduces new symptoms or limitations over time that affect ADL performance. New symptoms and limitations challenge individuals with progressive diseases to re-examine their previous expectations, belief systems, and values.

Progressive diseases impose distinct challenges for performing ADLs. Parkinson's disease, for example, is a progressive neurological condition that incrementally imposes physical limitations affecting ambulation, speech production, swallowing, and fine motor skills. Alzheimer's disease affects cognitive and social skills, including short- and long-term memory and reasoning skills. Cancer is progressive and imposes limitations on an individual's ability to perform ADLs. Cancers that metastasize to the brain also have a dramatic effect on cognitive abilities. Postpoliomyelitis syndrome is a late-onset condition that affects mobility, ambulation, and stair climbing (Jonsson, Moller, & Grimby, 1999). Uncontrolled diabetes reduces mobility and endurance. ALS is a fatal disease characterized by motor neuron lesions and bulbar palsy (T. Li, Alberman, Day, & Swash, 1986; Oliver, 1989) resulting in dysarthria, dysphagia, and a persistent decline of physical skills.

People with progressive illnesses use a variety of AT devices and tend to use them more as the disease progresses. Devices include AAC systems, electric wheelchairs, canes, and walkers; attendants are also employed (Dunne, Hankey, & Edis, 1987; Hornsey, 1994). People with progressive diseases, like people with congenital and acquired disabilities, assign their own meanings and expectations to AT. The different meanings and expectations regarding device performance arise because of the nature of each disease and the timing of the onset of the illness (Gitlin, 1999); in turn, expectations based on the type of disease and disease course affect the use of AT.

People with progressive diseases can experience value changes regarding health and well-being; the progression of the diseases makes this an ongoing process. The onset of a progressive illness often connotes a dramatic reduction in control over long-term health and pursuit of goals. Goals change from a focus on long-term health to control over disease symptoms. People with progressive diseases use AT to diminish the effect of disease on ADLs and to increase control over symptoms. Although they cannot control disease progression, they can reduce the consequences of symptoms by using AT (Jonsson, Moller, & Grimby, 1999; Wallhagen & Brod, 1997).

Nonuse of AT by people with disabilities due to progressive disease can arise from the social stigma attached to devices. Peace (1995) eloquently described Ms. Lipton, an older woman with Parkinson's disease. Ms. Lipton addressed the social stigma associated with her physical limitations and her AT devices by educating friends about her illness and what she could and could not do for herself. These explanations readily diffused the social stigma, but they gave rise to feelings of not fitting in. Ms. Lipton stated that she wanted to be treated normally, but she felt normal only with her grandchildren, who described their grandma to their friends as being "wibbly-wobbly."

Nonuse of AT devices by people with disabilities due to progressive, terminal diseases, such as ALS, is also attributable to what the use of AT symbolizes. AT may symbolize the "nearing of the end," or it may serve to make the disablement process more poignant. Jonsson and her colleagues (1999) reported that people with postpoliomyelitis syndrome typically use AT devices only after they have reached their physical limits. After the

AT devices were integrated into daily routines, people viewed them as solutions to problems. The meanings attached to these devices changed over time, with the progression of their disease, from serving as a reminder of the skills they have lost to a tool that allows them to maintain independence. Consequently, device use rates tend to increase over time as disease progressively limits individuals' functional skills; the meaning the individual attaches to the devices may or may not change over time.

People with progressive diseases use AT devices as a means of coping with symptoms and functional limitations. Device use tends to increase over time as disease progression continues. Nonuse can result from social stigma and, with terminal diseases, from reminders of future debilitation and ultimately death.

THE CASE OF KEN, WHO IS EMPLOYED AND TECHNOLOGICALLY SAVVY

Ken, age 35, is married with a 4-year-old daughter; he works full-time as a manager of training and development. He commutes to work 2 days per week and works from his home 3 days per week. He is married to an occupational therapist who specializes in AT. He has infantile spinal muscular atrophy, a degenerative condition.

Ken uses a power wheelchair that he operates with joystick commands. He uses a hydraulic Hoyer lift[1] and an environmental control system that operates a stereo, lighting, and other small appliances at home. He also uses a power door system that opens and closes the door to his condominium; the door is locked and unlocked automatically. He uses public transportation to commute to work, and he has a van equipped with a ramp, which his wife drives when they attend community activities. He uses a cordless telephone with a headset, preprogrammed dialer, and voice answering. He has a home office equipped with a PC that allows audio and video transmission and a wireless keyboard. He also has a laptop that he finds useful when he is away from home. He may, for example, look at the Web site of a local newspaper to check out movie times at their favorite theater. Ken owns and uses other AT devices, including a pedestal sink with a "pull out" faucet in his bathroom and a remote controlled audio–video unit in his bedroom. Ken does his own programming to individualize and personalize his AT systems.

Home activities enhanced by AT include the ability to enter his apartment independently, turn on lights and fans, watch television, and

---

[1] An assistive device that can be used to transfer a person from bed to chair and vice versa; it can be electronically or manually operated.

complete work tasks without assistance. Leisure activities are also enhanced by AT. Ken's laptop, for example, creates a social atmosphere and promotes interactions about some of his interests; Ken is a trainer, and his interests include seeking data and using on-line information services. He finds that his laptop is very useful for promoting social situations in which technology can be the topic of discussion. Technology can be the tool he uses to promote the subject matter and sharing of information with friends. His interests, for example, include digital photography, and he uses his laptop to show his in-laws his digital photographs. Ken also writes books about parental relationships with their children when one or both parents have a disability.

At work, Ken is assigned to an accessible cubicle. Unlike most mid-level managers at his company, he is assigned an administrative assistant. His assistant helps him perform job-related functions, such as photocopying, and this assistant was provided in lieu of adapting office equipment.

Ken defined coping as "focusing on building the strengths that you have while not letting any physical limitations prevent or inhibit your personal growth." He said that AT helps him minimize frustrating situations. He described how being able to enter and exit his apartment independently helps him cope with physical limitations. He explained that 10 years ago he had the strength to enter and exit his home but that he is no longer able to do so without an opener. Ken no longer uses an earlier version of commercially available speech recognition software. He described it as being difficult to use; his current software is more flexible. He has minimized purchasing AT devices that have not proven their potential longevity by investigating the suitability of equipment before purchasing it. He also uses an AT lending library to try out devices and described it as a great service; his network of peers who use AT also serve as resources regarding the suitability and longevity of AT devices. He communicates routinely with his peers by means of e-mail. Ken reports that his research reduces the likelihood of abandoning a device.

Ken offered this advice to others with his condition: "Don't be afraid of the computer, because it is nothing but a toaster with a keyboard, and hitting the wrong keystrokes will not launch anything toward a third world nation. Don't be afraid to try equipment. The worst excuse is fear."

PSYCHOSOCIAL ISSUES AFFECTING AT USE

AT is designed to reduce environmental obstacles to participating in valued activities, thereby maintaining valued relationships (Stineman, 1999). People use AT to gain access to, operate within, move through, and have an effect on their physical and social environments. The effectiveness of AT in reducing environmental obstacles is not, however, the sole determinant of whether devices are used or abandoned. Adaptation to or acceptance of disability plays a major role in the determination of AT use. In this section we summarize the literature on psychosocial issues in AT use; the key findings are summarized in the appendix.

Adaptation refers to a process by which people maintain and enhance valued relationships (Coelho, Hamburg, & Adams, 1974). Wright (1960) provided a framework for understanding the process of disability acceptance by conceptualizing acceptance of loss as a change in values. These changes involve a process by which individuals (a) enlarge their scope of values, (b) subordinate the emphasis placed on physical appearance, (c) contain the effects of disability "spread," and (d) minimize comparative values while emphasizing asset values. Enlarging one's scope of values involves valuing the activities and relationships that are not affected by disability. Subordinating the relative importance of physique allows people to focus on skills and relations that are intrinsic to one's self and not affected by disability. Containing the spread of disability effects to just those aspects of oneself affected by limitations assures that the entire self does not become equated with "disability." Asset values focus on "who I am" and "what I can do" rather than valuing oneself in terms of skills or abilities in comparison with others.

The process of disability acceptance can include a period of identity confusion as one comes to incorporate disability into one's experience of self. Cultural as well as individual values influence disability acceptance, which in turn affects the use and abandonment of assistive devices (Jonsson et al., 1999).

One's sociocultural context influences the development of values over a lifetime and, consequently, individuals' readiness to accommodate disability within their experience of self (Luborsky, 1993). The extent to which assistive devices are perceived as acceptable and useful tools will reflect the person's point in the life cycle, family life stage, cultural heritage, and the social consequences of AT use. Individuals' "script" of expected life states and transitions (e.g., childhood to young adulthood to parenthood to retirement) allow them to evaluate how "on time" their life events are (Boone, Roessler, & Cooper, 1978).

Several investigators have noted that although device use reduces environmental barriers and enhances functional independence and control it can threaten the user's identity or self-concept. Linkowski and Dunn (1974) examined two aspects of self-concept (self-esteem and social relationships) and found that acceptance of disability is related to the manner in which people view themselves as well as their relationships with others.

Stigma associated with AT use is a social phenomenon; the features that are often associated with this stigma and that inhibit use of AT devices include dishonor, disgrace, and embarrassment.

Disability acceptance and identity confusion are related. Social interactions provide a mirror that is used to shape identity. As do able-bodied people, people with disabilities define their self-concepts in part on the basis of social feedback. Over time, people modify or adjust their self-views according to ongoing social feedback and make efforts to realign this social image with the image of how they want to be seen. They make coping efforts to deal with the discrepancy between the feedback and their desired selves. AT can be used to support coping efforts so as to enhance congruence between feedback and the desired self.

Motivation is also related to disability acceptance. Boone et al. (1978) defined *motivation* in terms of levels of hope and anxiety. He found that moderate levels of each increase a person's motivation to adapt to disability consequences. These findings support Uhlig and Stevic's (1967) position that a moderate level of hope is conducive to disability acceptance. Boone's findings also provide support for McDaniel's (1969) theoretical position that moderate levels of anxiety facilitate acceptance. Boone used Stotland's (1969) operational definition of *hope* as positive expectations for successful goal attainment, and of *anxiety* as anticipatory fear of harm. Unrealistically high and excessively low levels of hope increase the likelihood of failure. Increasing levels of anxiety can limit a person's ability to realistically anticipate the future (Sullivan, 1953). Realistic expectations in conjunction with a moderate degree of anxiety or discomfort are essential for effective learning and asset valuation, both of which promote AD (Boone et al., 1978).

An example may illustrate how motivation is related to AD. A person with an SCI who has a reasonable level of hope for increasing participation in daily activities is apt to be more motivated to use an environmental control unit than is someone with a low level of hope. Someone with very high expectations is apt to experience disappointment and be more likely to discontinue use. A moderate level of anxiety about computerized technology might reduce the likelihood of AT use, but not to a degree that the person would avoid using devices altogether. A higher level of asset valuation increases individuals' emphasis on freedom of choice and coping, thus increasing the likelihood of using an environmental control unit so as to participate in valued activities.

The meanings people assign to AT are based on individual life experiences and the cultures in which they live shape these meanings (Spencer, 1999). George Covington, for example, eloquently explained how his life was shaped by his perception of using a white cane to diminish the effect of severely impaired vision. For years he perceived his white cane negatively, because it brought unwanted attention and threatened his value of fitting in. His experience of social stigma associated with the cane was derived from his individual and cultural values (Covington, 1999).

Covington (1999) explained how anxiety about fitting in played a role in shaping the meaning that he had associated with using a white cane. The humiliation associated with cane use was the consequence of anxiety regarding unwanted attention. He also had a low level of hope that the white cane would allow him to fit in. This high level of anxiety and low level of hope helped determine his decision not to use the cane. As Covington's vision worsened, he became increasingly aware of the effect on independent ambulation; his growing awareness intensified his desire to maintain independent and safe ambulation. He re-evaluated the meaning associated with the cane; in so doing, he transformed his values from comparative ones ("I want to fit in, and my cane excludes me") to asset values ("My cane helps me be independent"). His hope of maintaining independence began to rise, and his anxiety about not fitting in diminished. He came to perceive the cane as a tool without stigmatizing power. Hope and anxiety worked synergistically to increase his desire to use the cane. By 1998 he used the cane routinely to aid ambulation.

CONCLUSION

AT provides a means of reducing functional limitations resulting from impairment and illness, enhancing participation in home and community activities, and consequently enhancing quality of life. Adopting assets values (rather than comparative values) allows potential AT users to view devices as a means of enhancing function rather than as creating stigma. This chapter illustrates how AT can be integrated successfully into people's lives. Rehabilitation psychologists, working in collaboration with engineers and therapists skilled in AT prescription, can help potential users explore the meaning of devices, their expectations of AT benefits, the anticipated social costs, and ways to come to terms with disability as one of the features, but not the defining feature, of oneself.

REFERENCES

Balandin, S., & Morgan, J. (1997). Adults with cerebral palsy: What's happening? *Journal of Intellectual Developmental Disability, 22,* 109–124.

Boone, S., Roessler, R., & Cooper, P. (1978). Hope and manifest anxiety: Motivational dynamics of acceptance of disability. *Journal of Counseling Psychology, 25,* 551–556.

Buzolich, M., & Lunger, J. (1995). Empowering system users in peer training. *Augmentative and Alternative Communication, 11,* 37–48.

Coelho, G., Hamburg, D., & Adams, J. (1974). *Coping and adaptation.* New York: Basic Books.

Covington, G. (1999). Cultural and environmental barriers to assistive technology: Why assistive devices don't always assist. In D. Gray, L. Quatrano, & M. Lieberman (Eds.), *Designing and using assistive technology* (pp. 52–88). Baltimore, MD: Brookes.

Cushman, L., & Scherer, M. (1996). Measuring the relationship of assistive technology use, functional status over time, and consumer–therapist perceptions of ATs. *Assistive Technology, 8,* 103–109.

Dittuno, J., Stover, S., & Freed, M. (1992). Motor recovery of the upper extremities in traumatic quadriplegia: A multicenter study. *Archives of Physical Medicine and Rehabilitation, 73,* 431–435.

Dunne, J., Hankey, G., & Edis, R. (1987). Parkinsonism: Upturned walking stick as an aid to locomotion. *Archives of Physical Medicine and Rehabilitation, 68,* 380–381.

Forbes, W. F., Hayward, L. M., & Agwani, N. (1993). Factors associated with self-reported use and non-use of assistive devices among impaired elderly residing in the community. *Canadian Journal of Public Health, 84,* 53–57.

Garstecki, D. C., & Erler, S. F. (1998). Hearing loss, control, and demographic factors influencing hearing aid use among older adults. *Journal of Speech, Language, and Hearing Research, 41,* 527–537.

Gauthier-Gagnon, C., Grise, M.-C., & Potvin, D. (1994). Prosthetic profile of the amputee questionnaire: Validity and reliability. *Archives of Physical Medicine and Rehabilitation, 75,* 1309–1314.

Gauthier-Gagnon, C., Grise, M.-C., & Potvin, D. (1998). Predisposing factors related to prosthetic use by people with transtibial and transfemoral amputation. *Journal of Prosthetics and Orthotics, 10,* 99–109.

Gitlin, L. N. (1999). The role of social science research in understanding technology use among older adults. In M. Ory & G. Defriese (Eds.), *Self-care in later life research: Research program and policy issues* (pp. 142–169). New York: Springer.

Haas, U., Hakan, B., Anderson, A., & J. Persson (1997). Assistive technology selection: A study of participation of users with rheumatoid arthritis. *IEEE Transactions on Rehabilitation Engineering, 5,* 263–275.

Hanson, S., Buckelew S., Hewett, J., & O'Neal, G. (1993). The relationship between coping and adjustment after spinal cord injury: A 5-year follow-up study. *Rehabilitation Psychology, 38,* 41–52.

Hartke, R., Prohaska, T., & Furner, S. (1998). Older adults and assistive devices: Use, multiple-device use and need. *Journal of Aging and Health, 10,* 99–116.

Heinemann, A., Goranson, N., Ginsburg, K., & Schnoll, S. (1989). Alcohol use and activity patterns following spinal cord injury. *Rehabilitation Psychology, 34,* 191–206.

Heinemann, A., Magiera-Planey, R., Schiro-Geist, C., & Grimes, G. (1987). Mobility for persons with spinal cord injury: An evaluation of two systems. *Rehabilitation Psychology, 68,* 90–93.

Hornsey, J. (1994). Empowering patient and career through terminal MND. *Nursing Times, 90*(29), 37–39.

Jonsson, A., Moller, A., & Grimby, G. (1999). Managing occupations in everyday life to achieve adaptation. *American Journal of Occupational Therapy, 53,* 353–362.

Kelly, C., & Glueckauff, R. (1993). Disability and value change: An overview and reanalysis of acceptance of loss theory. *Rehabilitation Psychology, 38,* 199–210.

Li, L., & Moore, D. (1998). Acceptance of disability and its correlates. *Journal of Social Psychology, 138,* 13–25.

Li, T., Alberman, E., & Swash, M. (1986). Differential diagnosis of MND from other neurological conditions. *The Lancet, 2,* 731–733.

Light, J. (1988). Interaction involving individuals using augmentative and alternative communications systems: State of the art and future directions. *Augmentative and Alternative Communication, 4,* 66–82.

Linkowski, D., & Dunn, M. (1974). Self-concept and acceptance of disability. *Rehabilitation Counseling Bulletin, 18,* 28–32.

Luborsky, M. (1993). Sociocultural factors shaping technology usage: Fulfilling the promise. *Technology and Disability, 2,* 71–78.

Mann, W., Hurren, D., & Tomita, M. (1993). Comparison of assistive device use and needs of home-based older persons with different impairments. *American Journal of Occupational Therapy, 47,* 980–987.

Mann, W., Hurren, D., Tomita, M., & Barbara, C. (1995). The relationship of functional independence to assistive device use of elderly persons living at home. *Journal of Applied Gerontology, 14,* 225–247.

Mann, W., Hurren, D., Tomita, M., & Charvat, B. (1996). Use of assistive devices for bathing by elderly who are not institutionalized. *Occupational Therapy Journal of Research, 16,* 261–286.

Mann, W., Hurren, D., Tomita, M., & Charvat, B. (1997). A 2-year study of coping strategies of home based frail elder persons with vision impairment. *Technology and Disability 6,* 177–189.

Manton, K., Corder, L., & Stallard, E. (1993). Changes in the use of personal assistance and special equipment from 1982 and 1989 NLTCS. *The Gerontologist, 33,* 168–176.

McCall, F., Markova, I., Murphy J., Moodie, E., & Collins, S. (1997). Perspectives on AAC systems by the users and by their communication partners. *European Journal of Disorders of Communication, 32,* 235–256.

McDaniel, J. (1969). *Physical disability and human behavior.* New York: Pergamon Press.

Mechanic, D. (1995). Sociological dimensions of illness behavior. *Social Science Medicine, 41,* 1207–1216.

Moore, L. W. (1999). Living with macular degeneration: Creative strategies used by older women. *Journal of Ophthalmic Nursing and Technology, 18,* 200–206.

Nochajski, S., Tomita, M., & Mann, W. (1996). The use and satisfaction with assistive devices by older persons with cognitive impairments: A pilot intervention study. *Topics in Geriatric Rehabilitation, 12,* 40–53.

Oliver, D. (1989). *Motor neuron disease.* London: Royal College of General Practitioners.

Peace, G. (1995). Living with Parkinson's disease. *Nursing Times, 91,* 40–41.

Phillips, B., & Zhao, H. (1993). Predictors of assistive technology abandonment. *Assistive Technology, 5,* 36–45.

Sackett, D. L. (1989). Rules of evidence and clinical recommendation on the use of antithrombotic agents. *CHEST,* 95(2 Suppl.), 2S–4S.

Schaller, J., & Garza, D. (1999). "It's about relationships": Perspectives of people with cerebral palsy on belonging in their families, schools and rehabilitation counseling. *Journal of Applied Rehabilitation Counseling, 30,* 7–18.

Scheer, J., & Luborsky, M. (1991). The cultural context of polio biographies. *Orthopedics, 14,* 1173–1181.

Scherer, M. (1988). Assistive device utilization and quality of life in adults with spinal cord injuries or cerebral palsy. *Journal of Applied Rehabilitation Counseling, 19,* 21–30.

Scherer, M. (1990). Assistive device utilization and quality of life in adults with spinal cord injuries or cerebral palsy two years later. *Journal of Applied Rehabilitation Counseling, 21,* 36–44.

Scherer, M. (1996). Outcomes of assistive technology use on quality of life. *Disability and Rehabilitation, 18,* 439–448.

Singer, H. (1999). Success with low vision patients: Realistic prognosis, reasonable goals. *Journal of Ophthalmic Nursing and Technology, 18,* 65–67.

Spencer, J. C. (1999). Tools or baggage? Alternative meanings of assistive technology. In D. Gray & L. Quatrano (Eds.), *Designing and using assistive technology* (pp. 89–98). Baltimore, MD: Brookes.

Stewart, H., Noble, G., & Seeger, B. (1992). Isometric joystick: A study of control by adolescents and young adults with cerebral palsy. *Australian Occupational Therapy Journal, 39,* 33–39.

Stineman, M. (1999). The sphere of self-fulfillment: A multidimensional approach of assistive technology outcomes. In D. Gray, L. Quatrano, & M. Lieberman (Eds.), *Designing and using assistive technology* (pp. 30–51). Baltimore, MD: Brookes.

Stotland, E. (1969). *The psychology of hope.* San Francisco, CA: Jossey-Bass.

Sullivan, H. (1953). *The interpersonal theory of psychiatry.* New York: Norton.

Thyen, U., Kuhlthau, K., & Perrin, J. (1999). Employment, child care, and mental health of mothers caring for children assisted by technology. *Pediatrics, 103,* 1235–1242.

Uhlig, G., & Stevic, R. (1967). Client expectations and the rehabilitation process. *Rehabilitation Counseling Bulletin, 10,* 112–117.

Wallhagen, M., & Brod, M. (1997). Perceived control and well-being in Parkinson's disease. *Western Journal of Nursing Research, 19,* 11–31.

Watts, J., Erickson, A., Houde, L., Wilson, E., & Maynard, M. (1996). Assistive device use among the elderly: A national data-based study. *Physical and Occupational Therapy in Geriatrics, 14,* 1–18.

Weingarden, S., & Martin, C. (1989). Independent dressing after spinal cord injury: A functional time evaluation. *Archives of Physical Medicine and Rehabilitation, 70,* 518–519.

Wright, B. (1960). *Physical disability: A psychological approach.* New York: Harper.

Appendix
Summary of Published Evidence: Coping, Adjustment, and Assistive Technology (AT) Use

Study and journal	Population and sample	Measures	Class of evidence[a]	Did study report? AT Use	Coping	Adjustment	Values	Outcome	Principal findings
Balandin & Morgan (1997), J of Intellectual & Developmental Disability	N = 279 adults with cerebral palsy (CP)	Survey	V	Y	Y	Y	N	N	Aging with CP needs to be investigated further regarding needs for services because life span is increasing.
Boone et al. (1978), J Counseling Psychology	N = 48 rehabilitation clients with physical disabilities; 18–22 yrs	Self-Anchoring Scale (hope) Manifest Anxiety Scale	V	N	Y	Y	Y	Y[b]	Motivation = hope + anxiety; hope + anxiety + time since onset of disability predict AD; moderate levels of hope and anxiety predict better AD.
Buzolich & Lunger (1995), AAC	12-year-old alternative augmentative communication system user with mixed quadriplegic cerebral palsy	10-min videos of 3 conversational dyads with 3 classmates chosen by participant	III	Y	N	N	N	Y[c]	AT devices owned: motorized chair accessed with joystick and 128-location Light Talker accessed by infrared sensor. Before intervention: Used Light Talker more frequently with adults and peers in nondemanding settings/no time constraints. Rarely used Light Talker in classroom; used yes–no response (nonverbal) primarily in school setting. After intervention: Topic initiation increased from 20% to 35%; community breakdowns decreased from 4 to 1 in 10 min; turn taking increased.
Cushman & Scherer (1996), AT	N = 47 adults with a variety of disabilities	AT device predisposition assessment, Fone FIM	V	Y	N	N	N	Y[d]	Case series with follow-up; grooming aids most frequently abandoned; average 33% abandonment rate similar to other studies; most frequent reason: no need due to functional improvements. Functional gains correspond with device nonuse for about half of the devices. Study identified other multiple reasons for abandonment.

Reference	Sample	Measure							Comments
Dunne et al. (1987), *APMR*	3 persons with Parkinson's disease	Self-reports of effectiveness of up-turned walking stick	>	Y	N	N	N	N	Gait is facilitated by inverting a walking stick and using the handle as a visual cue or target to step over.
Forbes et al. (1993), *Canadian J Public Health*	Elderly people with impairments	Canadian Health and Activity Limitations Survey	>	Y	N	N	N	N	Nonuse of devices related to social isolation, education, and rural residence; relative risks reported for nonuse of hearing aids, visual aids, and mobility devices.
Garstecki & Erler (1998), *JSLHR*	131 adults with hearing impairments	Hearing Aid Management Questionnaire; Rotter's Internal–External scale; MMPI	>	Y	N	N	N	Y[e]	Older women who adhere to hearing aid use assume more responsibility for hearing loss management; greater levels of internal control among adherers was also found relative to nonadherers; nonadherers had higher external control.
Gauthier-Gagnon & Gire (1994), *APMR*	$N = 89$ adults with LE amputations	Prosthetic Profile of Amputee (PPA)	>	N	N	N	N	N	PPA measures factors potentially related to prosthetic use. Strong test–retest data demonstrated that the PPA was repeatable. Construct validity was demonstrated. Authors concluded that PPA is reliable and valid for clinical and research use.
Gauthier-Gagnon et al. (1998), *J of Prosthetics and Orthotics*	$N = 396$ adults with unilateral amputations	PPA	>	Y	Y	N	N	Y[f]	Adaptation to amputation was found to be the best predictor of prosthesis use.
Haas et al. (1997), *IEEE Transactions on Rehabilitation Engineering*	$N = 190$ persons with rheumatoid arthritis living in Sweden	Intervention: improving AT user knowledge through different mediums (workshops, group meetings, home visits, telephone interviews)	=	Y	N	N	N	Y[g]	Equipment selection process increased user participation, satisfaction, prescriptions, and costs, but the outcome measures showed small improvements; no improvement in pain and difficulty with ADLs; increased use of AT devices and improved health-related QOL for women 64 years or younger.

(continued)

Appendix
Summary of Published Evidence: Coping, Adjustment, and Assistive Technology (AT) Use (Continued)

Study and journal	Population and sample	Measures	Class of evidence	Did study report? AT Use	Coping	Adjustment	Values	Outcome	Principal findings
Hanson et al. (1993), *Rehabilitation Psychology*	N = 28 people with spinal cord injuries	Ways of Coping Scale, Symptom Checklist-90—Revised, Acceptance of Disability Scale, vocational data, medical data	V	N	Y	Y	Y	Y[b]	Investigated the relation between coping and adjustment 5–6 years post-SCI. Results suggest the importance of specific coping strategies to adjustment, changes over time, and support the belief that coping is a dynamic process.
Hartke et al. (1998), *J Aging and Health*	N = 14,210 noninstitutionalized people aged 65 years and older	1990 AD supplement to the NHIS	V	Y	N	N	N	N	Poorer health was associated with the use of AT, multiple device use, and expressed need.
Heinemann et al. (1987), *APMR*	N = 92 people with paraplegia due to SCI	Three-part survey	V	Y	N	N	N	N	Transportation and mobility needs in the sample were high. WCs were rated as having greater value compared to leg braces due to lower energy requirements. Nonuse of KAFOs was attributed to discomfort and pain.
Heinemann et al. (1989), *Rehabilitation Psychology*	N = 103 adults with SCIs	Activity Patterns Indicator, Acceptance of Disability Scale	V	N	Y	Y	Y	Y[b]	Coping categories/processes: direct action, emotional regulation, cognitive regulation, and maladaptive actions. Greater disability acceptance was associated with younger age, older injuries, and absence of maladaptive coping processes such as drinking. Self-blame was unrelated to AD.

Reference	Sample	Measures						Findings
Hornsey (1994), *Nursing Times*	N = 1 man with motor neuron disease and caregiver	Self-reports by patient and caregiver	V		Y	Y	Y	N — Impediments to AT use include viewing AT as a symbol of debility and death.
Jonsson et al. (1999), *Am J OT*	N = 22 persons with postpoliomyelitis syndrome	One to three structured interviews per participant	V		Y	Y	Y	N — Participants described 18 adaptive strategies that they use to deal with functional limitations; AT use was 1 of the 18.
Kelly & Glueckauf (1993), *Rehabilitation Psychology*				N	Y	Y	Y	N — Review article: basic tenets of Wright's acceptance-of-loss theory, particularly the value changes defining acceptance of disability.
L. Li & Moore (1998), *J Social Psychology*	N = 1,266 adults with disabilities residing in OH, MI and IL	Acceptance of Disability Scale, Self-esteem and investigator-designed emotional support scale	V	N	Y	Y	Y	Y[b] — Self-esteem and emotional support important to adjustment following disability. Perceived social discrimination had a significant impact on AD; acquired disability, multiple disabilities, and chronic pain were also important to AD.
Luborsky (1993), *Technology and Disability*	Two case studies of AT users			Y	Y	Y	Y	N — Two case studies illustrating the sociocultural dimensions of AT abandonment following polio. Cultural and social implications from using AT include: age-related psychological and physical capabilities, life cycle stage, family life stage, AD, social stigma, conflicting cultural expectations, ethnic differences, and personal biographies.

(continued)

Summary of Published Evidence: Coping, Adjustment, and Assistive Technology (AT) Use *(Continued)*

Study and journal	Population and sample	Measures	Class of evidence	AT Use	Coping	Adjustment	Values	Outcome	Principal findings
					Did study report?				
Mann et al. (1999), *OT J of Research*	N = 61 people aged 65 and older with arthritis living at home	Investigator-designed survey, FIM, Sickness Impact Profile (SIP), IADL section of Older Americans Resources and Services Program, Multidimensional Functional Assessment Questionnaire (OARS)	V	Y	Y	N	N	Y[h]	Survey found significant declines in health status and functional status at 3 years, a significant increase in number of AT devices owned and used; clear evidence of AT use as a coping strategy over the 3-year follow-up.
Mann et al. (1997), *Technology and Disability*	N = 38 elderly people with visual impairments	Older Americans Research and Service Center Instrument, Jette Functional Pain Index, SIP, FIM, MMSE, Rosenberg Self-Esteem Scale, CES–D, Social Resources Scale, Consumer assessments of AT devices used, Home Environment Scale	V	Y	Y	N	N	N	Needs of older persons (60+) with impairments were assessed initially and 2 years later. Results: Study participants owned an average of 19.1 devices and used 18.3 at first interview. About 75% of these devices addressed visual impairment. Two years later the number of devices owned increased to almost 24, and 90% were used. Vision remained stable. Authors concluded that AT represents a successful coping technique for the "frail elderly" with impaired vision. These results support Mann's (1993) previous report that older adults with visual impairments use more assistive devices than people with other impairments.

Citation	Sample	Measures						Comments
Mann et al. (1996), OT J of Research	Elderly 60+, noninstitutionalized	SIP: physical dysfunction, body care, and movement sections, motor FIM	>	Y	N	N	Yⁱ	Disability scores for satisfied and dissatisfied owners of bath devices were compared. Dissatisfied owners had greater disability, suggesting a benefit from a higher level device. Tested the Bath Device Prescription Model.
Mann et al. (1995), J Applied Gerontology	N = 117 pairs of elderly adults living at home; pairs were matched by age and predictor variables. Pairs were dissimilar on AT use.	OARS, FIM, MMSE, CES–D, Rosenberg Self-Esteem Scale, Responsibility Scale, AT Communication Needs Assessment, SIP, Jette Pain Index, Environment Survey	=	Y	Y	N	Yⁱ	Within most pairs, the participant with more devices was more independent in ADLs but less independent in IADLs. Results suggest that increased use of assistive devices relates to increased functional independence.
Mann et al. (1993), AM J OT	N = 157 noninstitutionalized people aged 60 years and older	SIP, OARS, OMFAQ, MMSE, AT use survey	>	Y	N	N	Yᵏ	Significant differences among impairment groups regarding number of devices owned and used and in satisfaction. Need for more devices for balance and mobility expressed.
Manton et al. (1993), The Gerontologist	1982: N = 26,924, 1989: N = 30,871 Medicare-enrolled people with chronic disabilities who reside in a community	National LTC Survey: 1982, 1984, and 1989	>	Y	N*	N	N	Reliance on personal assistance has declined while AT use combined with personal assistance has increased. Reliance solely on AT was prevalent for people with only IADL or 1–2 ADL impairments. AT use was higher for women. For people with 5–6 ADL limitations, AT supplemented personal assistance.

(continued)

Appendix
Summary of Published Evidence: Coping, Adjustment, and Assistive Technology (AT) Use *(Continued)*

Study and journal	Population and sample	Measures	Class of evidence	Did study report? AT Use	Coping	Adjustment	Values	Outcome	Principal findings
McCall et al. (1997), *European J of Disorders of Communication*	89 adolescents with cerebral palsy who use alternative and augmentative communication systems (AAC)	Structured interview regarding communication functions	V	Y	N	N	N	N	Vocabulary use rates, single-mode use rates; use rates of non-AAC mode; reasons for nonuse of AAC; 3 main areas of concern with AAC systems identified.
Mechanic (1995), *Social Science Medicine*				N	N	N	N	N	Examined the disability process. Discussed approaches to patient assessment and intervention. Argued for the need to extend traditional differential diagnosis to include an assessment of individual illness behavior in the primary medical care model.
Miedaner & Finuf (1993), *Pediatric Physical Therapy*	12 children aged 17–58 months with cerebral palsy	Bayley Scales of Infant Development	II	Y	N	N	N	Y[i]	Adaptive positioning has positive impact on standard cognitive tests for children 17–30 months. Cognitive tests specifically designed to accommodate neuromotor disabilities still recommended as cognitive level of functioning was not revealed.
Nochajski et al. (1996), *Topics in Geriatric Rehabilitation*	20 (from CAS sample) elderly people (65+) with cognitive impairments due to Alzheimers, MR, stroke, alcohol abuse	MMSE, FIM, OARS, Care Provider Burden Scale, Environment Survey, Activity Performance Worksheet, Assistive Device User Survey	V	Y	N	N	N	N	People with cognitive impairments use devices, but at a lower rate than people without cognitive impairments. Following assessment, AT devices were provided or existing devices were adapted. Training on use of AT and follow-up support were provided. 74% of the devices addressed physical impairments, and 22% addressed

Citation	Sample	Method						Findings
								cognitive impairments. Devices addressing physical impairments were more readily accepted and used than the devices that addressed cognitive impairments.
Peace (1995), *Nursing Times*	1 caregiver, 1 friend, 1 adult with Parkinson's disease	Structured interviews with patient, friend, and caregiver	>	Y	Y	Y	N	Patient, close friend, and daughter discussed meanings attached to functional limitations, social stigma. "Fitting in" identified as an important value.
Phillips & Zhao (1993), *AT*	$N = 227$ adults with disabilities	Survey	=	Y	N	N	N	29% abandonment rate reported. Strongest influences were change in needs, consumer involvement in device selection, device performance, expectations, device reliability, durability, comfort, and ease of use.
Scheer & Luborsky (1991), *Orthopedics*	7 case studies of persons with polio-related experiences	Structured interviews	V	Y	Y	Y	N	Cultural context of postpolio adaptation illustrated in case studies.
Scherer (1990), *J of Applied Rehabilitation Counseling*	$N = 5$ women with cerebral palsy and $N = 5$ men with spinal cord injuries	Personalities Capacity Questionnaire, Taylor–Johnson Temperament Analysis, Qualitative assessment of AT	V	Y	Y	Y	Y	Functioning and temperament improved over 2 years but adjustment of people with SCIs declined with time. AT users with SCIs displayed best functional skills, and nonusers with SCIs reported the most functional declines. Conclusions: People with congenital disabilities have different values and expectations.
Scherer (1996), *Disability and Rehabilitation*	Literature synthesis		V	N	N	N	Y[m]	Literature review of influences on AT use. Matching person to technology, environment/social setting, personality, and device characteristics are synthesized.

(continued)

Appendix
Summary of Published Evidence: Coping, Adjustment, and Assistive Technology (AT) Use *(Continued)*

Study and journal	Population and sample	Measures	Class of evidence	Did study report?					Principal findings
				AT Use	Coping	Adjustment	Values	Outcome	
Stewart et al. (1992), *Australian OT J*	5 adults aged 16–43 years with cerebral palsy	Displacement joystick and isometric joystick, response time accuracy	III	Y	N	N	N	Y[n]	Comparison of isometric and displacement joysticks on response time and accuracy. No difference was observed between the 2 types of joysticks with regard to performance.
Wallhagen & Brod (1997), *Western J of Nursing Research*	N = 101 people with Parkinson's disease, N = 45 spousal caregivers	Structured interview, mailed questionnaires, MOS 32	V	N	Y	Y	Y	N	Participants were interviewed two times; the second interview was 1 year after the initial interview. Findings indicate that an individual's locus of control shifted from controlling disease to controlling symptoms during this year. Symptom management became important to the patient and the caregiver.
Watts et al. (1996), *Physical & OT in Geriatrics*	N = 3,297 elderly adults (65+) that participated in the 1990 Assistive Device Supplement to the NHIS	NHIS 1990	V	Y[o]	N	N	N	N	Secondary analysis to evaluate the associations between self-reported health status, activity limitation, number of devices "used," and demographic characteristics. 23% of respondents reported owning an assistive device. African Americans reported more activity limitations. More women than men reported having activity limitations. People not living with a spouse reported owning more than one device.

Study	Sample	Method						Comments
Weaver et al. (2000), *Medical Care*				N	N	N	Y[p]	SCI is an important topic for the Department of Veterans Affairs (DVA); the authors reviewed the objectives of the SCI Quality Enhancement Research Initiative (QUERI). These objectives include identifying knowledge gaps. One topic under investigation includes the use of AT.
Weingarden & Martin (1989), *APMR*	10 persons with C_6 quadriplegia who were able to self-dress at discharge	Questionnaire at discharge, OT follow-up home visit	V	N	N	N	Y	Examined relation between time to complete self-dressing and decision to retain, modify, or delegate the activity after rehabilitation. None of the participants self-dressed (20–60 min for task completion). Respondents stated that it took "too much time and too much work," implying that a functional skill must be accomplished within an individually defined time frame.

Note. J = *Journal*; AD = acceptance of disability; AAC = *Augmentative and Alternative Communication*; FIM = Functional Independence Measure; *APMR* = *Archives of Physical Medicine and Rehabilitation*; *JSLHR* = *Journal of Speech, Language, and Hearing Research*; MMPI = Minnesota Multiphasic Personality Inventory; LE = lower extremity; ADLs = activities of daily living; QOL = quality of life; SCI = spinal cord injury; NHIS = National Health Interview Survey; WC = wheelchair; KAFOs = knee-ankle-foot orthoses; *AM J OT* = *American Journal of Occupational Therapy*; *OT J Research* = *Occupational Therapy Journal of Research*; MMSE = Mini Mental State Examination; CES-D = Center for Epidemiological Studies Depression Scale; IADL = independent ADL; OARS = Older Americans Research and Service Center Instrument; OMFAQ = Older Americans Resource and Service Program Multidimensional Functional Assessment Questionnaire; LTC = Long-term Care; CAS = Consumer Assessment Study; MR = mental retardation; MOS 32 = Medical Outcomes Study 32

[a]Classes of evidence (Sackett, 1989) are as follows: I = large, randomized trials with clear-cut results (and low risk of error); II = small, randomized trials with uncertain results (and moderate to high risk of error); III = nonrandomized trials with concurrent or contemporaneous controls; IV = nonrandomized trials with historical controls; V = case series with no controls. [b]Outcome = AD. [c]Outcome = interactional style changes and conversational control. [d]Outcome = AT use. [e]Outcome = adherence versus nonadherence. [f]Outcome = prosthetic use or nonuse. [g]Outcome = functional ability; pain, and ADL difficulty; AT device use; health-related QOL. [h]Outcome = changes in health, functional status, psychosocial status, and coping strategies. [i]Outcome = disability as measured with FIM. [j]Outcome = functional independence. [k]Outcome = satisfaction with AT. [l]Outcome = functional improvement. [m]Outcome = AT use or nonuse. [n]Outcome = performance as measured by speed and accuracy. [o]NHIS does not define AT use: Ownership and use were not distinguished. [p]Outcome = identifying outcomes of importance to providers and people with SCIs is another objective of the DVA SCI QUERI.

9

EDUCATING THE CONSUMER AND CARETAKER ON ASSISTIVE TECHNOLOGY

JAN C. GALVIN AND CHANDRA M. DONNELL

The challenge before us is to find creative and culturally appropriate ways to meet the needs of individuals with disabilities by providing knowledge and information that will enable them to achieve their aspirations for self-direction, independence, inclusion, and functional competence. In the past 20 years, technology has greatly enhanced the accommodation of disability, self-awareness has raised expectations of and for people with disabilities, and advocacy has resulted in the recognition of the rights of people with disabilities to societal access and reasonable accommodations. The past 20 years have also witnessed the emergence of new vulnerable populations where disability is coupled with conditions such as constantly changing health policies, poverty, enthnicity and culture, and the age continuum. In response to efforts to point out of challenging attitudinal and institutional barriers by people in the disability community, policymakers around the world have slowly begun to react. They have rejected the old paradigm of dependence and segregation and have begun to move toward a new paradigm that considers disability a natural and normal part of the human experience (Schriner & Batavia, 1995; Silverstein, 2000).

As the 21st century begins, this new paradigm is reflected in the *International Classification of Functioning, Disability and Health* (ICF; World Health Organization, 2001) reclassification of disability. The ICF includes terminology that is more positive and addresses factors such as the environment and personal issues. This new paradigm maintains that disability is a product of an interaction between characteristics (e.g., conditions or impairments, functional status, or personal and social qualities) of the individual and characteristics of the natural, cultural, and social environments.

Within this newer "sociopolitical" paradigm considerably more attention can be paid to public policy and societal barriers and their potential impact on people with disabilities (Bickenbach, 1999). This new paradigm is integrative and holistic and focuses on the whole person functioning in an environmental context, as reflected in the Americans With Disabilities Act (1990). For this new model to work successfully for consumers who use assistive technology (AT), service practitioners themselves must be educated and must be advocates of and partners with consumers in their joint mission. As a consequence, consumers will have access to critical information. They thus will become empowered, educated consumers who will be more involved, integral participants and members of the team in determining the most appropriate and effective AT devices to meet their individual needs.

In this chapter we provide information regarding the relevance and importance of education and training in the selection and use of AT devices for service providers and consumers. It is imperative that all people involved with AT devices are educated and trained. This includes the service providers, the consumer, and the consumer's family or caregiver. Appropriate education and training on the correct functional and environmental evaluation, selection, and use of AT devices not only will ensure that the appropriate device is chosen, but it could also be the difference between successful and unsuccessful rehabilitation. The purpose of this chapter, therefore, is to provide readers with an awareness of the importance of educated service providers and consumers and to describe some of the social and cultural factors that may affect successful interventions.

In this chapter we highlight the potential consequences of noneducation and the effect it can have on the consumer. We also offer several practical considerations for rehabilitation professionals as they work with consumers to select AT devices and as they train consumers to use AT devices. This combination of education and training will surely enhance the overall rehabilitation process.

Other chapters highlight the importance of psychological, social, and cultural factors that can hinder the rehabilitation process. These factors cannot be emphasized enough. No matter how thorough a practitioner may be in working with the individual to identify goals and needs, and no matter how well rehabilitation professionals do in developing creative materials and methods to assist individuals in the AT selection process, they have to understand and take into consideration the pertinent psychological, social, and cultural factors. The need for this consideration further stresses the importance of individualized service approaches. The educated consumer, the trained service provider, and the appropriate AT device are all integral components in creating successful outcomes.

PROVIDER EDUCATION, SERVICES, AND SUPPORT OF AT

Advances in technology and the rapid growth of AT devices offer the potential to help people maintain or regain independence and, for elderly people, AT devices may prevent or postpone institutionalization (Mann, 1997). However, advances in technology alone do not create people's access to it. The success of technology has more to do with people than with technology. People make the technology powerful by creatively using it to fulfill their dreams. Therefore, advances in technology also increase the demand for greater professional expertise in AT evaluation, selection, and ongoing training support. Individuals with disabilities and their families have expectations that professionals—such as educators, therapists, and rehabilitation counselors—have current knowledge about AT devices and services. "Creating true access ... means building in training, ongoing support, and building in opportunities for self-instruction and troubleshooting, both for the individual relying on the device and his/her caregivers" (Williams, 1995, p. 5).

Fifield and Fifield (1997) asserted that no service or support can be better than the skills and preparation of the professionals who have been trained to provide such services and support. Thus, it is necessary that competent professionals be involved in the delivery of AT devices and services and that such professionals come from a variety of clinical and technological disciplines. Technology has traditionally not been included in most discipline-specific curricula. In fact, according to the Institute of Medicine (Brandt & Pope, 1997), there is an increased need for rehabilitation-related education in and across all existing health care professions so that knowledge pertaining to AT can be integrated into the knowledge base of all general and primary care providers. Despite this need, there appears to be hesitancy among some professionals to actively seek out the needed training. The literature suggests that one possible explanation for such hesitancy is the misconception that "assistive technology is a highly specialized and technical process requiring intensive training" (as seen in Justesen & Menlove, 1994, p. 253; see also Bellamy, Newton, LeBaron, & Horner, 1992; Jaskulski, Metzler, & Zierman, 1990; Matson & Rusch, 1986). In some respects, AT is complex and challenging. Constant change and increasing advances make it difficult for even professionals in the field to be kept abreast of delivery methods (Somerville, Wilson, & Shanfield, 1989). However, proponents of AT are not suggesting the creation of "technological geniuses" but rather professionals educated in regard to the capability of technology to help increase disabled people's participation in society as well as how to efficiently access available resources (Mueller, 1989). Fifield, in testimony presented in 1990 to the U.S. House of Representatives, asserted that allowing untrained professionals to provide the services of sophisticated technology to consumers who are equally untrained in proper usage is setting the stage for failure.

The lack of effective collaboration between service providers and consumers continues to be a shortcoming of AT service delivery in most settings (Scherer & Galvin, 1994). The Assistive Technology Funding and Systems Change Project published one parent's frustrating dilemma of working with a school that provided computer software as AT for her son, only to find that the teachers themselves did not know how to use it (Goodman, 1999). This lack of sophistication on the part of service personnel is also apparent in maintenance and use of AT. Recent testimony at a National Institute on Disability and Rehabilitation Research (NIDRR) hearing told of one group home staff shelving a device as broken when all it needed was a recharged battery (NIDRR, 1998). Expanding training activities was identified as a critical need by the Coalition on Technology and Disabilities more than 10 years ago. "The most critical need at this time is for inservice training of consumers and of individuals who are already in the field providing services to people with disabilities" wrote T. Beattie, in a statement prepared for a public forum in 1990. This lack of knowledge is having an obvious impact on consumers who are not receiving basic information regarding AT devices from providers (Justesen & Menlove, 1994). The effect of this is profound, because consumer knowledge and training are considered to be the elements most imperative to successful AT use.

Another barrier to consumer empowerment is that AT services, for the most part, are components of other human services delivery systems (education, rehabilitation, health, and social services). Each of these programs presents a maze of problems. Requirements and bureaucratic obstacles—including separate intake systems, eligibility determination processes, and payment structures—represent just a few. Furthermore, even after being deemed eligible by an agency or service provider, the consumer is empowered with little leverage to participate in decision making about the services he or she will receive (National Council on Disability, 1996).

A consumer's interest in and acceptance of an AT device are not always consistent or predictable. Technology affects people in different ways. Some are excited and fascinated by the advances in technology, whereas others are threatened and alienated by it. As expressed by staff at a local school district, "All of us are so carried away by the adaptive computer technology that we are not doing appropriate assessments. . . . We may assess the developmental level of the child, but we do not assess the child's readiness or computer literacy." This technology lust can cause one to forget that there is a process for selecting a device, a process that involves the consumer in identifying his or her goals, the tasks to be accomplished, and his or her attitude toward technology. The result, if the assessment is conducted appropriately, may be an item of high technology or one of low technology—or, perhaps most important of all, no technology—rather than an alternative method of accomplishing the task.

Therefore, the real focus for rehabilitation practitioners should be on updating skills and information rather than technology. Many of the skill training models that are very effective in teaching human services skills (i.e., counseling, resource management, or advocacy) fall short in teaching skills concerning AT. AT competence clearly requires a hands-on, problem–solution, and trial-and-evaluation approach. Fifield and Fifield (1997) maintained that "skill training takes awareness beyond information and familiarity toward the acquisition of skills and competence necessary to achieve desired outcomes." (p. 78).

The importance of the participation of individuals with disabilities and their caregivers in the service delivery process is recognized by the various amendments to the Rehabilitation Act of 1973 and the Individuals With Disabilities Education Act (1991). However, there is still a lack of effective involvement by individuals with disabilities and their caregivers in the provision of AT devices and services (Galvin, 1997). Several studies of AT users have indicated that such lack of involvement often results in the consumer receiving inappropriate technology (Corthell, 1986; Grady, Kovatch, Lange, & Shannon, 1991; Phillips & Zhao, 1993; Rodgers & Holm, 1992). In a study conducted by Trivelli (1993), in which 1,949 people with disabilities were examined, more than half the respondents (56%) reported not having the AT they needed. This lack of availability can trigger other issues with AT, more specifically, abandonment. If an AT device is abandoned, this can have serious repercussions, from wasted resources to the person's inability to perform at his or her functional best. Nonuse of an AT device may decrease functional abilities, freedom, and independence while increasing monetary expenses for caregivers. On a service delivery level, device abandonment represents an ineffective use of limited funds (Scherer & Galvin, 1996). Reasons for abandonment include

- changes in consumer functional abilities or activities
- lack of consumer motivation to use the device or to do the relevant task
- lack of meaningful training on how to use the device (especially for individuals who are elderly or have cognitive impairments)
- ineffective device performance
- environmental obstacles to use, such as narrow doorways
- lack of access to and information about repairs and maintenance
- minimal or no need for the device
- device aesthetics, weight size, and appearance.

On the basis of these reasons one can assume that technology use is high when it meets the person's own need, he or she believes the technology is useful, he or she believes that he or she is personally capable of learning how to use the device, it increases meaningful experiences, or the risks of failure in learning to use the device are minimal. One can inversely assume that whenever these factors are not present, nonuse will occur.

Family and Caretaker

There are many situations in which family involvement is crucial to the success of the rehabilitation process. Indeed, the Individuals With Disabilities Education Act has given parents a critical role in the development of the child's individualized education plan. For young children with disabilities, AT and play are intricately involved in parents' search for toys that the children can hold or operate. Once such a child goes to school, a completely new range of technologies enters the picture: learning technologies. The emphasis today is on equipping schools with computers. Students are encouraged to use these computers for every facet of learning, from studying basic literacy skills to searching the Internet for up-to-the-minute data. In many cases students with disabilities are using highly sophisticated computer adaptations for access, from word prediction programs, voice input, or output software to refreshable Braille overlays and magnified screens. However, many parents are not as computer literate as their children; as technology in the schools becomes more sophisticated, parents can be left behind.

The Research Institute for Assistive and Training Technologies in Albuquerque, New Mexico, uses a family systems approach to educating consumers (Kroth & Bolson, 1996). It is within this systems approach that pertinent information can be gathered regarding the consumer to facilitate a stable and effective treatment program. The consumer's strengths, struggles, and efforts can then be closely monitored, which in turn may prevent some instances of abandonment. An informed and educated family is a great source of information to service providers. "A comprehensive, consumer-directed approach which takes a long-term view of an individual's assistive device use can improve efficiency and lessen the likelihood of abandonment" (Scherer & Galvin, 1994, p. 129). With potentially limited professional resources to provide individualized assistance, an educated and trained family can then become a valuable resource in the rehabilitation process. Kroth and Bolson (1996) asserted that oftentimes the training of family members and support professionals and caregivers on the intended use of AT devices is disregarded.

Educating the family can also provide an added support to a consumer who may not be totally adjusted to the device. This added support not only will promote continued use of the device, but it may also increase the consumer's usage of, positive attitude toward, and comfort in using the needed device. After all, Langton (1993) considered the most important factors in determining the successful rehabilitation of a consumer to be attitude and motivation. These are pertinent as well concerning the use of AT.

Including the family or using a family systems model of training calls for increased attention to be paid to current education models for AT—they would certainly require more individualized training be done. Although this thought is definitely not new, it is contrary to the typical approach. As Justesen and Menlove (1994) found, "the practice of fitting the consumer to the available services—versus designing and delivering individualized services—is the norm rather than the exception" (p. 253). If improvement in services is to be realized, then accepted practice must evolve into more individualized programs, to the ultimate benefit of consumers.

Caregivers of adults and older disabled people may find that some tasks are made easier with the use of an assistive device. In some circumstances AT may replace assistance provided by individuals. Finding the balance between the facilitation of independence by means of AT devices and the interactions provided by human help is critical to making an appropriate decision.

Social and Cultural Factors

Training practitioners in the appropriate evaluation, selection, and use of AT is in itself a challenging task. Establishing appropriate and usable AT training mechanisms for consumers and caregivers is proving to be very difficult. Providing individualized services to widely diverse groups is never an easy task. Ethnic minority groups in the United States continue to be underserved while they continue to experience the highest rates of health, mental health, social, and economic problems as well as disproportionally high rates of disabling conditions. Numerous barriers to services exist for all ethnic minority groups in the United States, especially for children. Service delivery practitioners must consider language, culture, and other significant barriers in serving any ethnic group, and they must develop specific programs to address these barriers. In some cultures the use of mechanical or electronic AT devices may be viewed very differently from the way they are in the United States. Therefore, service providers need to be aware of the cultural aspects of various groups (i.e., ethnic minorities, people who live in rural areas, and older people) and how one's culture may influence acceptance of disability as well as adaptation to AT. The need to implement effective minority outreach programs is critical: The U.S.

population is projected to be more than 300,000,000 by 2010, with 1 in 3 persons being a member of an ethnic minority (Day, 1996).

African Americans

Data have consistently shown, through census bureau reports and state–federal rehabilitation program statistics, that the population of the United States and of rehabilitation counseling clients is rapidly changing (Davis & Rubin, 1996). Statistics show that currently a disproportionate number of African American adults (14.1%) have some sort of disability as compared to European American adults (8.4%; "Statistical abstract," 1995). Alston and Turner (1994) asserted that African Americans incur disabilities almost twice as frequently as do White Americans.

Hispanic Americans

Statistics appear to be the same for other racial–ethnic minority groups in the United States. It is anticipated that the Hispanic population will soon exceed the African American population and become the largest ethnic minority group in the country, at 38 million people (Day, 1996). People of Hispanic origin make up 11.6% of all people with significant disabilities and 6.5% of working-age people with significant disabilities (U.S. Bureau of the Census, 1993). This information causes concern among rehabilitation professionals who are already well aware of the disproportionate number of ethnic minorities in the United States with disabilities. The most explicit implication of this "demographic destiny" is the urgent requirement to address the specific service needs of these populations.

Native Americans

Today, of 1.9 million American Indians and Alaskan Natives, an estimated 26% live with a significant disability—including about 94,000 with a mobility or self-care limitation (Fowler, 1999).

There are 312 federally recognized Native American tribes or nations in the United States and 500 tribal villages in Alaska. In these, more than 250 native languages are spoken. Forty-six percent of Native Americans live in rural areas. Congenital disabilities or disabling conditions at birth occur for Native Americans at three times the rate of all other births in the United States. They have a far greater rate of babies born with fetal alcohol syndrome and fetal alcohol effects than other ethnic minority groups do. Native Americans have a rate of visual impairment that is three times the rate of the general population in addition to a rate of hearing loss that is four times that of the general population. They often experience extreme poverty, lack of access to health care, high unemployment rates, poor housing, and poor nutrition.

Rural Americans

Approximately 53.3 million Americans reside in rural areas. A higher rate of serious functional limitations exists among rural populations. Approximately 12.5 million of these rural Americans have disabilities, and 6 million have severe disabilities. Living in an isolated rural area with a disability presents many barriers to finding appropriate AT devices and services. The major problems are scarcity of qualified providers and geographic distance from medical specialists in urban centers. Many rural residents do not have access to transportation, and according to a 1998 study by the University of Montana's Rural Institute on Disabilities, poor rural households are less likely than their urban counterparts to own telephones or computers with on-line access ("An update," 1998).

Older Americans

If current trends continue, Americans ages 65 and older will make up 20% of the total population by 2030 (U.S. Bureau of the Census, 1997) Also, the NIDRR (1998) predicted that, by 2010, when the baby boomer generation begins to retire, the demand for AT and related services will be even greater than it is now. It is currently estimated that 80% of elderly people have chronic medical conditions, and about 45% have some form of activity limitation because of such conditions (National Coalition on Aging and Disability, 1995). To maintain independence in their homes, older Americans require an approach that considers the environment as well as task specific assistive devices (Mann, 1997). An essential factor in training consumers and caretakers in appropriate evaluation, selection, and use of AT is finding the optimal mix of AT and personal assistance so that independence can be maintained but human contact is not lost.

Practice Implications

For successful interventions to occur—meaning that if a device is required, the appropriate device is selected, and the device is used by a knowledgeable and satisfied individual—multiple issues and strategies have to be considered in relation to subjective, social, cultural, and lifestyle dynamics. Remember also that some AT devices require a long learning curve before they can be assimilated into an individual's life, making it even more crucial that the person and the technology be appropriately matched. It would be shortsighted to treat the question of device acceptance as if it is independent from the social consequences and individual concerns of the user (LaBuda, 1990). Table 9.1 includes several practical strategies service providers may wish to consider that can facilitate successful outcomes for AT users.

TABLE 9-1
Strategies for Successful Consumer and Caretaker Education

Strategy	Hints for implementation
Never assume anything.	You may know more; you may know less. Unless you ask questions and listen carefully, you will never know.
Treat the individual as a customer.	Show the consumer respect and treat him or her with courtesy.
Understand that families may have to contend with other overwhelming needs.	Selecting an AT device may be only one of myriad concerns the family may be dealing with. Timing is important.
Understand the individual's, family's, and caregiver's experience with technology.	Never assume a level of knowledge or interest in technology. The individual may be knowledgeable and interested, family members might not be, or vice versa.
Understand your own biases when working with someone from a different socioeconomic or cultural group.	Find out all you can about the individual, the immediate and extended family, customs, and culture. Do not make assumptions or generalizations. Be open to learning and providing information and services in a different manner than you are accustomed to.
Develop local community information networks, linkages, and expertise.	Use trusted individuals, who have knowledge of local culture and who speak the language.
Materials need to be developed across the life span, from infants to older Americans. Develop audience-specific materials according to age, educational level, language, culture, and level of technology awareness.	This is more than just simplifying language or translating materials into another language. Make sure you know your audience and what your audience needs before you start.
Develop training mechanisms that can be individualized.	No cookie cutter training—use multiple methods. Develop training modules that vary by method, time, and level.
Develop outreach to remote locations and in community locations, such as Meals on Wheels and senior citizens centers.	Find creative ways to overcome distance. Always look for ways to go "there" rather than have individuals come "here."
Mobilize schools to provide more technology information and support.	Schools have a great need for information and education. Train school staff, and they become part of your expanding network.
Increase on-line options.	Make as much information available as possible on the Internet in accessible formats.

Research and Education Implications

Batavia and Hammer (1990) asserted that the best evaluation of an AT device is whether it satisfies the needs of the disabled consumer. For this satisfaction to happen, the consumer must be involved, the consumer must be educated, and the practitioner must be trained.

Considerable rethinking of curriculum design and of continuing education for much of the allied health care and human services professions is needed to enable the medical, social services, education, and geriatric care systems to respond effectively to the growing AT needs of people with disabilities. The literature contains several suggestions of the means by which to accomplish these goals. For example, Justesen and Menlove (1994) suggested that long-term AT training programs are needed. It would be beneficial if such programs included interdisciplinary experiences with consumers. They also suggested that the Commission on Rehabilitation Education should include AT training for their accredited programs.

Research in AT training needs to maintain a hands-on focus that deeply involves the consumer. Practicum courses in graduate training programs can provide students the opportunity to observe various training methods to find one that is best suited to provide them with a basic knowledge that will be helpful to the consumer. One possible arena to locate such trainings is the Internet. The Web page for the Rehabilitation Engineering and Assistive Technology Society of North America lists the growing number of AT/rehabilitation science graduate education programs (http://www .resna.org). Several videodisc and Internet-based training programs have been used and proved useful in educating professionals. For example, the Center for Persons with Disabilities at Utah State University and California State University—Northridge's Center on Disabilities both cover a wide range of issues relating to AT. It is important to note that any AT training program must include a hands-on, consumer-focused component. This greatly enhances the training and facilitates individualized provision of services.

Outside of curriculum-based instruction and practicum experiences there are many resources through which training in AT can be achieved. Professional organization affiliation is one example. Most organizations provide regular training opportunities that may include education in AT. The Rehabilitation Engineering and Assistive Technology Society of North America has developed a credentialing process for practitioners and suppliers. In addition, all states have received grants for Title I of the Technology Related Assistance for Individiuals with Disabilities Act. These state programs have the responsibility of increasing awareness of AT and providing training or technical assistance for professionals who provide services to people with disabilities. Many of these states have developed excellent AT training materials for professionals and consumers.

There are many excellent resources available on the Internet that may assist professionals and consumers in their search for AT devices and services. This information goes far beyond listings of devices to specific information for families with young children and families with aging parents, information that is disability specific, and information on issues such as relevant legislation and funding. One of the most interesting aspects of accessing Web resources is that an individual with a disability can find peers with whom he or she can discuss AT needs and find out more about selected devices.

Regardless of the method by which one attains knowledge, one thing is certain: A number of changes need to take place, facilitated by policymakers, payers, service providers, and consumers. Policymakers need to ensure that laws and subsequent regulations appreciate the unique needs of individuals with disabilities and provide for sufficient funding for training of service providers and consumers. Third-party payers need to understand the long-term implications of inappropriate AT selection and use and be prepared to pay for individualized training of consumers and caretakers. Service providers need to be educated about and trained on the appropriate selection and use of AT and work with funding sources to ensure culturally appropriate outreach to underserved communities and individuals. They also need to be trained to work with consumers to determine their readiness to be equal partners in the process.

Consumers and caretakers need training as well. Consumers need to be committed to the process of selecting and using AT, aware of their own needs, and be prepared to take an active role in evaluating their needs and the available technologies. This may include training family members to help them make informed decisions.

Finally, services must be individualized. The cookie cutter mentality must be abandoned if effective and appropriate individualized services are to be provided. When these matters are considered and acted on, the potential end result is enhanced, yielding successful rehabilitation interventions and outcomes.

REFERENCES

Alston, R., & Turner, W. (1994). A family strengths model of adjustment to disability for African American clients. *Journal of Counseling and Development, 72,* 378–383.

Americans With Disabilities Act of 1990, Pub. L. No. 101-336.

An update on the demography of rural disability. (1998). University of Montana, Rural Institute on Disabilities. Retrieved from http://ruralinstitute@umt.edu/rtcrural.

Batavia, A. I., & Hammer, G. S. (1990). Toward the development of consumer-based criteria for the evaluation of assistive devices. *Journal of Rehabilitation Research and Development, 27,* 425–436.

Bellamy, G. T., Newton, J. B., LeBaron, N., & Horner, R. H. (1992). Quality of life and lifestyle outcomes: A challenge for residential programs. In R. L. Schalock (Ed.), *Quality of life: Perspectives and issues* (pp. 123–144). Washington, DC: American Association on Mental Retardation.

Bickenbach, J. E. (1999). *ICIDH–2* and the role of environmental factors in the creation of disability. In C. Buhler & H. Knops (Eds.), *Assistive technology on the threshold of the new millennium* (pp. 7–12). Amsterdam: IOS Press.

Brandt, E. N., & Pope. A. M. (Eds.). (1997). Enabling America: Assessing the role of rehabilitation science and engineering. Committee on Assessing Rehabilitation Science and Engineering, Division of Health Sciences and Policy, Institute of Medicine (pp. 217–243). Washington, DC: National Academy Press.

Corthell, D. W. (1986). *Thirteenth institute on rehabilitation issues: Rehabilitation technologies.* Menomonie, WI: University of Wisconsin—Stout Research and Training Center.

Davis, E. L., & Rubin, S. E. (1996). Multicultural instructional goals and strategies for rehabilitation counselor education. *Rehabilitation Education, 10,* 105–114.

Day, J. C. (1996). Population projections of the United States by age, sex, race, and Hispanic origin: 1995–2050. In U.S. Bureau of the Census, *Current population reports* (pp. 25–1130). Washington, DC: U.S. Government Printing Office.

Fifield, M. G., & Fifield, M. B. (1997). Educating and training of individuals involved in delivery of assistive technology devices. *Technology and Disability, 6,* 77–88.

Fowler, L. (1999). *American Indian elders and people with disabilities: Common threads.* American Indian Disability Legislation Project, University of Montana, Rural Institute on Disabilities.

Galvin J. C. (1997). Consumerism and outreach to underrepresented populations. *Technology and Disability, 6,* 49–61.

Goodman, S. (1999, June). What does this have to do with assistive technology? Assistive Technology Funding and Systems Change Project [On-line]. Available: http://www.ucpa.org/html/innovative/atfsc/whatat.html

Grady, A., Kovatch, T., Lange, M., & Shannon, L. (1991). Promoting choice in selection of assistive technology devices. *Proceedings of the Sixth Annual Conference on Technology and Persons With Disabilities* (pp. 315–322). Los Angeles, CA: California State University, Northridge.

Individuals With Disabilities Education Act of 1991, Pub. L. No. 101-476.

Jaskulski, T., Metzler, C., & Zierman, S. A. (1990). *The 1990 reports: Forging a new era.* Washington, DC: National Association of Developmental Disabilities Councils.

Justesen, T. R., & Menlove, M. (1994). Assistive technology education in rehabilitation counseling programs. *Rehabilitation Education, 7*, 253–260.

Kroth, R. L., & Bolson, M. D. (1996). Family involvement with assistive technology. *Contemporary Education, 68*, 17–20.

LaBuda, D. (1990). The impact of technology on geriatric rehabilitation. In B. Kemp, K. Brummel-Smith, & J. Ramsdell (Eds.), Geriatric rehabilitation (pp. 57–72). Boston: College Hill Press.

Langton, A. J. (1993). Making more effective use of assistive technology in the vocational evaluation process. *Vocational Evaluation and Work Adjustment Bulletin, 26*(1), 13–19.

Mann, W. (1997). Aging and assistive technology use. *Technology and Disability, 6*, 63–75.

Matson, J. L., & Rusch, F. R. (1986). Quality of life: Does competitive employment make a difference? In F. R. Rusch (Ed.), *Competitive employment issues and strategies* (pp. 311–337). Baltimore, MD: Paul H. Brookes.

Mueller, J. (1989). Technology: Training awareness and needs. In L. G. Perlman & C. E. Hanson (Eds.), *Technology and employment of people with disabilities* (pp. 32–37). Alexandria, VA: National Rehabilitation Association.

National Coalition on Aging and Disability. (1995, March). National Summit on Aging and Disability. Washington, DC: Author.

National Council on Disability. (1996, July 26). Achieving Independence: The Challenge for the 21st Century, 15. Washington, DC: Author.

National Institute on Disability and Rehabilitation Research. (1998). *Blueprint for the Millennium: An analysis of regional hearings on assistive technology for people with disabilities*. Washington, DC: U.S. Department of Education.

Phillips, B., & Zhao, H. (1993). Predictors of assistive technology abandonment. *Assistive Technology, 5*, 36–45.

Rehabilitation Act Amendments of 1973, Pub. L. No. 99-506.

Rodgers, J., & Holm, M. (1992). Assistive technology device use in patients with rheumatic disease: A literature review. *American Journal of Occupational Therapy, 46*, 120–127.

Scherer, M. J., & Galvin, J. C. (1996). An outcomes perspective of quality pathways to most appropriate technology. In J. C. Galvin & M. J. Scherer (Eds.), *Evaluating, selecting, and using appropriate assistive technology* (pp. 1–25). Gaithersburg, MD: Aspen.

Scherer, M. J., & Galvin, J. C. (1994). Matching people with technology. *Rehabilitation Management, 7*, 128–130.

Schriner, K. F., & Batavia, A. (1995). Disability law and social policy. In E. dell Orto & R. P. Marinelli (Eds.), *Encyclopedia of disability and rehabilitation* (pp. 260–270). New York: Macmillan.

Silverstein, R. (2000). Emerging disability policy framework: A guidepost for analyzing public policy. *Iowa Law Review, 85*, 1691–1751.

Somerville, N. J., Wilson, D. J., & Shanfield, K. S. (1989). Identifying the technology training needs of occupational therapists. In *Proceedings of the 12th Annual RESNA Conference.* Washington, DC: RESNA.

Technology-Related Assistance for Individuals with Disabilities Act of 1988, Pub. L. No. 100-407.

Trivelli, L. (1993). 1991 Consumers and technology survey: The results are in! *AT Quarterly, 3,* 10–11.

U.S. Bureau of the Census. (1993). Poverty in the United States: 1992. In *Current Population Reports* (Series P60-185, pp. 91–96). Washington, DC: U.S. Government Printing Office.

U. S. Bureau of the Census. Statistical abstract of the United States: No. 12. Resident population characteristics—Percent distribution [On-line]. (1995). Available: http://www.medaccess.com/census/census_s.htm. Washington, DC: Author.

U.S. Bureau of the Census. (1997). Disabilities affect one fifth of all Americans (Report No. CENBR/97-5). Washington, DC: U.S. Government Printing Office.

Williams, B. (1995). Assistive technology: Building a national commitment to liberation. *Impact: Institute on Community Integration Newsletter, 8*(1), 1–22.

World Health Organization. (2001). *International classification of function, disability and health* (prefinal draft). Geneva, Switzerland: Author.

10

ENHANCING THE APPROPRIATE USE OF ASSISTIVE TECHNOLOGY AMONG CONSUMERS AND CARETAKERS

DENISE G. TATE, BARTH RILEY, AND MARTIN FORCHHEIMER

Since the early 1980s there has been an explosion in the number and types of medical, assistive, and learning technologies developed to help people with physical and cognitive limitations related to illness and disability. Accompanying the increased availability of these technologies has been a steadily growing concern about the their appropriate use by consumers. Whereas prosthetic devices, such as artificial limbs, replace or substitute a part of the body, assistive technologies (ATs) or assistive devices (ADs) are tools designed to enhance the independent functioning of people who have physical limitations or disabilities. An AT device, as defined by the Technology-Related Assistance for Individuals With Disabilities Act of 1988 (P.L. 100-497), refers to any item, piece of equipment, or product system, whether acquired commercially off the shelf, modified, or customized, that is used to increase, maintain, or improve functional capabilities of individuals with disabilities.

Such tools vary widely depending on the type of functional impairment they are designed to address. More common devices include wheelchairs, canes, walkers, and hearing and optical aids, whereas less common (and often considered more technologically advanced) devices include electronic communicators, teletype phones for people who are deaf or hearing impaired, speech processors, and computer-controlled environments.

Recent technological advancements have contributed to the promise of ADs in enhancing the functional independence of individuals with disabilities. In fact, the positive effects of various types of ADs on improving functional independence and quality of life has virtually been taken for granted (Scherer, 1988). Yet not all individuals with physical limitations decide to use ADs, and others who initially accept a device may later abandon it.

We have designed this chapter to help rehabilitation psychologists and other health care professionals who work with people with disabilities gain knowledge about key issues regarding the use of AT by consumers. Our main objective is to provide an understanding of the underlying reasons why people with disabilities may choose to accept or reject—use or abandon—AT. We also discuss the need for educating health professionals, caregivers, families, and consumers themselves about the appropriate use of AT and how to enhance such use. In doing so, we have focused on the cultural, social, and psychological reasons associated with the nonuse of AT. Last, implications for the advancement of science and research in this area are described. Information provided here is complementary to that discussed in chapter 9 regarding the appropriate selection and use of AT.

FACTORS ASSOCIATED WITH THE NONUSE OF AT

AT includes devices that are technologically complex, involving sophisticated materials and requiring precise operations—often referred to as "high tech"—and those that are simple, inexpensive, and made from easily available materials, commonly referred to as "low tech." Low-tech devices, for example, are often used by older people with disabilities to compensate for age-related functional losses.

On the other hand, discarding or not using AT devices may be the result of a variety of factors (Gray, Quatrano, & Lieberman, 1998). Some people with disabilities feel stigmatized if they are seen using AT devices. As one polio survivor put it, "it signals that I am broken to others and I just can't do it" (Tate, 1999). Sense of self and the role of AT in life are key considerations in developing rehabilitation plans that address physical and psychological needs. The functional limitations that each person perceives as essential need to be addressed and prioritized, taking into consideration the person's social and cultural environment as well as his or her psychological and emotional needs for comfort, acceptance, self-dignity, and self-respect.

Stiens (1998) addressed the importance of integrating the use of mobility devices into the lives of people with mobility impairments in the context of their self-concepts. Adjustment can be difficult for those who are injured or have a condition that impairs their mobility after they have developed skills, expectations, and relationships. Stiens recommended that rehabilitation goals and programs focus on these issues if they are to become successful in promoting adjustment, community reintegration, and enhanced overall quality of life. Often psychologists play a role in assessing a person's history, current capabilities, and plans for future activities. This information can give the rehabilitation team useful insight as the team members develop suggestions for appropriate AT. The aesthetic and functional aspects of AT devices are of primary importance in making choices that will result in a person returning to effective interactive relationships with the environment.

Brooks (1998) proposed that acceptance or rejection of AT is influenced by the understanding of disability by one's culture. The challenge for rehabilitation professionals is to incorporate AT into their existing conceptual models of disability and to provide their clients with the current information on AT that meets their specific needs (Gray et al., 1998). Many of these models of disability (such as the Institute of Medicine's model and the *International Classification of Functioning, Disability, and Health;* World Health Organization, 2001) currently encompass the concept of AT because they focus on environmental accessibility, which can readily be addressed with AT. According to these models, *technology* has been defined as the system by which a society provides its members with developments from science that have practical use in everyday life (National Institute on Disability and Rehabilitation Research [NIDRR], 1998).

Yet the meaning of devices in terms of how they affect self-concept may be of more importance than the devices' intrinsic capabilities, in terms of whether they will be accepted and incorporated into the lives of the people for whom they are prescribed, and how much benefit the people will obtain from such devices, assuming that they do derive some benefit. Spencer (1998) postulated three fundamental elements of understanding the role of AT in the lives of people with disabilities. First, AT devices are tools that are given meaning by the intentions that individuals have for their use, both personally and in the context of their culture. Second, adapting to the use of AT requires building new skills, developing positive emotional responses to the devices, modifying one's self-perception of AT use, and including the use of AT in daily life activities. Third, changes in life circumstances may require a flexible, individualized approach to considering the selection of AT. Although using a generic approach may appear attractive, practical, and cost effective for rehabilitation professionals and providers, this approach runs the risk of providing the wrong AT at the wrong time to the wrong person. Personal dynamics, including issues of functionality and psychological adjustment, must be considered first.

Vash (1993) believed that the pivotal issue determining whether an AT is used is "the degree to which the device promotes accomplishment of life tasks that the consumer sees as important" (p. 43). As Vash suggested, before AT use can enhance a person's quality of life there must be a social climate that values enhanced capability and a psychological readiness for use of technology on the part of the individual with a disability.

Self-concept, motivation, and personal aspirations may be shaped by social interactions that influence positive personal regard, resources, and opportunities. One's willingness to use or accept the use of AT is directly related to these personal concepts and external influences, which then serve to reinforce or diminish these self-perceptions. Thus, accepting the use of AT symbolizes acceptance of one's limitations and being ready to move beyond them. This concept is applicable to all people with disabilities but is especially salient for older adults. Older adults with disabilities often have difficulty incorporating AT use into their standard behavioral repertoire, because they need to adjust to their new limitations emotionally, physically, and socially.

An example highlighting this adjustment issue comes from work by Creange and Bruno (1997) about the effect of personal, family, and social self-concept on compliance with treatment by postpolio survivors (PPSs). Creange and Bruno concluded that treatment noncompliance is related to polio survivors' excessive Type A behavior as well as their heightened sensitivity to criticism by others and their belief that they must not appear to be "disabled." This conclusion is supported by a previous finding of abnormally elevated "sensitivity to criticism and failure" scores among post-polio survivors discharged from hospitals for noncompliance and the 1985 National Postpolio Survey, which found that embarrassment about having a disability was significantly correlated with refusal to use ADs (Bruno & Frick, 1990).

In a review of 11 studies concerning the frequency of AT use among older people with disabilities, Gitlin, Levine, and Geigger (1993) reported that the frequency of AD use ranged from 35% to 82%, with research participants owning an average of 6.8 ADs. Gitlin (1995) examined factors predictive of AT use following hospital discharge among elderly people. In her study, AT use in the home was examined during Months 1, 2, and 3 after hospital discharge. During the first month, AT use was highest among individuals who during hospitalization had a positive orientation regarding AT use and who expected to use the AT on returning home. AT use during the first month postdischarge was the best predictor of AT use during the second month. In the third month, AT use was best predicted by AT use in the second month in combination with the type of impairment experienced.

Gitlin's (1995) research showed that individuals with limb amputation tended to use their devices more than those with orthopedic or cardiovascular conditions. Stroke patients (usually elderly people) were found to have highly negative views of both their disability and the use of ADs. This study highlights the effect of individual factors, such as attitudinal factors and disability-related characteristics, in predicting device use. Individuals with disabilities may view AT as either a tool to increase independence or as a symbol of lost function or ability. Yet to ascribe these varying perceptions of AT solely to the individual would overlook the presence of these opposing values within the culture at large. Nowhere is this more evident than in the area of wheelchair use. Whereas Campbell and Ross (1990) concluded that wheelchairs are merely "a practical solution to a practical problem" (p. 23), negative attitudes toward wheelchairs and wheelchair users among nondisabled people have been well documented (Fewster, 1990; Fichten & Ansel, 1988; Fichten, Robillard, Tagalakis, & Ansel, 1991; Phillips, 1990; Wright, 1983). Interactions of nondisabled individuals with wheelchair users have been characterized by brevity and excessive physical distancing (Dawson, 1990; Fichten & Ansel, 1988; Hastorf, Wildfogel, & Cassman, 1979; Kleck, 1968).

Negative views concerning wheelchairs and their owners are not limited to nondisabled people. Research in this area suggests that whereas people with mild disabilities view wheelchairs as a temporary solution to a temporary problem, like nondisabled people, people with more severe and chronic disabilities held the most negative attitudes toward wheelchairs (Campbell & Ross, 1990). Similarly, Fichten et al. (1991) found that wheelchair users preferred the company of nondisabled individuals to that of other wheelchair users. Hence, rather than viewing their wheelchair as a tool to foster independence, people with chronic disabilities appear to adopt the negative views of the larger culture concerning wheelchair use, viewing them as symbols of disability, weakness, and personal failure (Bates, Spencer, Young, & Rintala, 1993).

The double-edged nature of AT as both tool and symbol of disability has important ramifications for the education of individuals with disabilities in the use of ADs. This perspective may help to explain why people with disabilities often accept but later abandon the use of ADs, as Gitlin (1995) described. Chapter 9 provides readers with a comprehensive list of reasons for AD abandonment. Whereas people with disabilities may have mixed or ambivalent feelings concerning AT, rehabilitation professionals, in their desire to help the consumer increase functional independence, may place a primary focus on ADs as solutions to various functional limitations. This disparity in the perceptions of consumers and clinicians can result in arguments and conflicts during the selection process and training of consumers in the use of ADs.

Scherer (1993) observed that many people with disabilities feel that ADs are forced on them, either by rehabilitation professionals or by family members. It is not uncommon for consumers to feel left out of the selection or decision-making process and, therefore, be less likely to comply with AD use. A more detailed discussion of this issue is provided in chapter 9, in which Galvin and Donnell point out that consumers often have little or no leverage to participate in the decisions made about the services or disability benefits (i.e., AT) they will receive. Feeling powerless about their lives creates an enormous sense of personal alienation, disinterest, and lack of personal commitment on the part of consumers.

Bates et al. (1993) provided a case summary that aptly illustrates the conflicts and difficulties inherent in educating consumers, caretakers, and team members about AD use. The consumer was a 30-year-old White man with acquired paraplegia undergoing acute rehabilitation. His initial goal for rehabilitation was to be able to use a wheelchair and return home. Early in rehabilitation, the patient was fitted with a high-back reclining chair. The occupational therapist prescribed a sitting schedule for the patient to increase his ability to tolerate the chair. Once he could sit in the chair at a 90-degree angle, the patient would be given a one-arm driving chair that he could propel. As rehabilitation progressed, however, the patient became increasingly frustrated and noncompliant with the sitting schedule. At times, he would make comments to the effect that he would not want to be "stuck in that chair" or that he would prefer death to being "crippled" (p. 1017). In this case, this patient felt powerless and disrespected and misunderstood by the rehabilitation professionals. Unfortunately, his feelings of frustration and noncompliance were interpreted by rehabilitation professionals as a covert prejudice toward the wheelchair and a reluctance to accept the need for one.

Disparities in communication and differences of opinion can be extremely detrimental to patient care. Advocating for patients' needs while respecting both their perspective and that of experienced professionals in rehabilitation is a delicate task. Psychologists, social workers, and other team members can facilitate this process by serving as good listeners and skillful translators between the patient and the team. Simply acknowledging the patient's needs and wishes is half of the task required for success.

ROLE OF THE REHABILITATION PSYCHOLOGIST

As Bates et al. (1993) concluded, rehabilitation professionals involved in the education of consumers in AT use, including occupational therapists, mobility instructors, and rehabilitation engineers, need to be aware that acceptance and use of ADs involve a process requiring considerable time for emotional adjustment. The process often involves a cognitive and emotional reorganization of one's life to accommodate the device. By nature of their training, psychologists are well equipped to help people with disabilities with this accommodation process. As the case described in the previous section illustrates, ambivalent feelings toward ADs can seemingly hinder or even stop the rehabilitation process, yet one should keep in mind that what rehabilitation professionals observe is only the initial pragmatic adaptation to ADs; emotional adaptation to ADs most likely will occur well after the consumer's discharge from acute or even subacute rehabilitation settings.

Even well after the initial, extreme emotional reactions to an AD have passed, it is likely that people with disabilities will continue to experience occasional negative emotions in response to their use of these aids, particularly when confronted by the prejudicial attitudes or behaviors of others. It is important for rehabilitation professionals to be aware of and sensitive to the intense negative and threatening emotional reactions people with disabilities may experience when first introduced to ADs. In light of these intense and often ambivalent feelings, the rehabilitation psychologist needs to continually monitor the extent to which the activities subsumed within rehabilitation are meaningful to the consumer. When reluctance or resistance to AD are observed, it may be necessary to stop the more pragmatic elements of AD training to talk with the consumer about his or her feelings regarding device use and whether the use of the device is consistent with his or her personal goals.

It is also important that the rehabilitation psychologist be flexible during the process of educating the consumer in the use of an AD. It may at times be appropriate to suspend training activities to allow the consumer to consider various AD alternatives. This step will provide the consumer with a greater sense of control over his or her life, body, and autonomy and will help minimize friction between clinicians and the consumer. In addition to flexibility, it is important that professionals who work with consumers of ADs be familiar and comfortable with a wide variety of products and product manufacturers to avoid imposing arbitrary limits on the consumers' device choices. It is desirable for the professional to take a "back seat" approach when the consumer is considering various device alternatives. In this respect, Post (1993) recommended a "consumerism" approach, in which people with disabilities are first given access to information sources, such as the ABLEDATA computer database, allowing them to make informed and independent AD choices.

Highlighting the positive contributions of using AD while downplaying issues of physical limitations and body image are also key to educating consumers and caregivers. Exploring the latter issues with an open mind may help consumers and their families adjust to these personal losses. In addition, feeling at ease with an AD and making it part of one's daily routine are important factors in compliance with AD use. Getting used to physical dependence on AD use can help a person build a new self-image and self-concept that include ADs as part of the self. Psychologists' role is to help people with disabilities minimize negative emotions such as shame and guilt and begin developing new self-identities based on acceptance. This process of personal growth involves accepting one's limitations and finding ways to effectively compensate for them in a positive manner, such as through the use of AT to enhance functional or cognitive independence and control.

Scherer and Cushman (1995) explained that patients and therapists often have different expectations and views of the benefits of AT. These differences need to be reconciled before progress can be made. Sensitivities experienced by consumers of rehabilitation services need to be clearly communicated to the various people intimately involved in the health care and personal lives of those for whom AT is being prescribed, including clinical members, insurers, family members and caregivers, employers, and educators. Educated family members and caregivers can facilitate personal acceptance and the development of positive self-esteem in people with disabilities. Vash (1981) advised rehabilitation counselors that each individual will react differently to this adjustment and that coping with AT may result in occasional anxiety about being seen as "different," appearing "freaky" or comical. Interactions with others may become difficult or avoided because of these fears. Asking for help if AT fails or breaks down is also another common problem for people with disabilities and their families. These fears are heightened by continued feelings of guilt or shame about having physical limitations.

Demonstrating personal assertiveness is difficult for people who have low self-esteem and concerns about their body image, as is the case for many people who use AT. The use of peers as role models can facilitate the adjustment process, reassuring consumers of their abilities and rights and providing information that is key to learning how to best use ADs to address personal needs.

It is also important that caregivers and family members are patient and demonstrate respect for feelings of guilt, low self-esteem, and ambiguity about the value of AT. Often family members tend to think that AT will enhance function and result in a stronger self-image for the person with a disability, yet they need to understand the true feelings, fears, and concerns of the disabled family member regarding AT. Both empathy and patience are key in this process.

For all involved, getting to know the consumer provides direction in determining how AT will be used to establish or re-establish life's balance. First, focusing efforts on the needs and problems that will affect life activities will help with the appropriate choice of AT and will enhance compliance. Second, facilitating empowerment and feelings of personal control by AT users will restore their sense of dignity, facilitating acceptance, self-efficacy, and compliance.

EDUCATING THE CONSUMER

As Post (1993) explained, "we should approach the provision of [AT] goods and services by examining how we can empower persons with disabilities to seek out and acquire the technology they need independently" (p. 1046). The process of buying AT devices differs markedly from how other material objects are normally purchased. There are many differences; they include the setting in which AT purchases are made, the attitudes and expectations of the professionals and consumers involved, and the manner in which the AT device is paid for. As Post (1993) emphasized, "everyone plays a role in perpetuating this model, and everyone can introduce a change." (p. 35). The consumer will need training, support, or assistance, and therapists and caregivers must be comfortable sharing or passing along responsibilities or risk fostering continued dependence.

The extent to which consumers receive useful information concerning AT devices as well as effective training in their use depends on several factors. Obtaining a thorough and accurate assessment of the individual's goals, needs, and capabilities (both strengths and weaknesses) is crucial. According to Scherer (1993), practitioners who work with AT consumers need to mutually and jointly assess the short-term, intermediate, and long-term goals of the consumer. Asking questions such as "What would you like your life to be like 1 and 5 years from now?" may elicit useful information as to whether and what type of AD will be most appropriate for the person. It is also important during the assessment process to differentiate between the needs of the consumer and what others think he or she will need.

Family members, for instance, may have their own ideas concerning what types of AD would be most helpful to the consumer, ideas that may or may not be consistent with the consumer's goals or needs. Psychologists can help consumers and their families by enhancing and clarifying this communication and promoting a healthy dialogue.

Once the need for AD has been established, the rehabilitation practitioner, with the consumer's input and consent, should establish a plan for AD training, outlining the goals of training as well as the specific activities involved in reaching those goals. This plan of action is created with the mutual understanding that the goals and steps involved in AD training can at any time be reviewed and reconsidered by the consumer or end user. Once an AD has been introduced to a consumer, it is important to provide adequate time, not only for the individual to learn how to use the device but also for family members to feel comfortable with the use and become supportive to the consumer. Scherer (1993) recommended providing repeat or follow-up visits for the consumer to give the device a "dry run" in his or her own environment. Moreover, informing the consumer that an immediate decision concerning selection of a device is not necessary, even after training begins, helps to alleviate feelings of anxiety.

AD training should be divided into a series of sessions, and each session should address a particular feature or aspect of operating the device. This is particularly true with more complicated devices, for which multiple steps or tasks are involved in operating the device, or when the device can be used in a variety of different situations. Each session should build on the tasks or skills acquired in previous training sessions and should end on a successful note to build the consumer's confidence in using the device.

A final comment should be made with respect to significant others (SOs) learning about the use of AD. As mentioned previously, SOs may carry ideas concerning the types of devices that would be most helpful to the person with a disability. Underlying the SO's attempt to direct the consumer toward a particular AD is the notion that the device will result in the consumer returning to fully independent functioning. This expectation, although well intentioned, can cause the consumer to make device choices that are not consistent with his or her goals or, worse, lead to unrealistic expectations and a sense of failure regarding functional recovery. It is important that practitioners educate both consumers and their family members or SOs about what the AD will enable the person with a disability to do, and in what situations. Limitations and benefits should be equally discussed as to provide a realistic view of the potential of the AD to enhance one's quality of life.

IMPLICATIONS FOR FUTURE RESEARCH

Scientific research has generated information that has enhanced greatly the lives of people with disabilities. However, little is currently known about the concerns, perceptions, and beliefs of people with disabilities regarding AT use. Much of the available literature lends support to a model of matching person and technology that considers environments of device use, characteristics of the user's preferences and expectations, and devices' features and functions. To ensure that AT enhances users' quality of life, future research will need to focus on consumer involvement in the selection and evaluation of appropriate AT and ways to make technologies more widely available and affordable (Scherer, 1997).

The complex processes involved in determining whether an AD is justified and what type of device will enhance which function are matters that need to be addressed by the research community in the very near future. Even now, health insurance companies have begun to restrict the purchase of AT in their zeal to streamline reimbursements and reduce costs. Empirical findings are needed to discriminate ADs that can facilitate enhanced functional independence and well-being from those that have little or no influence on the lives of disabled people (Spiegle & Abdelhamied, 1998).

Tate et al. (1994) investigated this issue when examining the effects of insurance benefits coverage on independent-living outcomes of 198 people with spinal cord injuries. In their study AT included environmental control units, computers, and intercom systems. Other benefits included durable equipment, such as wheelchairs, hospital beds, lifts, and rolling shower chairs. Results showed that sources of insurance sponsorship significantly differentiated subjects for both AT and other durable equipment along two dimensions: what was received versus what was perceived as needed by the consumer. Consumers with catastrophic insurance received three times as many ATs as did those whose primary insurance was Medicaid. Those with private, noncatastrophic insurance stated that they had the fewest unmet needs, followed by those with catastrophic insurance. Individuals with Medicaid had by far the most unmet needs. Satisfaction with life was similarly directly associated with the number of AT needs experienced and the number of unmet needs. Unlike with AT, unmet needs for durable equipment were not associated with life satisfaction.

The role of AT in promoting a sense of personal empowerment and greater self-reliance should be investigated further, because it has the potential to affect treatment outcomes significantly. Personal satisfaction may prove key to AT use and compliance, for example.

Research into the psychological factors that explain an individual's experience of disability may prove itself of unquestionable value in educating and training professionals and caretakers who work with disabled people. Furthermore, the social environment has a profound influence on how people with disabilities interpret their experiences. The ways in which rehabilitation professionals and caregivers or family members define their experience with disability have potent environmental influence on people with disabilities (Scherer, 1993). Research focusing on the interactions of the person–environment exchanges and resultant outcomes can help rehabilitation professionals to better understand the role of AT in the lives of people with disabilities and, therefore, promote and enhance its appropriate use.

Future research agendas by federal agencies sponsoring rehabilitation-related studies, including those focusing on technology and AT, should incorporate several cross-cutting issues, including the problem of small markets and the need for reliable outcome measures. Both the NIDRR and the National Center for Medical Rehabilitation Research at the National Institutes of Health have focused their research agendas on a number of AT-related topics, including biomedical engineering innovation; AT that promotes independence, function, and employment outcomes; and technologies that enhance mobility and cognitive function and promote better access to the built environment (Alexander, 2000; Seelman, 1999). See chapter 9 for a more detailed description of NIDRR's plan.

Most important, research on AT must result in useful knowledge for consumers: It must benefit the consumer. Such benefit may be in the form of long-term cost savings, enhanced quality of life, and consumer satisfaction. In addition, rehabilitation engineers must develop products that are safe, durable, marketable, and affordable. A similar perspective is offered by Galvin and Donnell's description of research and education implications in chapter 9. As in any product development line, the design and development of AT require the direct input of consumers or users of AT (Tate, 2000). According to Glaser and Taylor (1973), researchers who actively solicited input from consumers during the early stages of product development were most successful in creating a useful product.

Last, the larger gap between knowing what works in AT and finding evidence-based interventions suggests a need for AT interventions that are easily applied to routine settings and for research on how to introduce these findings into practice and service settings for rapid adoption. Both research and education can play important roles in answering questions about the efficacy and effectiveness of AT interventions and, thus, pave the way to more advanced scientific developments in this area.

REFERENCES

Alexander, D. (2000). *Director's report: National Advisory Child Health and Human Development Council*. Washington, DC: National Institute of Child Health and Human Development.

Bates, P. S., Spencer, J. C., Young, M. E., & Rintala, D. H. (1993). Assistive technology and the newly disabled adult: Adaptation to wheelchair use. *American Journal of Occupational Therapy, 47*, 1014–1021.

Brooks, N. A. (1998). Concepts, classifications, and categories of disabling conditions and assistive technologies. In D. B. Gray, L. A. Quatrano, & M. L. Lieberman (Eds.), *Designing and using assistive technology: The human perspective* (pp. 810–832). New York: Paul Brookes.

Bruno, R. L., & Frick, N. M. (1990). Psychologic profile of polio survivors. *Archives of Physical Medicine and Rehabilitation, 71*, 889.

Campbell, F., & Ross, F. (1990, October). Disability: Dealing with wheels. *Community Outlook*, 23–26.

Creange, S. J., & Bruno, R. L. (1997). Compliance for postpolio sequelae: Effect of Type A behavior, self-concept, and loneliness. *American Journal of Physical Medicine and Rehabilitation, 76*, 378–382.

Dawson, W. (1990). Spinal cord injury: A view from behind the wheel. *North Carolina Medical Journal, 58*, 397–399.

Fewster, C. (1990). Wheelchair apartheid. *Nursing Times, 86*(3), 49–51.

Fichten, C. S., & Ansel, R. (1988). Trait attributions about college students with a physical disability: Complex analyses and methodological issues. *Journal of Applied Social Psychology, 16*, 410–427.

Fichten, C. S., Robillard, K., Tagalakis, V., & Ansel, R. (1991). Casual interactions between college students with various disabilities and their nondisabled peers: The internal dialogue. *Rehabilitation Psychology, 36,* 3–20.

Gitlin, L. N. (1995). Why older people accept or reject assistive technology. *Journal of the American Society on Aging, 19,* 54–62.

Gitlin, L., Levine, R., & Geigger, C. (1993). Adaptive device use by older adults with mixed disabilities. *Archives of Physical Medicine and Rehabilitation, 74,* 149–152.

Glaser, E. M., & Taylor, S. H. (1973). Factors influencing the success of applied research. *American Psychologist, 28,* 140–146.

Gray, D. B., Quatrano, L. A., & Lieberman, M. L. (1998). *Designing and using assistive technology: The human perspective.* New York: Paul Brookes.

Hastorf, A., Wildfogel, J., & Cassman, T. (1979). Acknowledgement of handicap as a tactic in social interaction. *Journal of Personality and Social Psychology, 37,* 1790–1797.

Kleck, R. (1968). Physical stigma and nonverbal cues emitted in face-to-face interaction. *Human Relations, 21,* 19–28.

National Institute on Disability and Rehabilitation Research. (1998, October 26). Notice of proposed long-range plan for fiscal years 1999–2004. *Federal Register,* Part 5, 49–58.

Phillips, M. J. (1990). Damaged goods: Oral narrative of the experience of disability in American culture. *Social Science and Medicine, 30,* 849–857.

Post, K. M. (1993). Educating consumers about assistive technology. *American Journal of Occupational Therapy, 47,* 1046–1047.

Scherer, M. (1988). Assistive device utilization and quality of life in adults with spinal cord injuries or cerebral palsy. *Journal of Applied Rehabilitation Counseling, 19*(2), 21–30.

Scherer, M. (1993). *Living in the state of stuck: How technology affects the lives of people with disabilities.* Cambridge, MA: Brookline Books.

Scherer, M. J. (1997). Consumer subjective well-being and use of personal assistance and manual wheelchairs. *Archives of Physical Medicine and Rehabilitation, 78,* 909.

Scherer, M. J., & Cushman, L. A. (1995). Differing therapist–patient views of assistive technology use and implications for patient education and training. *Archives of Physical Medicine and Rehabilitation, 76,* 595.

Seelman, K. D. (1999). *The National Institute on Disability and Rehabilitation Research (NIDRR) long range plan: 1999–2003.* Washington, DC: Office of Special Education and Rehabilitative Services, U.S. Department of Education.

Spencer, J. C. (1998). When assistive technology is used and when it is not. In D. B. Gray, L. A. Quatrano, & M. L. Lieberman (Eds.), *Designing and using assistive technology: The human perspective* (pp. 975–1003). New York: Paul Brookes.

Spiegle, S., & Abdelhamied, A. (1998). Selecting, designing, and developing assistive technology for use by people with disabilities. In D. B. Gray, L. A. Quatrano,

& M. L. Lieberman (Eds.), *Designing and using assistive technology: The human perspective* (pp. 1010–1025). New York: Paul Brookes.

Stiens, S. S. (1998). Concepts, classifications, and categories of disabling conditions and assistive technologies. In D. B. Gray, L. A. Quatrano, & M. L. Lieberman (Eds.), *Designing and using assistive technology: The human perspective* (pp. 810–832). New York: Paul Brookes.

Tate, D. G. (1999). *Personal communication.* Unpublished manuscript, Department of Physical Medicine and Rehabilitation, University of Michigan, Ann Arbor.

Tate, D. G. (2000, September). *Participatory action research: Including consumers on your team.* Paper presented at the Assistive Technology Research and Development Conference, NIH/Whitaker Workshop, Chicago.

Tate, D. G., Stiers, W., Daugherty, J., Forchheimer, M., Cohen, E., & Hansen, N. (1994). The effects of insurance benefits coverage on functional and psychosocial outcomes after spinal cord injury. *Archives of Physical Medicine and Rehabilitation, 75,* 407–414.

Technology-Related Assistance for Individuals With Disabilities Act of 1988. Pub. L. No. 100-407, 29 U.S.C. 2202 (3).

Vash, C. (1981). *The psychology of disability.* New York: Springer.

Vash, C. (1993). Psychological aspects of rehabilitation engineering. In M. Redden & V. Stren (Eds.), *Technology for independent living II* (pp. 53–78). Washington, DC: American Association for the Advancement of Science.

World Health Organization. (2001). *ICF: International classification of functioning, disability and health, final draft.* [On-line]. Retrieved from http://www.who.int/icidh

Wright, B. A. (1983). *Physical disability—A psychosocial approach* (Vol. 2). New York: Harper & Row.

III

THE PROVIDER OF ASSISTIVE TECHNOLOGY DEVICES AND SERVICES

11

ASSISTIVE TECHNOLOGY AND RETRAINING UNDER THE REHABILITATION ACT

ROCHELLE BALTER

The role of rehabilitation psychologists in the 21st century will be very different from that of the rehabilitation psychologists of the 1970s. I hope that the focus of the discipline will change somewhat from the medical model to the wellness model and that rehabilitation psychologists will add the roles of educator and facilitator to their repertoires. To accomplish the aforementioned goals as well as those implicit in the Americans With Disabilities Act (ADA) of 1990, several skills need to be enhanced, such as

1. communications skills, including the use of assistive technologies (ATs) and alternative communication methods
2. knowledge of and familiarity with AT in rehabilitation, including how to introduce its use and help users become comfortable with AT devices
3. knowledge of and respect for multiculturalism, including perceptions of AT by different cultural groups
4. knowledge of legislative and advocacy issues, including legal aspects regarding the use of AT. The knowledge base should include seating and wheeled mobility, communication, computer access, environmental controls, work accommodation, transportation, recreation, and AT used by people with sensory disabilities.
5. skills training, including assertiveness with and without AT
6. advisement on educational access, including the use of AT.

In this chapter I focus briefly on each of these factors. Many of the suggestions I offer regarding the factors listed above are derived from my professional and personal experiences.

COMMUNICATIONS SKILLS

What is meant by the statement "the rehabilitation psychologist needs to be able to communicate with the consumer"? Have not psychologists always "communicated" with their clients? Most individuals with disabilities would respond in the negative. In the 1970s and 1980s, professionals were often seen as talking "at" clients, using approaches that were experienced by clients as condescending, patronizing, and simplistic. There was a definite separation between consumer and professional based on status and power, and the consumer and the rehabilitation psychologist were not viewed as working as a team; neither was the consumer involved in goal setting. The consumer was often told that he or she needed help and what kind of help that would be.

Rehabilitation psychologists in the 21st century will be expected to communicate and partner with consumers in a barrier-free, nondiscriminatory manner. Therefore, among the skills workshops offered under Title III of the Rehabilitation Act of 1973 should be some relating to the use of fair language. Language often mediates attitude and interaction. Person-first approaches help to create a level playing field. The individual is referred to as "having paraplegia or quadriplegia," not as "being a *para* or a *quad*." The individual with the disability should be encouraged to use a designation with which he or she is comfortable. The concepts of mutual dignity and respect need to be adhered to closely.

As part of communications skills, the arts of Socratic questioning and listening rather than lecturing, and of eliciting participation rather than obedience, need to be taught. The individual with a disability also has the right to be communicated with and assessed in each one's communication modality. Therefore, if a consumer is deaf or hard of hearing and uses sign language, a sign language interpreter or a professional trained in sign language needs to be available to facilitate communication. Such communicators may also have to be able to sign in a foreign language, because the stereotypic rehabilitation consumer is no longer a young, White male.

AT is playing a more important part in communicating with people with disabilities than ever before. This is especially true when dealing with individuals with sensory disabilities, such as blindness or deafness. For today's rehabilitation professional to be truly accessible to people who are deaf or hard of hearing, a TTY (text telephone) or relay system should be used. Knowing that such equipment exists and developing a level of comfort using it are the bare minimum needed for modern rehabilitation psychologists. When working with someone who is blind or visually impaired, rehabilitation psychologists should be familiar with other types of sensory assistive devices, such as computers that read to the consumer and into which information can be placed on diskettes. Machines can also be used to synthesize speech for people who have difficulty communicating. Rehabilitation psychologists do not need to be experts in the use of each type of equipment, but a knowledge of the existence of such equipment, and knowledge of its use and of resources where various ATs can be acquired, are the minimum rehabilitation professionals should have. Rehabilitation professionals also need to develop comfort in using such equipment with a client who needs assistive devices for primary communication.

Sensitivity training regarding disabilities may be helpful. This type of training existed in the 1970s and early 1980s but was dropped from many programs because it often resulted in negative rather than positive attitude change (Wright, 1980). When simulations such as wheelchair use and using colored filters to block vision or cotton to block hearing were included as part of training, participants revealed negative emotional reactions, such as loneliness, helplessness, fear of being talked about by others, embarrassment, and dependency (Wright, 1980). Wright pointed out that most people with disabilities would be quite resentful about having their lives seen in such a negative manner.

New methods are needed in which sensitivity training is included only after the professional has taken coursework or attended workshops on the medical and functional aspects of disabilities. Sensitivity training should then be conducted by qualified, competent, professionals who have the disability in question. The trainer can then properly instruct the trainee on the use of assistive devices and appropriate social interactions when using assistive devices (e.g., delaying one's response to an individual user of an electronic communications device, such as a relay system, when one must wait for the other individual to respond, rather than finishing the other person's sentence); accompany the trainee when the trainee is using a wheelchair or a cane; and debrief the trainee, pointing out problem-solving paradigms and strengths. If professionals with disabilities are not involved in this type of training, old negative attitudes are likely to resurface. Sensitivity training should also include fair-language reinforcement as well as an awareness of individual psychology and attitudes and beliefs concerning disability.

IMPACT OF AT

Unlike the AT devices that were used in the 1970s, today's list includes signaling devices; adapted telephones; sound amplification systems; myriad computer-based devices, especially in the area of communications; automatic feeding devices; and even environmental control systems (Scherer & Lane, 1997).

Almost every human being uses AT every day. Telephones; computers in all sizes and varieties; and other modern and not-so-modern accommodations, such as the carts that city dwellers use to transport groceries or laundry, are examples of this type of device.

The purpose of this chapter is not to discuss the benefits and problems associated with AT but to highlight the importance of including this topic in a discussion of new skills training necessary for rehabilitation specialists in the next century. Assistive devices are successful only when they are being used. No matter how technically sophisticated a particular device is, it is of no use if it is never taken out of its packaging. Acceptance of AT devices may depend on the devices' ease of use, comfort, and cost. Other factors that may influence acceptance and use are social practicability or, conversely, fear of stigmatization. "Devices open the door for social acknowledgment of a disability. A device announces the physical difference, facilitating social–psychological interpretations of that difference" (Brooks, 1991, p. 1418).

Brooks (1991) pointed out that assistive device use was not well integrated into the rehabilitation process and that "too often, professionals see devices as cures rather than as components of the total rehabilitation process" (p. 1419). Therefore, an integration of technologies into the rehabilitation process needs to be part of rehabilitation professionals' updated skills training. In coming years rehabilitation psychologists will be expected to understand the impact of a multiplicity of factors on the individual and to help the rehabilitation team suggest appropriate accommodations for the individual as well as assisting him or her in adapting to and growing comfortable with the appropriate assistive devices.

In the near future, rehabilitation professionals will find that they are taking on newer and more consumer-oriented roles. Scherer and Lane (1997) reported on the Consumer Ideal Product Study, a survey conducted by the Rehabilitation Engineering Research Center on Technology Evaluation Transfer through its 14 consumer agencies. The consumer agencies conducted focus groups in which they discussed a device category, such as walkers. The consumers were led through 11 evaluation criteria concerning the product in question (Scherer & Lane, 1997, p. 532). These criteria include categories such as effectiveness, affordability, durability, reliability, and operability. Consumer satisfaction was examined, and consumers were given an opportunity to suggest product improvements. Brooks (1991), in an earlier study, examined AT use among scientists with disabilities. Brooks found differences in employment and private use of ATs and found differences in public use of assistive devices among individuals with different disabilities. Studies conducted by researchers such as Brooks and Scherer and Lane should be made easily available to rehabilitation professionals, who in turn can advise consumers.

MULTICULTURAL ISSUES

When the Rehabilitation Act of 1973 was passed, the majority of consumers in rehabilitation settings were male and White. In the 1990s, the incidence of disabilities among African Americans (14.8%) was much higher than that among White Americans (Flack et al., 1995), because African Americans have higher incidences of cancer; diabetes; cardiac and vascular illnesses; and traumatic injuries, some resulting from criminal assault. Uswatte and Elliott (1997) reported a disproportionately high number of African Americans and Latinos among those with violent-onset spinal cord injuries. This could be attributed to living in high-crime areas.

Members of ethnic minority groups may have less access to health care and follow-up treatment, often have less trust in physicians and modern medical practice (Uswatte & Elliott, 1997), and sometimes have different cultural emphases and meanings attached to their disabilities. An ethnic minority individual living with a disability can be seen as multicultural, that is, as belonging to two minority groups, because the disability makes that individual a member of another minority group.

Disability can be seen as a distinct "culture" or minority group. Wirth (cited in Brooks, 1991) defined a *minority* as any group of people who "because of their physical or cultural characteristics are singled out from others in the society in which they live for differential treatment and unequal collective discrimination." (p. 1418). This is obviously true for people with disabilities because,

> socially and politically, people with disabilities share many common experiences of exclusion and discrimination that transcend ethnicity and gender. These may include physical, economic and attitudinal barriers to employment and services, denial of affection and sexual needs, and stereotyped assumptions about abilities and behaviors. (Hwang, 1996, p. 9)

Rehabilitation psychologists of the 21st century will require training in how to approach individuals from various minority groups. The idea of valuing the individual's experience without pathologizing it needs to be taught, and ideally this should be taught by a member of that specific group (Uswatte & Elliott, 1997). Other multicultural communication skills that need to be taught include using the consumer as an expert resource regarding his or her experience of the situation, learning about beliefs in various cultures and how these influence the consumer, and the consumer's changed lifestyle and emerging needs. An example of differences in beliefs about disability is highlighted in a study by Davis, Jackson, Smith, and Cooper (1999) in which the authors recruited groups of African American and White undergraduate women as participants. The authors had the participants judge slides of 10- to 12-year-old males of their own race, with and without hearing aids, on the basis of appearance, personality, assertiveness, and achievement. A semantic-differential scale was used. White participants exhibited a hearing aid effect across all categories, whereas African American participants exhibited such an effect only on the appearance dimension. This study indicates that ethnic differences exist, but the authors did not discuss AT use.

Rehabilitation psychologists of the 21st century also will need to know how to introduce the use of ATs to ethnic minority consumers in a manner that is culturally syntonic. The best technological assistance will be invisible (known only to the user).

Very few studies have examined the meaning of AT in ethnic minority groups. Pell, Gillies, and Carss (1999) conducted a study in Australia in which they looked at how people in Brisbane use technology, especially computer-associated devices. Pell et al. looked only at the use of technology in a national sample of people with disabilities and did not look at ethnic differences in comfort using the devices.

Silverman, Musa, Kirsch, and Siminoff (1999) compared ethnic groups (African American and White) on self-care activities during chronic illness by in-person interviews. They found some differences in illness monitoring and assistive device use between the ethnic groups. Rimmer, Rubin, Braddock, and Hedman (1999) studied physical activity patterns in African American women with disabilities but did not correlate their findings with other ethnic groups and did not include the use of assistive devices in their study.

A number of studies have examined the use of computer technologies (Web page accessibility, telehealth) in individuals with disabilities (Hufford, Glueckauf, & Webb, 1999; Larkin, 2000) but have not examined ethnic differences in their samples.

Because the literature on evaluating ethnic minority differences in response to AT is so sparse, it might be valuable to consider a possible study that would examine differences in the use of assistive devices between different ethnic groups when education, income, diagnosis, and prognosis are controlled for and the assistive devices used are identical. The participants in this proposed study would be patients at a number of rehabilitation centers with the same diagnosis (e.g., spinal cord injury) who are being given the same assistive devices. Giving participants the device eliminates the cost factor, which could be a controlling issue for low-income individuals. Family members and patients would be asked to volunteer to be consumer evaluators of the devices to be used. Each family member and patient would complete a questionnaire concerning his or her attitude toward assistive devices, such as the Assistive Technology Device Predisposition Assessment (Scherer, 1990), and a prediction form concerning how useful the patient believes the device will be. The patient and family member would then view a film in which a physician of their ethnicity extols the use of the device. All films and training materials would be in the patient's preferred language. Training materials would also be presented in a culturally sensitive context, and telephone help lines would be available in appropriate languages.

The patient and family member would each be given weekly evaluation forms to complete on which they would indicate the frequency with which the device is used and any problems the patient encounters with it as well as any features the patient or the family member believes are exemplary. Individual follow-up interviews would be conducted with each patient and family member by rehabilitation professionals at 3 and 6 months after the patient begins using the device. The Assistive Technology Device Predisposition Assessment would be completed again at the second interview. The interviewers would also preferably be from the same ethnic group as the participant and would explore any known cultural issues that might interfere with device use.

The data from the interviews and the evaluation forms would then be analyzed and compared according to all demographic variables, with special attention paid to ethnicity. Although this experiment would yield only some information, it might be a good first step toward exploring the interaction of ethnicity and assistive device use. This type of experiment could also be conducted with groups that have different disabilities and their disability-appropriate devices.

Ethnic minority rehabilitation psychologists are a minority within the profession; therefore, to make efficient of use of their time, we may need to use teleconferencing or videotaped modules in training. With interactive communication techniques, this will be a probability rather than a possibility.

To be culturally sensitive, rehabilitation professionals will need to know how different cultures evaluate and use ATs. Researchers will need to ask questions specifically geared toward cultural attitudes toward technology. For instance, it is considered disloyal in one culture for an individual to use an AT device such as transfer boards when traditionally a family member would assist with this activity. Brooks (1991) found that people with neuromuscular disabilities were most likely to use devices in all settings; however, those with sensory disabilities were less likely to use devices in intimate settings. Do devices indicate stigmatization? When a disability is incurred, do people in ethnic groups value access to the major culture, or do they value isolation? These questions can be answered only by members of the various ethnic groups concerned. One responsibility of rehabilitation professionals is to promote research on topics of ethnic minority responses to both disability and technology and to integrate this information into treatment paradigms.

KNOWLEDGE OF LEGISLATIVE AND ADVOCACY ISSUES

As has been indicated previously, it is hoped that rehabilitation psychologists will have a very different role in the 21st century, a role that will include different ways of working with consumers. The work will include educating the consumer as to his or her rights under the law, privileges granted by legislation, and how to advocate for needed services. In this age of economics-driven health care, consumers may become one of the major forces for funding through the avenue of their advocacy. Rehabilitation professionals will need to help consumers become advocates to obtain needed services and equipment.

The combination of statutory rights, such as those set forth in the ADA, and AT use are beginning to find a new and highlighted forum. One example is the case of Ryan Taylor (Boyd, 1999), a 9-year-old boy with cerebral palsy who uses a wheeled walker for ambulation. Ryan played youth soccer with the Lawton Evening Optimist Soccer Association, which leased a field from the Fort Sill Army Post in Oklahoma. Because a public facility was used for the games, Ryan's family was able to sue under the ADA when the president of the soccer league attempted to bar Ryan from playing in the last game of the fall season, explaining that Ryan's walker presented a safety hazard to himself and others on the field. When considering this controversy one needs to remember that the soccer league is a children's league. It is informal and a perfect setting for changing attitudes toward disability. No one had any problem with Ryan playing until the soccer official intervened. Ryan's comment of "I just wanted to play with my friends" put the whole case into perspective. U.S. District Court Judge David Russell ruled that Ryan could play in the game, even though he did suggest that some extra padding be added to the walker and that an official stay near Ryan to prevent injury.

This type of controversy is reminiscent of an incident that pitted Professional Golf Association officials against Casey Martin, a professional golfer with a mobility impairment (on May 29, 2001, the Supreme Court found that under the ADA Martin could use a golf cart to travel the distances between holes during play; P.G.A. v. Martin, 2001), and similar controversies may well increase in coming years as AT is used by more individuals with disabilities in public settings.

How do recent ADA rulings affect rehabilitation professionals? They probably mean that rehabilitation professionals will need to become familiar with legislative measures; case law to some extent; and rulings on AT use; as well as with legal resources, such as lawyers who are experienced in ADA litigation, as more and more consumers stand up for their rights.

Rehabilitation professionals need to be familiar with cases such as Ryan Taylor's and Casey Martin's, and it also is of primary importance that continuing education coursework in legal aspects of disability, legislative developments, and prevailing advocacy become requirements for recertification. Continuing education courses can be offered by state psychological associations in conjunction with their state bar associations to update rehabilitation psychologists. Alan A. Goldberg (private practitioner, Tuscon, AZ, personal communication, February 14, 2001) suggested that access to various Web sites, such as those of the ADA Disability and Business Technical Assistance Centers (see http://www.adata.org/) and the Center for Disability Law and Policy (see http://www.equalemployment.org/aguideto.html) would help accomplish this goal, as would access to *The Mental and Physical Disability Law Reporter*. Knowledge regarding the landmark legislation that directly affects consumers should be mandated as part of continuing education training and American Board of Rehabilitation Psychology (ABRP) requirements.

It is important that both continuing education requirements and ABRP requirements include the various areas in which AT is used. Rehabilitation professionals may also need to assist in consumer advocacy when negotiating for needed AT or when lobbying for improvements in AT and in funding to obtain them. This will allow rehabilitation psychologists to be a proactive force in the field of preventive medicine as well as a formidable advocate for consumer independence issues.

SKILLS TRAINING

The consumer with a disability, whether a member of a one or more minority cultures, will need to learn the skills to succeed in the workplace and deal with the various systems that may have to be negotiated. These skills, which many consumers may not have thought necessary prior to the onset of the disability, may be very necessary now. Possible skills that rehabilitation professionals may need to teach include assertiveness training (because individuals with disabilities are expected to be passive), social skills, conversational skills, and advocacy skills. It is also important when teaching assertiveness that the professional understand that assertiveness may also have an AT focus. The individual with a disability may need to learn assertiveness skills to negotiate the right to obtain and use AT in numerous settings, especially in the workplace.

Life span planning is an essential skill that must be understood by psychologists and taught to consumers. As a person with a disability ages, he or she may experience secondary complications. Life span planning is emerging as a necessary part of a holistic approach to working in the field of rehabilitation. Rehabilitation psychologists should preferably take the responsibility for teaching this skill and should also bear the responsibility for educating staff in the importance of this concept. The aforementioned skills may also be learned in workshops that grant continuing education credits.

EDUCATIONAL ACCESS

Title III of the Rehabilitation Act of 1973 provides for training and dissemination of information to individuals with disabilities and their families, advocates, and guardians. A consulting or rehabilitation psychologist is the most appropriate person to provide information regarding educational matters such as training or retraining for the individual with a disability. To fulfill this role, psychologists will need to know about accessibility, including what the consumer's rights are regarding physical accessibility as well as reasonable accommodations, assessment modifications and the reporting of assessment results, and the rights that a person with a disability has to educational accommodations and the use of AT.

To provide the aforementioned services, psychologists will need to learn about educational systems, reasonable accommodations, and assessment practices concerning both admissions policies and ongoing assessments as well as how to access educational resources. Psychologists will also need to know how to find information and gain expertise regarding educational matters, accessibility issues, and the types of assistive devices that are available to people with disabilities, as well as the use of AT devices and the impact they will have on the areas previously discussed.

Psychologists may be asked to consult with the facility the consumer chooses or to act as a facilitator by either the educational institution or the consumer. Psychologists may especially be expected to have current knowledge of AT devices and be able to advise consumers regarding their use in the educational process. This will be very important in dealing with sensory AT and various speech and recording technologies.

CONCLUSION

Psychologists working in the field of physical rehabilitation in the 21st century will have a role that is very different from that of rehabilitation psychologists in the past 25 years. This role will be redefined and expanded to include educator, coach, advocate, advisor, and facilitator. To meet these new role requirements, psychologists will need training in multiculturalism, current legislative and legal issues relating to disability, skills training, life span planning, and enhanced communications skills. Knowledge of all levels of AT will be vital, as will the skills needed to fully integrate AT into the rehabilitation process. It is hoped that Title III funding and specialty certification requirements will allow psychologists to meet these requirements.

REFERENCES

Americans With Disabilities Act of 1990, Pub. L. No. 101-336, 104 Stat. 327.

Boyd, D. (1999, November 4). *Boy barred from playing soccer with aid of walker. Corpus Christi Caller Times.*

Brooks, N. A. (1991). Users' responses to assistive devices for physical disability. *Social Science & Medicine, 32,* 1417–1424.

Davis, M., Jackson, R., Smith, T., & Cooper. W. (1999). The hearing aid effect in African American and Caucasian males as perceived by female judges of the same race. *Language, Speech & Hearing Services in the Schools, 30,* 165–172.

Flack, J. M., Amaro, H., Jenkins, W., Kunitz, S., Levy, J., Mixon, M., & Yu, E. (1995). Panel I: Epidemiology of minority health. *Health Psychology, 14,* 592–599.

Hufford, B., Glueckauf, R., & Webb, P. (1999). Home-based interactive videoconferencing for adolescents with epilepsy and their families. *Rehabilitation Psychology, 44,* 176–193.

Hwang, K. (1996, December). Disability as culture—Some personal reflections. *Focus,* pp. 8–9.

Larkin, M. (2000). Web gears up for people with disabilities. *The Lancet, 356,* 142.

Pell, S., Gillies, R., & Carss, M. (1999). Use of technology by people with physical disabilities in Australia. *Disability and Rehabilitation, 21,* 56–60.

P.G.A. Tour Incorporated v. Martin, 129 (S. Ct. 1879), 2001.

Rehabilitation Act of 1973, Pub. L. No. 93-112, 87 Stat. 355.

Rimmer, J., Rubin, S., Braddock, D., & Hedman, G. (1999). Physical activity patterns of African-American women with physical disabilities. *Medicine and Science in Sports and Exercise, 31,* 613–618.

Scherer, M. J. (1990). Assistive device utilization and quality of life in adults with spinal cord injuries or cerebral palsy: Two years later. *Journal of Applied Rehabilitation Counseling, 21,* 36–44.

Scherer, M. J., & Lane, J. P. (1997). Assessing consumer profiles of "ideal" assistive technologies in ten categories: An integration of quantitative and qualitative methods. *Disability and Rehabilitation, 19,* 528–535.

Silverman, M., Musa, D., Kirsch, B., & Siminoff, L. (1999). Self care for chronic illness: Older African Americans and Whites [Abstract]. *Journal of Cross-Cultural Gerontology, 14,* 169–189.

Uswatte, G., & Elliott, T. R. (1997). Ethnic and minority issues in rehabilitation psychology. *Rehabilitation Psychology, 42,* 61–71.

Wright, B. (1980). Developing constructive views of life with a disability. *Rehabilitation Literature, 41,* 274–279.

12

TELEHEALTH: THE NEW FRONTIER IN REHABILITATION AND HEALTH CARE

ROBERT L. GLUECKAUF, JEFFREY D. WHITTON,
AND DAVID W. NICKELSON

Over the past 15 years, telecommunications-mediated health care services (also known as *telehealth*) have grown substantially across the United States and other developed countries (Nickelson, 1996). There are currently more than 170 telehealth programs in the United States alone (Grigsby & Brown, 2000). Several proponents have argued that telehealth may resolve pressing national health problems, such as the provision of adequate access to health care information and reductions in the spiraling costs of specialty services to underserved areas, including rural communities, military bases, and correctional facilities.

Although telecommunications-mediated health services (TMHS) have expanded at a rapid pace, there is currently a substantial gap between the widespread demand for TMHS and the scientific evidence supporting its efficacy and cost effectiveness. There currently is only limited information about how and under what conditions telehealth leads to positive health outcomes for individuals with disabilities. Furthermore, research on consumer perceptions about the utility of TMHS and on cost effectiveness is in the early phase of development. This is especially true for applications to health care subspecialties, such rehabilitation psychology, health psychology, and clinical neuropsychology.

In the first section of this chapter we define the field of telehealth and its relation to assistive technology (AT) services as well as describe the background and rationale for the growth of telehealth services. In the second

This chapter was supported in part by grants from the National Institute on Disability and Rehabilitation Research and the Department of Veterans Affairs Rehabilitation Research and Development Service to Robert L. Glueckauf. The opinions expressed in this chapter are solely those of the authors and do not reflect the policies of the University of Florida or the American Psychological Association. We thank Tonia Lihatsh for her helpful comments on earlier drafts of this chapter.

section we provide a framework for categorizing the technologies used to deliver telehealth services, which is followed by a description of commonly used equipment and transmission networks. In the third section we review pertinent outcome research on telecommunication-mediated interventions in rehabilitation and health care. Finally, we propose future directions for telehealth research and practice.

DEFINITION OF TELEHEALTH AND ITS RELATION TO AT SERVICES

Our politically charged health care and telecommunications systems continue to evolve with almost blinding speed. Any definition of telehealth must be flexible enough to accommodate technological advances while acknowledging current clinical and political realities. This is why we have defined *telehealth* as the use of telecommunications and information technology to provide access to health information and services across a geographical distance (Nickelson, 1998). Put simply, telehealth is a tool for providing health information and services across a distance. Note that the information and service provided by a telehealth practitioner are basically the same as the information or service delivered by a professional in a clinic or office setting.

A wide range of telehealth services is currently offered, including (but not limited to) initial screenings, diagnostic exams, consultations, education, and short-term interventions. These services are performed by several types of professionals, such as nurses, physicians and, more recently, health care psychologists, each working within the scope of their license and professional competence (Glueckauf et al., 1999).

The relation between telehealth and AT services is intuitive and straightforward: Telehealth is a subset, or subspecialty, of AT services. AT service delivery includes a vast array of technological devices, product systems, services, and training programs, such as the development of easy-to-open door handles for individuals in wheelchairs, telecommunication devices for people who are deaf, and training in the use of environmental control units for those with spinal cord injuries. In contrast, telehealth focuses more narrowly on the use of information technology—especially two-way interactive audiovisual communications, computers, and telemetry—to deliver health information and services at a distance (Darkins & Cary, 2000). Note, however, that the overarching goals of the two fields are essentially the same. Both telehealth and AT strive to enhance the quality of life and independence of individuals with disabilities and chronic health concerns. They are also unified in their commitment to fit technology to the needs of consumers, their personal preferences, and their cultural milieu.

RATIONALE FOR THE GROWTH OF TELEHEALTH

Three pervasive problems in our nation's health care system have contributed significantly to the growth of telehealth: (a) uneven geographic distribution of health care resources, including health care facilities and health manpower; (b) inadequate access to health care for certain segments of the population, such as individuals living in rural areas and those who are physically confined; and (c) the spiraling costs of health and rehabilitation services, particularly specialty care.

First, most health services in the United States are centralized in metropolitan statistical areas, leaving a sizable segment of the population without adequate access to health services. Although a variety of outreach programs have been implemented, they have not succeeded in closing this resource gap. One of the most underserved constituencies are individuals living in rural areas. More than 60 million people—approximately 25% of the U.S. population—live in rural areas (Office of Technology Assessment, 1990). For these individuals, traveling to obtain needed health services, particularly specialty care, may require several hours and attendant financial loss.

Second, several populations have inadequate access to health care, primarily as a result of geographic isolation or physical confinement. For example, Native Americans often reside in geographic areas that are isolated from adequate health services. Military personnel have access to adequate health services while they are on base, but this situation can change dramatically when they are abroad. Physical confinement also represents a significant barrier to obtaining adequate health care. In 1994, more than 1.5 million men and women were incarcerated in various prisons across the United States. This population is particularly at risk for health problems, especially infectious diseases and psychiatric disorders.

Groups who are homebound, such as geriatric populations with severe neurological and mobility limitations, older people living in high-crime areas, and those with psychiatric disabilities such as agoraphobia, may encounter difficulties in obtaining adequate health care. Their medical problems make traveling even short distances difficult. In all these cases, telehealth may offer a means of closing the gap between limited provider resources and the health care needs of the population.

Third, one of the most pressing problems in health care is the escalating cost of specialty services. This is particularly the case for people with disabilities in rural areas, who may require treatment by specialists located in major metropolitan centers. Clients in rural areas frequently experience high transportation costs and concomitant loss of wages to obtain specialty health care that is unavailable where they live. Telecommunication-mediated specialty services delivered in the home or at a local medical facility have the potential of significantly reducing the economic hardship of rural citizens with disabilities. However, the key question is whether such services can be provided without significant reduction in quality of care. A recent report by Nancy Ellery, head of the Health Policy and Services Administration of Montana, offered preliminary support for the cost effectiveness of telehealth. Ellery estimated that Montana's telehealth network saved rural clients with psychiatric disabilities $65,000 in travel time, lost wages, food, and lodging in fiscal year 1995 (DeLeon, 1997).

TELEHEALTH TECHNOLOGY AND TELECOMMUNICATION SYSTEMS

The communication technologies used to provide telehealth services fall into two broad categories: asynchronous and synchronous. *Asynchronous communication* refers to information transactions that occur among two or more persons at different points in time. Electronic mail (e-mail) is the most common form of asynchronous communication and has been used in the delivery of a variety of health care services (e.g., Gustafson et al., 1993; Gustafson et al., 1999).

Synchronous communication refers to information transactions that occur simultaneously among two or more persons. Synchronous telecommunications include computer-synchronous chat systems, telecommunications devices for people who are deaf, telephones, and videoconferencing. Chat systems permit users to communicate instantly with one another through typed messages. Users can "chat" in two ways: (a) through channels, or "chat rooms" in which several individuals communicate simultaneously or (b) through a direct connection in which two persons hold a private conversation. During chat room discussions each person's contribution is displayed on screen in the order of its receipt and is read by all participants in the "room" (Howe, 1997).

Telecommunication devices for people who are deaf, or telecommunication display devices (TDDs), are instruments that facilitate text-based conversations through standard telephone lines. TDDs typically consist of a touch-typing keyboard; a single-line, moving-LED screen; text buffer; memory; and signal light. The entire unit is approximately the size of a laptop computer. In 1993 there were approximately 175,000 TDDs in use across the United States (Harkins, 1993).

The most common form of synchronous communication is the telephone. The major advantage of the telephone is its widespread availability and ease of access. The telephone has become the standard mode of communication in psychological practice for conducting preliminary screening interviews, follow-up sessions, and crisis intervention (Haas, Benedict, &

Kobos, 1996). Over the past few years, innovative, low-cost automated telephone technologies have become an increasingly viable option in treating people with chronic health conditions (e.g., Friedman et al., 1996) and in providing support to caregivers of individuals with severe disabilities, such as Alzheimer's disease (e.g., Mahone, Tarlow, & Sandaire, 1998).

Although at present the telephone is the most accessible form of communication technology, we anticipate that videoconferencing will become the modality of choice for delivering telehealth services in the 21st century. Public demand for interactive videocommunication services is expected to grow exponentially over the next 10 years. This surge of popularity is fueled by the declining costs of videoconferencing equipment and software, increased penetration of telecommunication services, and the broadening appeal of the World Wide Web as well as the anticipation of gigabit-speed Internet 2 (Davey, 1996; Finnerman, 1996; Mittman & Cain, 1999).

Three types of videoconferencing equipment currently are used to deliver telehealth services: (a) room or rollabout, (b) desktop, and (c) plug-and-play systems. Although room or rollabout systems (e.g., VCON's IP set-top) are available in several configurations, the basic setup consists of a rollabout cart; a single large-screen monitor; codec (i.e., a specialized computer program that reduces the number of bytes consumed by large files); a microphone or speakerphone; a set-top camera; and, frequently, an accompanying document camera. Many rollabouts use a second large-screen monitor to exhibit documents. This enables users on each end to view simultaneously both document displays and one another. Rooms or rollabouts are ideal for facilitating multipoint groups (i.e., groups in various sites) as well as person-to-person videoconferencing. The cost of room or rollabout systems varies from $14,000 to $50,000.

Desktop systems (e.g., Intel ProShare and VCON) offer a low-cost, high-quality alternative to room systems in a convenient smaller package. Desktop solutions can accommodate peripheral devices (e.g., document cameras and large-screen monitors) and are portable. The typical desktop videoconference unit consists of a standard desktop computer (e.g., Compaq Prosignia 6450X, Model-1000/SDM, 10GB Hard Drive, PII 450 CPU, 56K V.90 PCI modem, and a Compaq S900 19–in. [48-cm] color monitor), a videoconferencing software kit (e.g., Intel ProShare 500 or VCON Cruiser), digital camera, speakerphone, 19-in. (48-cm) color monitor, and a digital network interface. Transmission of simultaneous audio and video signals is accomplished through the use of Integrated Service Digital Network (ISDN) and, in certain cases, Internet Protocol. The current cost of a desktop videoconferencing system is $3,000 and up, varying with CPU speed, memory, monitor size, and the selection of peripheral devices.

Plug-and-play systems (e.g., TeleVyou and TeleEye) are currently the cheapest solution among the videoconferencing systems. These devices generally use plain old telephone service (POTS). Special telecommunication services, such as ISDN, are not required. Note, however, that these devices use a modem to transmit their information across the telephone network. As a result, images frequently can be jerky or grainy, and sound may be poor in quality. Furthermore, image-to-sound synchronization may be periodically inadequate, rendering verbal communications difficult to follow. The current costs of plug-and-play systems range between $200 and $1,000.

Turning to telecommunication networks, there are three basic telecommunication media currently used for videoconferencing: (a) POTS, (b) Internet protocol (IP) networks (including WideArea Network (WAN) and LocalArea Network (LAN) and (c) ISDN point-to-point as well as multipoint connections.

First, the POTS network is a circuit-switched service offered to homes and businesses by the local telephone company. A *switched circuit* is defined as a two-way connection that exists only for the time required to make a call. When the user completes a long-distance call, the circuit is broken, and the individual is no longer charged for the service. This is contrasted with a permanent, or "nailed-up" circuit, which is connected and usable at all times (e.g., a dedicated T1 line).

The major downfall of POTS is the local loop or the wire from the local telephone company's switch or pole to the user's facility. Transmissions within the local loop are analog in nature (i.e., electronic transmissions accomplished by adding signals of varying frequency to carrier waves of a given frequency of alternating electromagnetic current. Telephone has conventionally used analog technology). This is the reason why people use modems (that convert analog to digital signals and vice versa) to connect with the Internet. This analog local loop is slowly being replaced with digital technology. As this happens, the bottleneck of slow connectivity from the home to the Internet will diminish significantly.

To make a video call on the POTS network the sender dials the telephone number of the recipient videoconferencing user the same way he or she would dial a number for a regular phone call. Such videoconferencing interactions are termed *point-to-point connections*. A point-to-point call takes place when one user connects with another user. Multipoint video transmissions are also possible on POTS and involve simultaneous interaction among three or more parties.

Second, the IP network is a packet, switched service in which digital information (1s and 0s from the computer) are bundled into sets or groups called *packets*. These packets contain data, as well as transfer-formatting information to facilitate transmission from place to place on the Internet. Individuals typically gain access to the Internet at their work site (through the corporation's LAN or WAN) or at home through a local Internet Service Provider (ISP).

ISPs connect the consumer to the Internet using a router-based network. Routers are very fast computers whose sole job is to route or transfer IP packets to their destinations. These digital packets traverse the network directed by routers and bridges to the addresses contained in the packets. When the packets arrive at their destinations they are amalgamated and are then seen by the end-user as files, images, or text on the screen.

IP-based networks can experience transmission delays and sometimes lose information (i.e., data packets), particularly at times when the network is congested. This results in a degradation of image and sound quality as well as image-to-sound synchronization. However, the future of Internet videoconferencing appears especially promising. With advancements in router technology; improved protocols; and low-cost, high-bandwidth next-generation Internet, IP videoconferencing is likely to become the preferred mode of audiovisual interaction.

Third, ISDN is also one of several switched digital services on the market that can support high-quality, point-to-point or multipoint videoconferencing. The user pays an initial installation charge ($100–$200), a monthly service fee ($75–$100), a per-minute usage charge from the local provider of the service and, if applicable, long-distance charges. ISDN is offered at several different bandwidths ranging from 128 kilobits/s (kbps) to 1.56 megabits/s. Although somewhat expensive, ISDN provides an attractive high-speed (e.g., 128 kbps) alternative to slower analog modem transmission (56 kbps).

TELEHEALTH OUTCOME RESEARCH

Although telehealth holds considerable promise as a tool for reducing inequities in the allocation of health resources, access limitations, and escalating costs, evaluation of the benefits of telehealth has only recently begun. In keeping with the rehabilitation focus of this book, we have restricted our review of telehealth research to representative, controlled intervention studies involving people at risk for, or currently diagnosed with, chronic, disabling medical conditions. This body of research falls into four telecommunication categories: Internet, telephone, and videoconferencing investigations, as well as comparative studies across telephone, videoconferencing, and face-to-face modalities.

Internet Studies

David Gustafson and his colleagues at the University of Wisconsin have conducted several investigations (Gustafson et al., 1993; Gustafson et al., 1994) of the effects of e-mail interventions for adults with chronic disabilities. Their work has focused on the development and evaluation of the Comprehensive Health Enhancement Support System (CHESS), a home-based computer system that provides a variety of interactive services to individuals with life-threatening conditions, such as women with breast cancer and people with HIV/AIDS. CHESS users are able to communicate with others by means of typed messages in a discussion or chat group, type in questions for experts to answer, read articles about others with similar health concerns, monitor their health status, and gain information about coping techniques. Of the multiple CHESS options, Gustafson et al. (1993; Gustafson et al., 1999) reported that e-mail discussion groups were used most often. Such groups accounted for approximately 60% of uses across both their 1993 and 1999 investigations.

Gustafson et al.'s (1999) most comprehensive outcome study to date was a quasi-experiment in which 104 people with HIV/AIDS received CHESS in their homes for 3–6 months, as compared to 97 control individuals with HIV/AIDS who were not offered CHESS or other additional support services. Participants with HIV/AIDS selected the e-mail discussion option for 73% of the total number of CHESS uses. At the 2-month follow-up, Gustafson et al. found that CHESS participants rated their perceptions of quality of life significantly higher on five of eight quality-of-life measures (e.g., increased participation in their own health care and increased cognitive functioning) than did the 97 control participants who did not receive CHESS services.

In one of the few randomized controlled trials of Internet-based health education, Robinson (1989) evaluated the impact of the Stanford Health-Net in enhancing health-promoting behaviors. Stanford University undergraduate and graduate students ($N = 1003$) were randomly assigned to Health-Net, a computer network emphasizing specific self-care and preventive strategies, or to a standard treatment control condition. Robinson reported a 22.5% decrease in ambulatory medical visits in Health-Net users as compared to no change in standard treatment control participants. Furthermore, Health-Net participants reported significantly higher perceived self-efficacy in preventing sexually transmitted diseases (e.g., AIDS) than did control participants, who reported little change over time.

Telephone Studies

Telephone-based telehealth research can be classified into two major categories: (a) first-generation evaluations of telephone counseling and assessment procedures using standard POTS equipment and (b) second-generation studies of automated telephone systems that offer a variety of services, including access to health education modules, consultation with health care experts, and telephone support groups for peers with similar medical conditions or their caregivers.

First, Evans and colleagues have conducted the majority of first-generation telephone counseling studies (e.g., Evans, Fox, Pritzl, & Halar, 1984; Evans & Jaureguy, 1982; Evans, Smith, Werkhoven, Fox, & Pritzl, 1986). In one of the first controlled telephone studies, Evans and Jaureguy (1982) assigned veterans with severe visual disabilities to one of two groups: telephone group counseling ($n = 12$) or standard office-based treatment ($n = 12$). They found significantly lower levels of depression and loneliness, and higher participation in social activities, for counseling participants than for no-treatment control participants, who showed no change over time. The veterans' positive response to telephone-mediated counseling was consistent with findings from similar studies that relied on uncontrolled, single-group designs (Evans et al., 1984; Evans et al., 1986; Stein, Rothman, & Nakanishi, 1993).

Turning to second-generation studies, Friedman et al.'s (1996) randomized controlled trial of the effects of automated telephone technology on adherence to treatment of hypertension is one of the highlights of contemporary telehealth research. Friedman et al. randomly assigned 267 individuals with hypertension to a telephone-linked computer (TLC) system or to standard treatment over a period of 6 months. TLC interacted with home-based participants over the telephone by means of computer-controlled speech. The participants, in turn, communicated using a touchtone keypad on their telephones. The primary functions of the TLC system were to inquire about the health status of users and to promote adherence to the treatment regimen. During TLC conversations, patients reported self-measured blood pressures, data on adherence to antihypertensive medications and, if pertinent, medication side effects. This information was stored in a database and subsequently was transmitted to each patient's physician in printed form. Standard-treatment patients received the usual care from their health care providers.

Friedman et al. (1996) found that TLC patients reported significantly greater average adherence to treatment and lower diastolic blood pressure as compared to control patients, who showed little change over time on these measures. Note, however, that these effects were largely attributable to gains made by nonadherent patients in the TLC condition. TLC participants who were nonadherent prior to treatment (i.e., those who took less than 80% of their antihypertensive medications) showed significant improvements in mean adherence at the 6-month posttest, whereas nonadherent standard-treatment control participants showed no change over time. In contrast, adherent TLC and adherent control participants showed no significant between- or within-groups differences in adherence to treatment.

The authors reported a similar pattern of findings for diastolic and systolic blood pressure. However, they found only a trend in the predicted direction for the systolic measure ($p = .09$). Cost-effectiveness ratios also were calculated for the TLC use. The cost per 1 mmHg improvement in diastolic blood pressure across all TLC participants was approximately $5 and $1 for the non-adherent TLC group.

Other creative applications of telephone technologies, including voice bulletin boards and computer-based telephone integration systems, have been reported for people with severe asthma and caregivers of people with Alzheimer's disease (Bruderman & Abboud, 1997; Mahone et al., 1998). These telehealth initiatives appear quite promising and should provide a wealth of information on health outcomes and cost effectiveness as well as user perceptions of desirability and utility of telephone-based health care services.

Videoconferencing Studies

Two major types of controlled videoconferencing studies have been performed: (a) comparisons between closed-circuit television (CCTV) and face-to-face interviews and (b) evaluations of the reliability (e.g., interrater agreement) of videoconferencing-based mental status exams. Although the latter represent an important domain of research (see Ball & McLaren, 1997), we will not review these studies, because they are not in keeping with the telehealth intervention focus of this chapter. Furthermore, these studies generally make no explicit linkages between assessment and rehabilitation treatment.

In one of the larger videoconferencing studies, Dongier, Tempier, Lalinec-Michaud, and Meuneir (1986) assessed the perceptions of 50 clients with psychiatric disabilities who received CCTV interviews versus 35 matched control clients who received the standard, face-to-face approach. All interviewees were asked to rate various aspects of the interview, such as feelings of ease during the interview, ability to express oneself, feelings of ease following the interview, the quality of the interpersonal relationship, and the utility of the assessment interview in guiding treatment. In addition, the psychiatrists and other team members involved in the interviews were asked to rate the quality of the patient–consultant relationship; rate the quality of written conclusions for diagnosis, management, and treatment; and provide a global evaluation of the usefulness of the interview.

Dongier et al. (1986) found no significant differences in clients' satisfaction ratings between the CCTV and face-to-face conditions. In contrast, psychiatrists and team members rated CCTV as significantly inferior to face-to-face conditions in regard to written conclusions for diagnosis and global evaluations of the usefulness of the interview. Although the authors tended to minimize the psychiatrists' and their team's dissatisfaction with CCTV interviews, it is possible that professionals may be more skeptical about the validity of conclusions of audiovisually based modalities. They may tend to emphasize the importance of direct "social presence" in obtaining good interview data.

Although Dongier et al.'s (1986) study has not been replicated, we do have preliminary empirical evidence suggesting that health care professionals' judgments of the process and utility of clinical interviews may vary as a function of the availability of alternate telecommunication modes. Using participants as their own controls, Ball, McLaren, Summerfield, Lipsedge, and Watson (1995) exposed six psychiatrists and their patients to four interview modalities: (a) videoconferencing; (b) face to face; (c) speakerphone; and (d) standard, handheld telephone. In contrast to Dongier et al., they found no substantial differences between the face-to-face and videoconferencing conditions for physicians' and patients' evaluations of process dimensions, such as descriptions of the problem, clarity of explanations, disappointment with the interview, and overall satisfaction. However, psychiatrists noted differential and significantly higher levels of dissatisfaction with speakerphone and handheld telephones in which visual cues were absent.

Comparative Studies of Telecommunication Technologies

Glueckauf and his colleagues (Glueckauf, Whitton, Baxter, et al., 1998a; Glueckauf, Whitton, Kain, et al., 1998b; Glueckauf, Fritz, Dages, Liss, & Carney, in press; Hufford, Glueckauf, & Webb, 1999) have performed, to our knowledge, the only randomized, controlled study of the differential effects of video versus speakerphone versus face-to-face counseling for individuals living in rural locations with severe disabilities. This multisite investigation is still ongoing and will involve more than 95 families of rural teenagers with seizure disorders across five midwestern and three southeastern states.

Glueckauf's (2000) initial evaluation highlighted the broad utility and acceptability of disparate telecommunication modalities. They randomly assigned 39 teenagers with uncontrolled seizure conditions and their parents from the rural Midwest to one of three conditions: (a) home based, family videocounseling; (b) home-based speakerphone counseling; or (c) traditional, office-based family counseling. The differential effects of these counseling interventions on outcome were assessed 1 week after the six-session counseling program and 6 months following treatment.

Twenty-two families completed the six-session counseling program. Twelve families dropped out before the first assessment session, and 5 families dropped out after the initial assessment session. Dropout was differentially associated with office counseling that required long-distance travel. Glueckauf et al. used a multimethod approach in assessing key intervention and process variables. Their outcome measures were (a) problem-specific rating scales derived from the Family and Disability Assessment System (Glueckauf, 2000; Glueckauf et al., 1992) and (b) the Social Skills Rating System (Gresham & Elliott, 1990). Process measures included the Comfort and Distraction subscales of the Audiovisual Equipment Rating Scale (Glueckauf & Hufford, 1998), homework completion ratings, and missed appointments (Glueckauf et al., in press).

On the Family and Disability Assessment System measures, teenagers with epilepsy and parents reported significant reductions in both severity and frequency of identified family problems across all three modalities from pretreatment to 1-week posttreatment and from pretreatment to the 6-month follow-up. On the Social Skills Rating System scales parents reported significant reductions in problem behaviors at home from pretreatment to the 1-week posttreatment to the 6-month follow-up. In addition, parents reported significant improvement in their teenagers' social skills (e.g., doing chores) across all three assessment phases. Consistent with previous telehealth research, mode of transmission did not differentially influence the outcomes of treatment. Significant and similar treatment gains were found across home-based desktop video, home-based speakerphone, and face-to-face office counseling.

Turning to consumer perception of the use of telecommunication devices, teenagers and parents reported moderate to high levels of comfort in the use of audiovisual equipment for all three conditions. Family comfort with equipment also improved significantly from Sessions 2 to 5 across all modalities. (Note that "office" families were asked to rate their comfort with videorecording devices mounted on the walls of the family therapy room.)

A different pattern was observed for distraction in the use of telecommunication devices. Although teenagers and parents reported only slight to moderate levels of distraction in the use of audiovisual technology, their perceptions varied as a function of condition and time of assessment. Office and home-based speakerphone families reported increased levels of distraction from Sessions 2 to 5, whereas no changes in distraction over time were noted in the home-based videocounseling participants.

Contrary to prediction, no substantial differences were found across conditions on completion of therapy homework assignments and number of missed appointments. Glueckauf (2000) had anticipated that home-based video and home-based speakerphone would confer a substantial advantage in adherence to treatment as a result of their contextual proximity and high convenience. It is possible, however, that the delivery of telehealth services in the home as a stand-alone intervention (i.e., without the use of intensive monitoring strategies) does not lead to incremental improvement in adherence to treatment. Nonetheless, caution should be exercised in interpreting this current null result. Office-counseling control clients consisted only of those families who did not drop out as a result of lost wages or the inconvenience of long-distance travel, and thus they may have represented a more adherent and highly motivated subsample of families of teenagers with seizure disorders.

Glueckauf et al. also provided initial estimates of the costs of home-based video, home-based speakerphone, and office-based counseling for rural families. The per-family costs for six sessions of home-based videocounseling, home-based speakerphone, and office counseling were $3500, $1300, and $1900, respectively. Thus, the preliminary analysis suggests that the costs of home-based videocounseling are significantly higher than both home-based speakerphone and drive-in office counseling, approximately a 2:1 ratio. It is anticipated, however, that the costs of home-based videocounseling will decrease over the next few years as a result of market competition. Furthermore, point-to-point ISDN service may not be required to ensure good videoconferencing fidelity, data security, and privacy. With advances in codec technology, increased availability of high bandwidth from ISPs, and dynamic allocation of bandwidth over the Internet, the prospects for supporting low-cost Internet home-based videoconferencing are quite positive.

FUTURE DIRECTIONS FOR TELEHEALTH IN REHABILITATION AND HEALTH CARE SETTINGS

Outcome and Cost-Effectiveness

As discussed previously, telehealth holds considerable promise for resolving the access barriers of people with disabilities in rural areas and to homebound rehabilitation populations that may benefit from psychological services. However, we continue to lack basic information about how and under what conditions telecommunication-mediated services lead to positive psychological and health care outcomes. We also have limited information about the cost effectiveness of telehealth services. This is especially true for cost effectiveness of telehealth applications in rehabilitation and health psychology. In a rehabilitation marketplace increasingly focused on both the cost and quality of care, this research will be important to payers and policymakers and will ensure that rehabilitation psychology has a place in future technology-laden iterations of the health care system.

It is imperative that large-scale evaluations of the differential effects of telecommunications-mediated interventions become a funding priority for federal health care agencies, such as the National Institutes of Health and the Health Resources Services Administration. Although a substantial number of demonstration grants have been awarded over the past 10 years, funding for randomized, clinical trials of the benefits of telehealth for chronic medical populations (e.g., people with traumatic brain injuries and dementing disorders) has been slow to emerge. Rehabilitation professionals can no longer tout the benefits of telehealth services for people with chronic disabilities without solid empirical evidence for their effectiveness. If rehabilitation professionals are to advance as a responsible scientific enterprise, they must begin to subject to scientific scrutiny their basic assumptions about "what works" in telecommunications with their clients.

Cost-effectiveness studies are also an integral component of the acceptance of large-scale telehealth interventions (Bashshur, 1995). To become a viable health service option, telehealth networks must show that the costs of treatment are at least equal to or less than those of alternative approaches that produce similar outcomes. Although several studies have documented the cost effectiveness of psychotherapeutic interventions for psychiatric, substance abuse, and geriatric populations (see Glen, Lazar, Hornberger, & Spiegel, 1997; Krupnick & Pincus, 1992), there has been little published research on the cost effectiveness of telecommunication-mediated psychological interventions for people with chronic disabilities.

Process studies

Although randomized, controlled field studies are the litmus test of the effectiveness of telehealth, it is essential to understand the social–psychological mechanisms that link intervention and outcome. We currently lack basic information about the factors that both enhance and reduce the quality (clarity, ease of use, distractibility, and comfort) of telehealth communications across modalities, disabilities, age groups, minorities, and ethnic groups and, in turn, their relation with treatment outcome. We also have only limited knowledge about the impact of different telecommunication modalities (e.g., home-based videoconferencing vs. e-mail) on intervention adherence, attendance, and attrition.

Practice Guidelines and Client Training Material

Practice guidelines are potentially powerful tools to enhance quality control. Guidelines provide a method of determining the most effective treatment of a disorder and establish accepted treatment approaches and duration of treatment modalities. They are likely to be critical to the broad-based acceptance of telehealth interventions and may help to establish the appropriate level of expertise of telehealth providers (cf., DeLeon, Frank, & Wedding, 1995). The Joint Working Group on Telemedicine has outlined the critical questions that the health professions need to work together to answer in the development of practice guidelines for the delivery of tele-health services (Joint Working Group on Telemedicine, 1998; National Telecommunications and Information Administration, 1997). The time is ripe for developing and evaluating the use of practice guidelines in the delivery of telecommunication-mediated psychological services to persons with chronic disabilities and their families.

REFERENCES

Ball, C., & McLaren, P. (1997). The tele-assessment of cognitive state: A review. *Journal of Telemedicine and Telecare, 3,* 126–131.

Ball, C. J., McLaren, P. M., Summerfield, A. B., Lipsedge, M. S., & Watson, J. P. (1995). A comparison of communication modes in adult psychiatry. *Journal of Telemedicine and Telecare, 1,* 22–26.

Bashshur, R. I. (1995). Telemedicine effects: Cost, quality, and access. *Journal of Medical Systems, 19,* 81–91.

Bruderman, I., & Abboud, S. (1997). Telespirometry: Novel system for home monitoring of asthmatic patients. *Telemedicine Journal, 3,* 127–133.

Darkins, A. W., & Cary, M. A. (2000). *Telemedicine and telehealth: Principles, policies, performance, and pitfalls.* New York: Springer.

Davey, T. (1996). Telcos feel the heat, set to roll out new services. *PC Week, 13*(38), 1–3.

DeLeon, P. (1997, December 17). *Steadily evolving into the 21st century—Telehealth.* Available E-mail: federal-ppp@lists.apa.org. Subject: Division 29 column—December 1997.

DeLeon, P. H., Frank, R. G., & Wedding, D. (1995). Health psychology and public policy: The political press. *Health Psychology, 14,* 493–499.

Dongier, M., Tempier, R., Lalinec-Michaud, M., & Meuneir, D. (1986). Telepsychiatry: Psychiatric consultation through two-way television: A controlled study. *Canadian Journal of Psychiatry, 31,* 32–34.

Evans, R. L., Fox, H. R., Pritzl, D. O., & Halar, E. M. (1984). Group treatment of physically disabled adults by telephone. *Social Work in Health Care, 9*(3), 77–84.

Evans, R. L., & Jaureguy, B. M. (1982). Group therapy by phone: A cognitive behavioral program for visually impaired elderly. *Social Work in Health Care, 7*(2), 79–90.

Evans, R. L., Smith, K. M., Werkhoven, W. S., Fox, H. R., & Pritzl, D. O. (1986). Cognitive telephone group therapy with physically disabled elderly persons. *The Gerontologist, 26,* 8–10.

Finnerman, M. F. (1996). Sizing up the ISDN market. *Business Communications Review, 26*(11), 81–85.

Friedman, R. H., Kazis, L. E., Jette, A., Smith, M. B., Stollerman, J., Torgerson, J., & Carey, K. (1996). A telecommunications system for monitoring and counseling patients with hypertension: Impact on medication adherence and blood pressure control. *American Journal of Hypertension, 9,* 285–292.

Glen, G. O., Lazar, S. G., Hornberger, J., & Spiegel, D. (1997). The economic impact of psychotherapy: A review. *American Journal of Psychiatry, 154,* 147–155.

Glueckauf, R. L. (2000). The Family and Disability Assessment System. In J. Touliatos, B. F. Perlmutter, & G. W. Holden (Eds.), *Handbook of family measurement techniques* (Vol. 2). Newbury Park, CA: Sage.

Glueckauf, R. L., & Hufford, B. J. (1998). *Audiovisual equipment rating scale.* Department of Psychology, Indiana University Purdue University Indianapolis, Indianapolis, IN.

Glueckauf, R. L., Hufford, B., Whitton, J., Baxter, J., Schneider, P., Kain, J., & Vogelgesang, S. (1999). Telehealth: Emerging technology in rehabilitation and health care. In M. G. Eisenberg, R. L. Glueckauf, & H. H. Zaretsky (Eds.), *Medical aspects of disability: A handbook for the rehabilitation professional* (2nd ed., pp. 625–639). New York: Springer.

Glueckauf, R. L., Webb, P., Papandria-Long, M., Rasmussen, J. L., Markand, O., & Farlow, M. (1992). The Family and Disability Assessment System: Consistency and accuracy of judgments across coders and measures. *Rehabilitation Psychology, 37,* 291–304.

Glueckauf, R. L., Whitton, J., Baxter, J., Kain, J., Vogelgesang, S., Hudson, M., & Wright, D. (1998a). Videocounseling for families of rural teens with epilepsy: Project update. *TeleHealthNews* [On-line], *2*(2). Available: http://cybertowers.com/ct/telehealth

Glueckauf, R., Whitton, J., Kain, J., Vogelgesang, S., Hudson, M., Hufford, B., Baxter, J., Garg, B., & Herndon, M. (1998b). Home-based, videocounseling for families of rural teens with epilepsy: Program rationale and objectives. *TeleHealthNews* [On-line], *2*(1), 3–5. Available: http://cybertowers.com/ct/telehealth/

Glueckauf, R. L., Fritz, S., Dages, P., Liss, H., & Carney, P. (in press). Videocounseling for rural teens with seizure disorders: Phase I findings. *Rehabilitation Psychology.*

Gresham, F. M., & Elliott, S. N. (1990). *Social Skills Rating System manual.* Circle Pines, MN: American Guidance Service

Grigsby, B., & Brown, N. (2000). *The 1999 ATSP report on U.S. telemedicine activity.* Portland, OR: Association of TeleHealth Service Providers.

Gustafson, D. H., Hawkins, R. P., Boberg, E. W., Serlin, R. E., Graziano, F., Pingree, S., & Chan, C. (1999). Impact of a patient-centered, computer-based health information/support system. *American Journal of Preventive Medicine, 16*(1), 1–9.

Gustafson, D. H., Wise, M., McTavish, F., Taylor, J. O., Wolberg, W., Stewart, J., Smalley, R. V., & Bosworth, K. (1993). Development and pilot evaluation of a computer-based support system for women with breast cancer. *Journal of Psychosocial Oncology, 11*(4), 69–93.

Haas, L. J., Benedict, J. G., & Kobos, J. C. (1996). Psychotherapy by telephone: Risks and benefits for psychologists and consumers. *Professional Psychology: Research and Practice, 27,* 154–160.

Harkins, J. E. (1993). Ergonomic considerations for communication technologies for deaf and hard-of-hearing people. In M. J. Smith & G. Salvendy (Eds.), *Human–computer interaction: Application and case studies.* New York: Elsevier.

Howe, D. (1997). *Free on-line dictionary of computing* [On-line]. Available: http://wombat.doc.ic.ac.uk/

Hufford, B. J., Glueckauf, R. L., & Webb, P. M. (1999). Home-based, interactive videoconferencing for adolescents with epilepsy and their families. *Rehabilitation Psychology, 44,* 176–193.

Joint Working Group on Telemedicine. (1998, January 6). *Report of the Interdisciplinary Telehealth Standards Working Group* [On-line]. Available: http://www.arentfox.com/telemed/reports/telehlth.html.

Krupnick, J. L., & Pincus, H. A. (1992). The cost-effectiveness of psychotherapy: A plan for research. *American Journal of Psychiatry, 149,* 1295–1305.

Mahone, D. F., Tarlow, B., & Sandaire, J. (1998). A computer-mediated intervention for Alzheimer's caregivers. *Computers in Nursing, 16,* 208–216.

Mittman, R., & Cain, M. (1999). The future of the Internet in health care: Five-year forecast. *Hospital Quarterly, 3*(4), 63–65.

National Telecommunications and Information Administration. (1997, January 31). *Telemedicine report to Congress* [On-line]. Available: http://www.ntia.doc.gov/reports/telemed/

Nickelson, D. W. (1996). Behavioral telehealth: Emerging practice, research and policy opportunities. *Behavioral Sciences and the Law, 14,* 443–457.

Nickelson, D. W. (1998). Telehealth and the evolving health care system: Strategic opportunities for professional psychology. *Professional Psychology: Research and Practice, 29,* 527–535.

Office of Technology Assessment. (1990). *Health care in rural America* (OTA-H-434). Washington, DC: Government Printing Office.

Robinson, T. N. (1989). Community health behavior change through computer network health promotion: Preliminary findings from Stanford Health-Net. *Computer Methods and Programs in Biomedicine, 30*(2–3), 137–144.

Stein, L., Rothman, B., & Nakanishi, M. (1993). The telephone group: Accessing group service to the homebound. *Social Work With Groups, 16,* 203–215.

13

ASSISTIVE TECHNOLOGY ON-LINE INSTRUCTION: EXPANDING THE DIMENSIONS OF LEARNING COMMUNITIES

CAREN L. SAX

Distance education, or *mediated learning*, is changing how many teachers and learners access education. Faculty and administrators at universities and other institutions of higher education are struggling with the political, financial, and pedagogical implications of distance courses and are questioning existing policies that conflict with on-line parameters. Although it may not be the ideal learning mode for everyone, many students who have enrolled in Web-based courses appreciate the ease and flexibility of attending classes at their convenience. Professionals who enroll in courses for purposes of continuing education while working full-time value the opportunity to earn advanced degrees from universities that are located in other cities or states. In addition, accessing education via the Internet enables individuals who may have mobility, transportation, or physical or medical limitations to participate more fully. Courses offered by distance clearly can be as good (or as bad) as traditional campus courses. This chapter's description of a successful approach to on-line continuing professional education demonstrates important considerations in this new world of advancing technology.

> If we allow the information superhighway to bypass education—even for an interim period—we will find that the information rich will get richer while the information poor get poorer with no guarantee that everyone will be on the network at some future date. (Thornburg, 1994, p. 8)

Rapid advances in technology are shaping a new world in which lifelong learning means survival and where self-directed learners will have the advantage over others who rely on more traditional ways of learning

(Thornburg, 1994). These advances have compelled institutions of higher education to offer an increasing number of on-line courses and degree programs (Dringus & Terrell, 1999; Scollin & Tello, 1999; Smart, 1999). Technological innovations affect how instruction is delivered, how individuals access education, how resources are made available, and how students and instructors interact with each other. New ways of using technology may transform not only the way the curriculum is delivered but also how the learning takes place, emphasizing both the professional and personal skills that are necessary in today's world. Distance learning has introduced "a whole new set of physical, emotional, and psychological issues along with the educational issues" (Palloff & Pratt, 1999, p. 7) that differ from those encountered in the traditional classroom. Consider the following academic scenario:

> The class discussion was growing livelier. The professor presented several thought-provoking questions, and a number of students raised issues regarding traditional ways of thinking about assistive technology and the ways in which they related to rehabilitation services. Luis agreed with a premise from the week's readings and videotapes, adding his perspective about systems changing and how people tend to respond to those changes. Glenda responded, reflecting on her own approach to interacting with people with disabilities. She wondered if in helping or supporting an individual to find his or her balance of independence, interdependence, and dependence, it was possible to not impose personal prejudices. David agreed, adding that after reviewing the examples of people accessing assistive technology in innovative ways, his preconceived notions had been challenged. Others joined in, expressing opinions, providing examples from personal experience, and trying to convince one another of alternate perspectives.

This idea exchange took place not in a campus classroom but on the Internet, with students deciding when and where they accessed instruction. In addition, each student felt reassured that before hitting the "send" button the responses could be reviewed and edited. Welcome to the world of distance learning!

THE EVOLUTION OF DISTANCE LEARNING

> We are witnessing the most profound change to affect our society and our corporate and professional lives since the Industrial Revolution and the advent of the nationwide rail system: the information-technology revolution. (Foa, Schwab, & Johnson, 1996, p. 41)

Technological innovations historically have been introduced slowly and too often have perpetuated traditional curricula. Before the 1970s, the concept of distance learning referred primarily to correspondence courses that provided materials to read and tests to submit by mail. The scope of distance learning in the 1970s and 1980s included viewing programs on public television or, more recently, on cable access channels, with or without a professor available for discussions (Deloro, 1997). One of the main advantages to accessing lectures in this context was the ability to not only videotape a session and watch it at a convenient time but also to have the option of fast-forwarding or reviewing the material at will. The format was typically the same: a "talking head" on the screen, occasional bulleted highlights and, all too seldom, guest interviews or panels of experts. The course assessment procedure was similarly predictable, that is, multiple-choice tests that could be scored electronically. Students sat at home watching hours of videotaped instruction rather than sitting in classrooms listening to hours of lecture. Although arguably more accessible to students unable to attend classes because of scheduling, transportation problems, or other restrictions, distance education implemented in this manner offered limited interaction between professors and students and no opportunities for interaction among students. Current distance education efforts are incorporating strategies for delivering content effectively, engaging students in active learning, and offering an approach that is "flexible, multiple-perspective, experiential, project-based, and holistic—what is often referred to as student-centered" (Berge, 1998, p. 21).

Distance education now incorporates electronic mail (e-mail), the World Wide Web, on-line resources and materials, and a range of formats that provide unique opportunities for instructors to increase interactions with and among students. Furthermore, creative instructors arrange meaningful activities that relate to the students' daily experiences (Berge, 1996) and introduce students to learning without boundaries as they communicate with peers and experts around the world (Meyen, Lian, & Tangen, 1997). Students discuss readings and assignments using small-group or whole-class listservs, post comments on a discussion board, and participate in real-time conversations in "chat rooms." In addition, students can communicate privately with instructors by means of e-mail messages to ask questions or clarify assignments. Given these obvious advantages, are there drawbacks? Does instruction become more homogeneous? Are effective models of teaching and learning compromised? How much enthusiasm and participation can be generated on-line? Do students feel isolated? Instructors and students, as well as technical support staff, all have roles and responsibilities in maximizing learning opportunities as well as creating a sense of community in "virtual" environments, just as they do in physical classrooms.

In this chapter I describe a Web-based graduate course, "Applications of Rehabilitation Technologies," which is offered as part of an on-line master's degree program in Rehabilitation Counseling at San Diego State

University (SDSU). This class was originally designed and taught as a traditional one-semester on-campus course, but the content and instruction were reconsidered, revised, and reconstructed to best meet the needs of the students and the demands of the distance learning environment. The challenges included maintaining individualized aspects of instruction, using effective models of teaching and learning, and generating the enthusiasm on-line that had been featured in the face-to-face course. The newly designed class offered benefits beyond the academic content. The students and professors developed trust, communication, and mutual support that resulted in a virtual learning community.

CONTEXT OF THE COURSE

SDSU's on-line rehabilitation counseling graduate program was designed in response to the professional development needs of the California Department of Rehabilitation (CaDR). CaDR, in trying to comply with the educational requirements of the Rehabilitation Act Amendments of 1992, interpreted the law to mean that newly hired counselors should be required to have a master's degree, and current counselors who did not have this degree could receive state assistance to earn one (Warn, Compton, Levine, & Whitteker, 1998). Although some university programs existed across the state, they were geographically accessible to only a small percentage of counselors. If CaDR were going to offer opportunities for continuing education, other options also had to be considered. Distance education offered the accessibility and the flexibility that counselors sought. A needs assessment indicated that at least 200 counselors were interested in pursuing a master's degree on-line. Negotiation among the university and CaDR stakeholders was required to finalize approvals, procedures, safeguards, and accountability (see Warn et al., 1998, for procedural details). A pilot group of 34 students began the 30-month master's-degree program in 1997.

This diverse cohort of students hailed from as far south as Los Angeles to the northernmost Humboldt County. English was a second language for many of the students, and 15% of them had a disability, including physical and sensory limitations. Instruction was provided in accessible formats to meet the range of student needs. Before the sequence of courses began, all students were invited to San Diego for a hands-on orientation to distance learning strategies. Each professor was provided technical training as necessary and teamed with an instructional designer to prepare his or her course for on-line delivery. The curriculum content helped direct the methods and media for each course, and a range of pedagogical approaches was used. These approaches included, but were not limited to, instructional strategies that were learner centered, context oriented, collaborative, experiential, and designed to encourage lifelong learning. In addition to on-line teaching, other interactions were engineered through videoconferencing, audioconferencing, and face-to-face meetings.

Roles and responsibilities of students as well as those of the professors were redefined as everyone learned about the challenges and benefits of the distance media. As Sacks (1996) suggested in his commentary on members of Generation X attending college, professors must learn to apply new technologies that reinforce postmodern arrangements. There is little need for professors to merely disseminate information that can be accessed more easily and quickly by means of the computer and the Internet. Rather, Sacks perceived the professor's role emerging as an "expert consultant" who has two main responsibilities:

> 1) guiding students in the use of information-gathering tools, i.e., helping them learn how to learn; and 2) helping students imagine new ways of looking at knowledge, while prodding them to appreciate subtle complexities about a discipline not obtainable from machines and databases. (p. 180)

LEARNING ENVIRONMENTS

"Applications of Rehabilitation Technology" was third in the sequence of the master's courses. As the professor, I was welcomed into what was already developing as a learning community. Determined to play an active role in becoming part of this community and nurturing it further, I included aspects of the three learning environments that Thornburg (1994) described using the archetypes of the campfire, the watering hole, and the cave. First, the campfire was the place where people gathered to learn wisdom from their elders through storytelling. In the rehabilitation technology course, accessing information and knowledge from the experts was an important component of learning about the world of assistive technology (AT). When teaching the campus course I regularly invited local AT users to share experiences and offer advice to students as the students began their class projects. In the distance course I invited experts to present written "Web-lectures" and follow them up with on-line discussions with students. This practice expanded my list of guest lecturers to individuals living across the United States, without incurring travel expenses. Second, Thornburg distinguished the watering hole from the campfire by emphasizing the teaching and learning that occurred among peers in an informal setting. "Just as water is necessary for survival, the informational aspect of the watering hole is necessary for cultural survival" (p. 167). Because these graduate students were practicing rehabilitation counselors, they had a great deal of information and experience to share with one another, and they soon learned that they had more familiarity with ATs than they originally stated. I discovered that the brainstorming activities I conducted in my campus course could be duplicated on-line. Presenting scenarios on the discussion board about people with disabilities stimulated students to explore Web resources and encouraged creative thinking about AT solutions. Each comment built on a previous response, similar to a classroom discussion. The third environment, the cave, represents the setting in which people reflect on what has been learned and incorporate knowledge into their personal belief systems. Students were urged not only to share reactions through their on-line responses but also to reflect on how they were using this knowledge on a daily basis. Given that the on-line students were practicing professionals, they had immediate opportunities to translate theory to practice and apply their new skills in their work environments. Feedback throughout and at the end of the course reflected the effectiveness of this learning process.

Transferring curriculum to this new medium was challenging. I was initially apprehensive about whether I could adequately convey my passion for AT on-line. I found out that by using videotapes, audiotapes, and writing as enthusiastically as I speak my students clearly sensed my level of interest and commitment. Activities that I did in my campus class to encourage interaction and spark creativity could be accomplished on-line but required a slightly different approach, such as setting up small groups that could meet for synchronous or asynchronous discussions. Integrating opportunities for students to learn from the experts, to learn from one another, and to have time to become reflective practitioners were important strategies used throughout the courses. Moreover, I have been able to introduce on-line resources and guest speakers to on-campus students, enhancing their use of instructional technology.

TEACHING AND LEARNING MODELS

A number of teaching and learning models were used to engage students as active participants in the learning process and that added to the richness of the learning community. Experiential learning, learner-centered education, lifelong learning, and cooperative learning were all integrated into SDSU's on-line master's program.

Experiential Learning

Learning about ATs by means of instructional technologies presented the cohort with the unique opportunity to experience firsthand the challenge of integrating technology into one's lifestyle. This type of experiential learning helped to familiarize students with some of the psychological aspects of becoming comfortable with technology. Many innovative programs incorporate a number of strategies to enhance experiential learning. For example, cohorts are often organized to help establish a learning community (Bullough & Gitlin, 1995), an approach that was embraced by SDSU in creating this degree program. In addition, mentoring was provided in a variety of ways. Students from this cohort were mentored and supported by other graduate students who had taken the campus version of the course and likewise, students in the course were expected to provide mentoring to students in future cohorts.

Learner-Centered Education

> The focus on individuality, on the personal benefits and the utility of education, has a rich tradition in American higher education. (Boyer, 1987, p. 67)

Given this interest in meeting the individual interests of students, it might seem logical that education be learner centered. History tells us otherwise. By the end of the 1980s, lecture was still the most preferred method of instruction, according to the Carnegie Foundation's extensive studies of undergraduate education (Boyer, 1987). Paulo Freire's (1970) description of the *banking* concept of education defines the limitations of this approach. A banking approach to education positions the teachers as the depositors and the students as depositories. The danger, Freire argued, is that "knowledge is [seen as] a gift bestowed by those who consider themselves knowledgeable upon those whom they consider to know nothing" (p. 58). This unidirectional approach in which the control of information belongs to the instructor does little to motivate most learners.

A learner-centered approach is more likely to address motivational questions as well as issues of power and control. With the advancement of technology and increase in teaching by distance communication modes, research is emerging about learner-centered education. "Teaching through discussion relies on a learner-centered approach, whether the participants meet face to face, or on the computer screen. It rests on principles of collaborative learning and egalitarian relationships" (Rohfeld & Hiemstra, 1995, p. 1). Studies have indicated that placing students in the center of the learning process encourages active participation, increased self-esteem, and improved interpersonal relationships (Jones & Young, 1997). Furthermore, enabling students to become more active in guiding the learning process may uncover "the hidden power faculty exert when they claim responsibility for guiding and teaching knowledge" (Jones & Young, 1997, p. 100). Students in this cohort commented repeatedly on the learner-centeredness of this program. They felt that their voices were heard, whether the communication was by means of e-mail, telephone, fax, or in person.

Lifelong Learning

As early as 1931, Alfred North Whitehead proposed that "education must now be defined as a lifelong process of continuing inquiry. And so the most important learning of all—for both children and adults—is learning how to learn, acquiring the skills of self-directed inquiry" (as cited in Knowles, 1990, p. 167). His insights were based on the increasingly rapid cultural changes that people were experiencing in their lifetimes. Moreover, if humans were going to be prepared to continually face new situations and conditions, they must be educated to do so. Some 40 years later, Faure and his associates observed that "education was preparing men for a type of society which does not yet exist" (as cited in Knowles, 1990, p. 168), reaffirming the concept of lifelong learning. Many other educational thinkers followed suit, offering the support of such approaches as "innovative learning" versus "maintenance learning" (Botkin, Elmandjra, & Salitza, 1979) and "systems theory and holistic thinking" (Capra, 1983). Knowles (1990) proposed a complex system of lifelong learning in the context of a learning community that suggested identifying new roles and competencies for learners and instructors as well as tapping other potential learning resources in a community.

Distance education is well suited for encouraging the pursuit of lifelong learning. Throughout their courses, students were provided with strategies to find resources, scenarios to develop problem-solving skills, and opportunities to challenge traditional perspectives in light of new knowledge. Geographical boundaries no longer limited their ability to find solutions. Expertise was made available beyond the duration of the course through continued networking and electronic communication.

Cooperative Learning

The essence of community lies in collaboration, with people working together and sharing responsibility that requires everyone's unique and individual talents (McKnight, 1995). Cooperative learning is based on this concept; that is, each person assumes specific responsibilities toward an identified goal. Institutions, organizations, and other programs that promote collaboration do not always model it themselves, as it is often easier to talk about than to practice. The distance program modeled collaboration in a number of ways. The state and the university developed cooperative agreements to establish the degree program on-line; state administrators collaborated with district offices to support the employees who became part of the cohort; and instructional designers and professors worked together to design and implement the coursework. Collaboration across a variety of disciplines is even more challenging but may offer potential for new thinking and innovative approaches that result from the cross-fertilization of ideas (Helgesen, 1995). In the "Applications of Rehabilitation Technology" course students were required to develop interdisciplinary tech teams to address AT needs (Sax, Fisher, & Pumpian, 1996). Students interacted with local experts, including rehabilitation engineers, physical and occupational therapists, speech and language specialists, employers, and coworkers, and they interacted by distance with experts through the professional networks identified by the professor. Collaboration benefited all participants, especially the focus individual (i.e., person with a disability interested in AT) who played a key role in the assessment process and in identifying possibilities for AT equipment, services, or both.

MODELS IN PRACTICE

These teaching and learning models were central to the rehabilitation technology course (Sax, 2000). Designing the class to meet the needs of the students was the first step in ensuring that the instruction would be learner centered. Because the students were all full-time rehabilitation counselors, they were provided readings, videos, and assignments that related directly to their professional responsibilities. They were offered names of local AT or rehabilitation engineering experts and encouraged to find generic resources available in their communities. The flow of the course was also modified as necessary. For instance, before the third week of class, the use of a discussion board was introduced as an alternative to sending e-mail messages on the class listserv. Although most students felt that the number of e-mail messages was becoming increasingly cumbersome, other formats were unfamiliar. The generally positive mood of the class changed drastically when the new format was presented. "That @#$#$% Message Board" became the most frequently used title in e-mail messages as students rebelled against the new strategy. It was likely that, given more time, students would realize the advantages to using the board. At that point, they were obviously feeling overwhelmed by yet another new phase of this technology. Not only were they learning unfamiliar content, but they were also expected to master new ways of class participation essentially on their own, albeit with on-line instructions. A "deal" was offered to the students. If they would give the board another chance, their course requirements would be reduced. The response was reassuring. Luis wrote,

> I haven't made up my mind about the Message Board yet, since I know that I personally need time to "warm up" to new changes. I'm willing to continue the trial run, and I'm thankful for your "spirit of cooperation." One of the strongest aspects of this program is the staff's willingness to

listen to feedback from the students and to work with it in making the program as user friendly as possible. Thanks for the concession!

David agreed but acknowledged that others were not feeling comfortable with the changes.

Again, just for the record, I really like the message board. I think it has a lot more positives then negatives. But, as our [former] President might say, "I feel your pain," and I can understand some of the frustrations.

Glenda explained her perspective next:

Your diplomacy is extremely effective, I feel like I am getting used to the new wrinkle in how we do business, and I know the bugs will get worked out soon . . . However, as any good Teamster, I will go with the crowd for the benefit of happy campers all around? Hang in, we whined about fieldwork too!

After this trial by fire, the class rallied and mastered the use of the board over the next several weeks. The technical support staff played an important role in building the level of skill and comfort and often guided individuals through the process over the telephone. Meanwhile, the students felt acknowledged and respected, and the community feeling grew as they first commiserated about their frustrations and later celebrated their accomplishments. The bargaining chip was secondary to the "spirit of cooperation" that led to a solution.

SIGNS OF A LEARNING COMMUNITY

The unique culture of the group included good-natured bantering and shared stories about prior courses and work-related events; however, not everyone reached the same comfort level at the same speed. Although some students used terms such as "incredible" and "amazing" to describe the knowledge and resources they were accessing, other students described their initial experiences as "overwhelming," "terrifying," and "intimidating." One phrase that was already becoming legendary was the ending disclaimer, "it's just my opinion, I may be wrong," revealing a sense of humor, humility, a spirit of cooperation, and a request not to be judged, all at the same time. In the context of this collegial atmosphere, two other dimensions of community were noted: building professional and personal relationships.

Building Professional Relationships

Students in distance courses have a great deal of control over their learning (Rohfeld & Hiemstra, 1995). They decide when to log on and how much they want to participate. In the "Applications of Rehabilitation Technology" course students also determined how they were going to complete group work with their colleagues. They had the choice of using real time—that is, synchronous—interactions (e.g., a chat room) or asynchronous interactions, which enabled each person to log on at his or her convenience (e.g., the group listserv). Students had mixed reactions to the group experiences. Some felt that, as in any group work situation, the workload was often difficult to share equitably. A number of assignments seemed to be better suited for group work, such as the task of compiling a list of questions for guest lecturers. Interaction with the guest lecturers expanded their professional network and lent more professionalism to the class in general. The students welcomed the guests and offered advice to help them learn about the distance learning strategies.

The community spirit continued to grow as students tried more problem solving and brainstorming on-line. They shared secrets of acquiring supports and services for their constituents and offered suggestions for tapping into community resources. Their respect for one another on a professional level increased. Several students collaborated outside of class to submit a proposal to initiate a peer mentoring program, based on information from a guest lecturer. Discussions at a meeting held several weeks after the course ended also revealed the strength of these professional relationships. Several students commented on their increasing confidence in approaching their jobs and their interactions with people with disabilities. Although they were frustrated about not having enough time to share what they were learning with their coworkers and supervisors, they claimed to have experienced a new level of awareness in self-evaluation and recognized the value in what they were accomplishing.

Building Personal Relationships

The increase in electronic communication has led to new rules for interaction in cyberspace. Although electronic communication can offer a sense of security and anonymity to those who might otherwise "sit quietly in the back of the room," personal relationships form just as they would in a physical classroom. Students clearly developed friendships with people in the class. During the series of courses, students shared news of births, deaths, promotions, conferences, and suggestions of places to go for dinner in each others' cities. Students in the class who had disabilities themselves had the option of sharing that information if and when they chose to do so. As the students began to trust one another, several shared personal experiences related to their disabilities and to the accommodations that they required for full participation in the class.

The majority of class interaction took place in writing, but additional opportunities for "face-to-face" time occurred in all of the courses. Each instructor prepared videotaped instruction for students to view. In addition, some courses included desktop videoconferences, where students gathered at four sites designated in the state to communicate with the instructor and each other via the computer screen. All four sites were linked to the main site, and each computer featured each group in a quarter of the screen. Researchers are investigating interpersonal connections via computers (Eastmond, 1992; Florini, 1989), raising the notion that more efforts should be focused on how to use computers to improve and expand on human contact rather than negating it (Phillips, 1995). The kind of camaraderie displayed in this program does not develop on its own but rather must be purposefully nurtured to foster the high quality of personal interactions. Once again, everyone has a role to play in building a feeling of community. When cohort members met in person, it seemed that many personal relationships transferred from virtual space to real space. Although not everyone felt the same level of trust in person that they had on-line, the overall atmosphere was friendly, supportive, and respectful, and contradicted the criticism that distance education is impersonal.

REFLECTIONS FROM A DISTANCE

Since this first cohort of students graduated in spring 2000, more than 200 students, representing 18 states and 3 Pacific jurisdictions, have enrolled in this on-line graduate program. This called for new organizational and administrative structures and strategies. The percentage of students with disabilities participating in these courses remains consistent at about 15%. Accommodations provided for students include, but are not limited to, the following:

- Videotapes are captioned and transcribed, with transcriptions posted on the Web site.
- Videotapes are copied to audiotapes for students with visual impairments.
- Materials are labeled in Braille.
- Web site information, including course readings and presentations, are screen reader accessible.
- Streaming videos on the Web site are open captioned.
- Interpreters are hired as necessary for special assignments.

Research that goes beyond merely addressing the comparison of distance programs with on-campus programs is beginning to emerge (Eldredge et al., 1999; Smart, 1999). As Smart wrote in a special issue of the journal

Rehabilitation Education that featured distance learning, "distance education is a model that demands serious study, more than just simply comparing it to on-campus education" (p. 201). At the time of this writing, follow-up surveys to determine the extent to which students have integrated the approaches to AT assessment and service delivery into their job responsibilities have been designed to investigate further implications of the students' experiences. Overall, reactions from students in the online "Applications of Rehabilitation Technology" course have been overwhelmingly positive and demonstrate the potential impact of this medium. One student, who noted that she had been a counselor for 25 years, wrote the following:

> This course opened the door to my transformation into a different counselor. I have a list of tools at my fingertips so that I stop the dependence that has, heretofore, been a burden on me. I will give the honor of managing the details to my clients so that they do not see this journey as welfare. I have gotten much friendlier with the computer, and hence, a new world.

Creating a sense of belonging, or community, in education sets the stage for the development and support of new perspectives (Sergiovanni, 1994). "Community is the tie that binds students and teachers together . . . to something more significant than themselves: shared values and ideals" (p. xiii). Furthermore, Sergiovanni suggested that becoming a community of learners can be an "adventure in shared leadership and authentic relationships" (p. 155). If continuing education is designed to produce better educated professionals who are capable of improving the services that they provide and changing the larger system in which they work, then students must feel that their contributions are recognized and valued. It is clear that shared leadership and authentic relationships can happen on-line as well as in the classroom. In this degree program, instructors and students alike have taken responsibility, and can take credit, for strengthening their learning community, virtual and otherwise.

REFERENCES

Berge, Z. (1996). *The role of the online instructor/facilitator* [On-line]. Available: http://star.ucc.nau.edu/~mauri/moderate/teach_online.html

Berge, Z. (1998). Conceptual frameworks in distance training and education. In D. A. Schreiber & Z. L. Berge (Eds.), *Distance training: How innovative organizations are using technology to maximize learning and meet business objectives* (pp. 19–36). San Francisco: Jossey-Bass.

Botkin, J. W., Elmandjra, M., & Salitza, M. (1979). *No limits to learning.* New York: Pergamon Press.

Boyer, E. L. (1987). *College: The undergraduate experience in America*. New York: Harper & Row.

Bullough, R. V., Jr., & Gitlin, A. (1995). *Becoming a student of teaching: Methodologies for exploring self and school context*. New York: Garland.

Capra, F. (1983). *The turning point: Science, society, and the rising culture*. New York: Bantam Books.

Deloro, J. (1997). *Web school: Interactive distance learning puts college and corporate classrooms online* [On-line]. Available: http://www.eyemedia.com/backissues/1997/0897/9708distmain.htm

Dringus, L. P., & Terrell, S. (1999). The framework for DIRECTED online learning environments. *The Internet and Higher Education, 2*(1), 55–67.

Eastmond, D. V. (1992). Effective facilitation of computer conferencing. *Continuing Higher Education Review, 56*, 155–167.

Eldredge, G. M., McNamara, S., Stensrud, R., Gilbride, D., Hendren, G., Siegfried, T., & McFarlane, F. (1999). Distance education: A look at five programs. *Rehabilitation Education, 13*, 231–248.

Florini, B. (1989). Teaching styles and technology. In E. R. Hayes (Ed.), *Effective teaching styles: New directions for adult and continuing education* (pp. 41–53). San Francisco: Jossey-Bass.

Foa, L., Schwab, R. L., & Johnson, M. (1996, May 1). Upgrading school technology. *Education Week*, pp. 40–41.

Freire, P. (1970). *Pedagogy of the oppressed*. New York: Continuum.

Helgesen, S. (1995). *The web of inclusion*. New York: Doubleday.

Jones, T., & Young, G. S. A. (1997). Classroom dynamics: Disclosing the hidden curriculum. In A. I. Morey & M. Kitano (Eds.), *Multicultural course transformation in higher education: A broader truth* (pp. 89–103). Boston: Allyn & Bacon.

Knowles, M. (1990). *The adult learner: A neglected species* (4th ed.). Houston, TX: Gulf.

McKnight, J. (1995). *The careless society: Community and its counterfeits*. New York: Basic Books.

Meyen, E. L., Lian, C. H. T., & Tangen, P. (1997). Developing online instruction: One model. *Focus on Autism and Other Developmental Disabilities, 12*, 159–165.

Palloff, R. M., & Pratt, K. (1999). *Building learning communities in cyberspace: Effective strategies for the online classroom*. San Francisco: Jossey-Bass.

Phillips, G. (1995). Creating a real group in a virtual world. *Interpersonal Computing and Technology: An Electronic Journal for the 21st Century, 3*(4), 42–56.

Rehabilitation Act Amendments of 1992, Pub. L. No. 102-336, § 101 (a)(7)(B).

Rohfeld, R. W., & Hiemstra, R. (1995). *Moderating discussions in the electronic classroom* [On-line]. Available: http://star.ucc.nau.edu/~mauri/moderate/rohfeld.html

Sacks, P. (1996). *Generation X goes to college: An eye-opening account of teaching in postmodern America*. Chicago: Open Court.

Sax, C. (2000). Distance education: Taking it to the next level. In *Proceedings of the RESNA 2000 annual conference* (160–162). Arlington, VA: RESNA Press.

Sax, C., Fisher, D., & Pumpian, I. (1996). Outcomes for students with severe disabilities: Case studies on the use of assistive technology in inclusive classrooms. *Technology & Disability, 5,* 327–334.

Scollin, P. A., & Tello, S. F. (1999). Implementing distance learning: Frameworks for change. *The Internet and Higher Education, 2*(1), 11–20.

Sergiovanni, T. (1994). *Building community in schools.* San Francisco: Jossey-Bass.

Smart, J. (1999). Issues in rehabilitation distance education. *Rehabilitation Education, 13,* 187–206.

Thornburg, D. (1994). *Education in the communication age.* San Carlos, CA: Starsong.

Warn, M. M., Compton, C., Levine, S., & Whitteker, S. (1998). Graduate programs at a distance: A partnership between the California Department of Rehabilitation and San Diego University. In D. A. Schreiber & Z. L. Berge (Eds.), *Distance training: How innovative organizations are using technology to maximize learning and meet business objectives* (pp. 155–184). San Francisco: Jossey-Bass.

14

THE COUNSELING PROCESS IN ASSISTIVE TECHNOLOGY EDUCATION AND SELECTION

SERENELLA BESIO

All the actions that might be described as "transfer of knowledge" about assistive technology (AT) to end users have, over time, shifted from a technology-centered approach toward a user-centered one. In the wake of recent epistemological reflections, the carers' objective and external position toward their object has been definitively called into question (Gadamer, 1994). Indeed, scholars have stressed the special position of carers "inside the system" (Cecchin, 1987), with a specific accent on the influence exerted by their prejudices, knowledge, feelings, opinions, reactions, and personal stories.[1] The carer's description of the user's situation and the "punctuation" he or she establishes are connected in a special way to his or her own world of ideas, feelings, and perceptions. This description can no longer be considered objective and identical for all.

Consequently, help, care, and cure relationships have acquired a less deterministic perspective, becoming more open to discussion and continuous redefinition of their objectives, purposes, and results. At the same time, the user has become a fully fledged protagonist in this relationship, a source of knowledge and possibilities, a partner in the decision-making process.

KNOWLEDGE TRANSFER PROCESSES AND THE END USER'S ROLE

The European project EUSTAT (Empowering USers Through Assistive Technology)—financed within the Telematics Application Programme

---

[1] The notion of prejudice is essential in the recent development of the systemic approach (Cecchin, Lane, & Ray, 1994).

—has just come to an end.[2] The project participants developed ideas and materials directed toward the empowerment of people with disabilities and elderly people, helping them to become the protagonists of their own pathways toward autonomy and independent living (Neath & Reed, 1998; Singers & Powers, 1993; Thomas & Velthouse, 1990). EUSTAT explored the role of AT in this pathway. The different methodologies of transferring AT knowledge to the end user have been classified in three main typologies: counseling, education, and information.

Information (including awareness campaigns) plays a major role in notion and competence dissemination while not seeking to increase the individual's ability to take initiative. Counseling, on the other hand, is a well-defined set of actions aimed at changing something in a person's life. Education lies between the two, having a balanced interest in both objectives (increasing competence and initiative).

In these processes the actors differ, as do the relationships that are established among them during the knowledge transfer process. Nonetheless, they can be placed along a continuous line, as in Figure 14.1.

Although the main relationship between the professional (or the peer counselor) and the end user is formally defined and structured, in any informational activity this relationship is more informal and less dependent on specific rules. These processes also differ in the kind and number of people to whom they are mainly addressed: Whereas the counseling process is generally addressed to a specific individual, information can be addressed to a large and undetermined public. In both cases (target group and relation), the educational process is situated in the middle.

No magazine, newspaper, or communication medium will underestimate the end user's importance; no information service will disregard customer approach techniques. The role of the user (in the guise of consumer) is even more evident in the case of advertising.

During the past few years, the AT user's decisive role has been recognized by the pedagogical sciences, where an unquestionable shift has occurred from a behavioral methodology of knowledge transfer to a cooperative one (Duffy, Lowick, & Jonassen, 1993; Slavin, 1990).[3]

Methodological models, as well as theoretical reflections and practical examples, are being proposed for the knowledge transfer process across Europe, but comparing them proves difficult. Furthermore, the

---

[2] The project involved five European partners (from Italy, Belgium, France, Portugal, and Denmark) representing research institutions and associations of people with disabilities, under the guidance of SIVA in Milan, Italy. For more information, visit the Web site http://www.siva.it/research/eustat.
[3] The European project HEART Project Consortium has produced interesting materials in this field (HEART project Consortium, 1994).

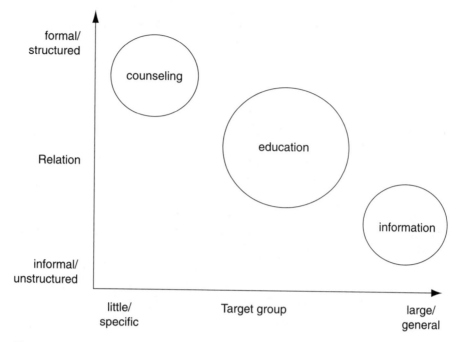

Figure 14.1. From *Deliverable D03.2: Critical Factors Involved in End-Users' Education in Relation to Assistive Technology* (p. 37) by EUSTAT Consortium, 1998, Brussels, Belgium: European Commission DG XIII, Telematics Application Programme. Copyright 1998 by European Commission DG XIII, Telematics Application Programme. Adapted by permission.

lack of a common language and terminology does not make dialogue any easier.[4]

SOME REFLECTIONS ABOUT THE COUNSELING PROCESS IN AT CHOICE

The user-centered approach has also been gaining ground, although with difficulty, within the counseling process. In this context a special relationship is established between a professional and an end user; problems are considered in detail and, whenever possible, solved. Information given in counseling should be tuned to the client in terms of content, modalities, and typology, but it should also involve all the right, possible, and needed

---

[4]The EUSTAT D04.2 study has been totally devoted to in-depth investigation of the educational initiatives in the field of AT already under way both inside and outside Europe (Besio & EUSTAT Consortium, 1998).

partners. The counselor should be able to understand the specific moment in the end user's life in which the request is expressed and to catch the right moment and the right ways to deliver the information. This should be done without saying too much or too little, without giving rise to fears or underestimating difficulties, without taking sides when the decision is up to the end user. If and only if all these conditions—and some others— are fulfilled can knowledge transfer trigger a process of individual change toward autonomy and independent living. The authors of the EUSTAT study (EUSTAT Consortium) proposed a representation of the decision-making process that leads the individual to identify, choose, and obtain the AT appropriate to his or her level of autonomy (see Figure 14.2).

Each of the stages depicted in Figure 14.2 can take place within a negotiation process, a constructive dialogue between one or more professionals (or peer counselors) and the end user. This clearly shows how the whole

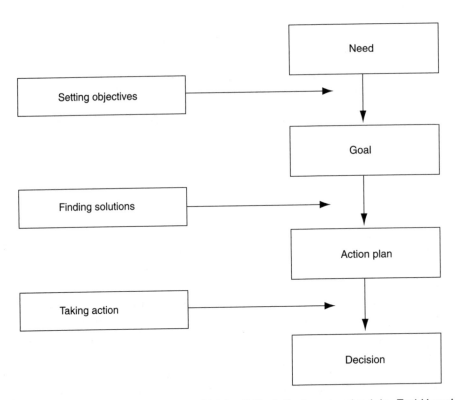

Figure 14.2. From *Deliverable D03.2: Critical Factors Involved in End-Users' Education in Relation to Assistive Technology* (p. 43) by EUSTAT Consortium, 1998, Brussels, Belgium: European Commission DG XIII, Telematics Application Programme. Copyright 1998 by European Commission DG XIII, Telematics Application Programme. Adapted by permission.

process needs to be grounded on equality and coparticipation among the actors involved. There is general recognition in the field of rehabilitation psychology of the strong, direct connection between the decision process leading to the acquisition of AT and the sciences of human relationships and dialogue: in short, the psychological sciences.

In this chapter, instead of considering the many different action models, I present a reflection, following the systemic approach (Hershenson, 1998; Hoffman, 1981; Malagoli Togliatti & Telfener, 1983). Through this reflection I examine the contribution that psychological thought may offer to the AT counseling process (Besio, 1997).

A Simple Addition?

Consider the process of AT identification, choice, and counseling from an essentially psychological perspective. On the one hand, many international-level studies and initiatives have linked the concept of autonomy for people with disabilities to their human relationships.[5] On the other hand, the role of AT in favor of the autonomy of people with disabilities is being ever more widely recognized and seen as incontrovertible.[6] To complete the picture, it is worth mentioning that personal autonomy is the main goal of many psychological therapies regardless of the chosen approach.

Consequently, things might seem quite simple. A person with a disability wants to achieve a more satisfactory level of autonomy, so he or she needs information. In his or her research this person is supported by a widespread social movement that claims full independence for people with disabilities as a civil right. In addition, social and health services are likely to be available, along with helping and supportive professionals who possess information, know methodologies, adopt a user-centered perspective, and agree on the goal of individual autonomy.

In this way, the decision process might simply seem to be the result of a sum of addends—but the sum does not always add up. This process does not always unfold in a plain and painless way, as if it were a flowchart on paper.

---

[5]Two action programs of the European Commission promoting equal opportunities and the integration of people with disabilities, namely HELIOS I (1988–1991) and HELIOS II (1992–1996), proposed a definition of the concept of *autonomy* as a dynamic process that includes the individual's point of view, the family's viewpoint, the immediate outer circle, and society. Consequently, four domains of autonomy were described: body and mind, home and family, community, and society (Andrich & Porqueddu, 1990).

[6]This matter is amply covered in the international literature in the field; here I cite only Swain, Finkelstein, French, and Oliver (1993).

Giving Meaningfulness to Life Systems: Whom to Involve

Obviously it is not possible to provide an exhaustive review of all the personal variables that might have a significant influence on clinical counseling in the field of AT. However well-prepared a counselor may be, however detailed the information file is on the end user, the actual meeting with the real system[7]—with the group of people who, here and now, are present in the session—is always a different matter. There are thousands of details that cannot possibly be foreseen a priori. Thousands of variables may influence the relationship climate, the mood of the meeting, its success, the released emotions. Some issues will be explicitly expressed, whereas others, although momentous, will be barely perceptible; others will be just waiting for somebody to bring them to light, and speaking about them will be resolutive.

The main problem is that counseling never involves only one person, only one user, as if he or she were an island disconnected from its surroundings, as Figure 14.2 might suggest. On the contrary, counseling involves the user as a system and therefore as a part of many intertwined life environments and relationships. At the very moment counseling is requested, and on the basis of the kind of request, only some of these environments and relationships will acquire meaningfulness, that is, acquire the characteristic of a significant figure set against the background of a rich and complex life.

The nuclear family, or the extended family, or more than one family unit, might be involved in the process; it might also be useful to involve the rehabilitation system, the health care system, or school system. Sometimes the request for counseling does not come from the person with a disability but from someone related to him or her—for example, teachers or a rehabilitation professional; in this case, the person with a disability remains in the background.

The choice of meaningful systems is to some extent arbitrary, because it is based on diagnostic and prognostic hypotheses, general ideas, and prejudices that the counselor may use from time to time. For this reason, the counselor's knowledge and control of his or her own work methodology, adopted choice criteria, and the project to be developed take on a crucial level of importance.

There are two key moments for deciding which systems should be involved in the counseling session. The first concerns the data collection that precedes the session itself. The main aim of this is to investigate (a)

---

[7]The definition of *system* used in the approach of the same name derives, with further elaboration, from the general system theory. From a historical perspective, the family has been the most exhaustively studied system in psychology. It has been said of the family (although the same might be true of any human system) that each member influences the others and in turn is influenced by them; each member acts on the system but is influenced by the communication received from the system itself (Selvini Palazzoli, Prata, Boscolo, & Cecchin, 1975; Minuchin & Fishman, 1982).

what exactly is being requested; (b) who is making the request; (c) how many and to which systems the request belongs; and (d) how many and what systems the request involves, even if not directly.

This analysis allows the counselor to decide not only whom to invite to the counseling session but also who cannot be invited. It indicates whether there is general agreement or conflict regarding the request and has the additional purpose of determining which professionals will participate in the counseling session.

The second key moment takes place during the counseling itself. When the skein begins to unravel, and the counselor begins to find his or her way through the various facets of the request, the picture of the user's significant relationships becomes increasingly clear, as does their relative importance to the request being discussed. During the data collection phase, some of them might have been overlooked. It also becomes clearer whether there is a need to involve yet other systems or to reduce the total number of systems involved in the decision.

Adopting a systemic perspective means, at the very outset, investigating life systems, their relations, and their ethical and ideal values, as well as their prejudices. Neglecting a significant system might lead a project to failure; underestimating an important member's opinion might result in the planning of unfeasible actions.

By placing full trust in the systems and their possibilities of self-fulfilment (Cecchin, Lane, & Ray, 1992), the relationship between the user and the counselor becomes clearly defined. This relationship connects the constraints and possibilities each one is able to evaluate and describe; in any case, it implies a prospect of change.

Constraints and Possibilities: Toward the Future

By itself, a knowledge transfer process can trigger a change (in accordance with Figure 14.2, one ought to say "produce a decision") only when the recipients of this information are to some extent ready to enact that change, when their perceptions of ways of life, human relationships and their own possibilities and abilities, as well as their awareness of their own needs, allow them to accept new ways of thinking.

If this is the case, a situation considered unsatisfactory can be modified by any of several options: a technical journal, a television program, word of mouth, a telephone information service, a rehabilitation professional's suggestion. The same role can be performed by an educational activity, which can give rise to specific individual interests and can suggest new ideas and solutions.

Sometimes, however, a person's situation in life and human relationships, his or her self-perception and self-esteem, personal view of future possibilities, and evaluation of his or her own potential and abilities may not allow any prospect of change. In these cases information alone is absolutely ineffectual in bringing about modification. On the contrary, it can become counterproductive, strengthening the individual's self-perception of being defeated and unable to change. In these cases the counseling session brings into play the building (or rather, the cobuilding between the systems involved) of a feasible future (Boscolo & Cecchin, 1988). This is a difficult and unpredictable task.

At the end of the counseling process there will no longer be simply the end user's idea of his or her own future and the counselor's idea of the end user's future. Rather, a third idea (or, more exactly, a group of third ideas) will be built out of the dialogue between the two (or among all the systems involved), a result of the logical—and emotionally expressed—analysis of the system's real developmental possibilities.

Of what, exactly, does this work consist? Actually, a change comes into play anyway in the user–counselor relationship; this may happen precisely as a consequence of the introduction of new information by the counseling professional (Dell, 1980).

What kind of new information is introduced? One example is technical information about one or more ATs that might make some daily activities easier. If correctly presented, this information allows the user to outline the scenario of a feasible future, one in which his or her personal and relational daily life differs from the present one (Boscolo & Cecchin, 1981). This kind of information may offer a new sort of lifestyle, disclose secret hopes, or reveal an idea of the world.

By using the idea of the future, the information throws the user into a hypothetical world that seems feasible, near at hand, and achievable but, in some cases, the acceptance of new theories and new concepts of the world is needed (Caillé, 1981).

So, the counselor outlines a possible scenario, triggers some hopes, suggests some desirable possibilities for the user's life. These possibilities are firmly linked to the counselor's analysis of the user's situation as the counselor evaluates it—the constraints, in the counselor's view (Ceruti, 1996).

But this scenario may conflict with the user's deeply rooted perception of his or her own situation as a constraint: "Oh yes, it would be wonderful, but it will never be for me." Evidently, the possibilities the user is able to make out are very different. The counselor knows that change cannot be pushed in the desired direction: Change can be hypothesized, not directed (Dell, 1980).

The user may feel oppressed by a difficult situation that he or she considers more arduous and intolerable than ever before, now that he or she has found a touchstone. However, the user can be helped to describe these constraints in detail and can make them explicit, analyze them, and weigh them up. Furthermore, an analysis of the systems involved in his or her perception of the constraints and the feasible possibilities may give rise to new information. The user system can be extended toward the outside, by including other ones, thus introducing new perspectives. During the discussion, the user system itself (or the family system) can discover new, heretofore unseen resources and new energies for working toward the solution. Or it can discover that the perception of insuperable constraints is due to a faulty or inaccurate picture of the situation or to the lack of sharing of awareness within the system itself.

During the conversation that takes place in the counseling session, the perceived constraints may be understood differently because they are set against a new background and compared. They involve new perspectives on life and new systems; they assume different shapes, weights, and values, revealing themselves to be resolvable or not. By comparing the ideal dreamed-of possibility on the one hand, and the reshaped constraints on the other hand, by confronting the counselor's and the user's ideas, the concrete project will emerge: the possible possibility.

SOME CLINICAL CASE STUDIES

Next I present some cases from the work experience of Servizio Informazione Valutazione Ausili (SIVA), an AT consulting service in Milan, Italy.[8] These cases illustrate, in the traditional pathway of case narration, how a systemic approach can prove fruitful in making decisions regarding AT and how the dialogue between constraints and possibilities can be conducted, with a different shape and different solution being found on each separate occasion.[9] I also comment on each case, seeking to stress the development of the decision-making process in accordance with the graph presented in Figure 14.2.

---

[8]The SIVA consulting service is run by a multidisciplinary team that includes physiotherapists, occupational therapists, a computer technician, and a psychologist. It is run as a daily service that provides advice on AT matters for users, families, professionals, teachers, and so on. This is done by means of appointments and via telephone and mail. The service does not offer diagnosis, prescription, or psychological therapy but rather advice and information. In some cases it fulfills the functions of counseling, supervision, and evaluation. The SIVA team makes use of its own computerized information system on technical aids, other national and international databases, and an AT device exhibit, in which end users try out technical devices. The organization's working methodology, already described at the international level (Andrich, 1993), is still undergoing experimentation and research (Andrich, 1996; Besio, 1997).

[9]The clinical and health aspects of the cases presented, as well as the technical solutions singled out, have been deliberately outlined rather than described in detail, because the emphasis here is on the development of the counseling session as a process between the poles in dialogue.

Why Am I Here? The Real Problem Lies Elsewhere

Anna, age 7, sees a speech therapist who believes that Anna has a reading and writing impairment. The speech therapist would like to know if suitable educational software might be useful in rehabilitation. She would also like to discuss Anna's use of the computer as a technical aid for writing.

During the counseling session the therapist's diagnostic hunches will need to be clarified; consequently, the role of the computer and the educational software, as well as their usefulness for remedial school learning, might be considered and discussed.

Anna's father, her speech therapist, and her class teacher all attended the meeting, bringing with them many of Anna's exercise books. When the counselor asked for a description of the problem, the father called on the two women to speak. The teacher and the speech therapist described the situation in detail, showing Anna's spelling mistakes and explaining their efforts at remediation. A diagnosis has not yet been made, but the two professionals are worried: Anna is clever, but she has difficulty in learning to read and write, and she makes too many mistakes. While they speak, the speech therapist and the teacher repeatedly look at Anna's father, seeking confirmation and trying to obtain his approval. During this presentation the father sits side on in a serious pose and takes a lot of notes in a little notebook. When asked by the counselor whether he agrees with the description, the father answered in a professional tone, adding some more details about Anna's study skills. The teacher adds a point that the counselor considers enlightening: The father is a teacher, too; he works in Anna's school and is well known for his professional competence.

The counselor decides to allow Anna's father to show his parenting skills, leaving his professional role behind. She asks him about his daughter's activities at home: her games, interests, likes, and dislikes. The father is reluctant at the beginning but outlines the picture of a girl always on the point of being happy, without actually managing to be. She likes somebody to read stories to her but is always afraid that the story won't have a happy ending. She adores flying kites but has asthma and is unable to run for a long time. She is jealous of her sister, so she tries to separate herself, but she is really only happy when the two of them are playing together. She wakes up very often during the night because of bad dreams; she wants to get into her parents' bed but subsequently gets out by herself and goes back to her own bed. All the attempts to help her have been unsuccessful, the father says in a resigned tone; even if the school problem really exists, he and his wife consider it a side issue.

The counselor, realizing the weight these problems pose for Anna's father, agrees with him and suggests deeper examination of this situation with a developmental psychologist or a family therapist; afterward, the learning problem will be reconsidered.

A short time later, the speech therapist calls with an update on the situation. Anna and her family have begun family therapy, and for the moment the girl has stopped attending the rehabilitation service, but according to the teachers she is more relaxed.

Sometimes the needs underlying the received request have yet to be clearly defined, requiring an investigation at the initial stage of the decision process. In this case the family system, with its priorities and expressed suffering, acquires prevalence over the rehabilitation system from which the request first came, as do the needs expressed during the counseling. Was the problem described by the speech therapist negligible? Does Anna present a learning impairment or not? At this moment, from the perspective of the system that has gained greatest significance, these are not the "real" problems. This realization will lead to new solutions, both for the family and Anna.

What Is the Problem? Determining the Diagnosis

The mother of 8-year-old Stefania called for a meeting: She wanted to discuss with some counselors the usefulness of computers for improving Stefania's grades. The mother is quite vague when describing Stefania's problems, saying she has a general developmental delay and has regular sessions with two speech therapists. The telephone interview arouses some perplexities. A clinical investigation was determined to be necessary to understand exactly the problems faced.

Only Stefania's father attends the meeting. The initial conversation serves to sum Stefania's unusual clinical history. According to her father, all the girl's difficulties originated during a period of illness when she was 11 months old. She was admitted to hospital with a severe state of undernourishment, and this caused a delay in her development: She began walking unaided when she was 2 years old and started to speak when she was 5. Her movement and speaking are still somewhat impaired; what's more, she experiences severe obstacles in learning. Her parents have tried a lot of different rehabilitation methodologies and numerous therapies. Now they are wondering if computers and educational software might be useful. They own and use a computer, and Stefania is curious about it, so perhaps this might be a good idea, the parent suggest. The counselor has the feeling that the parents consider the computer an additional therapy to insert into a hectic daily routine.

The long conversation that follows is totally devoted to focusing the father's attention on the possible objectives of computer work. But this matter raises a question: Which of Stefania's problems should be addressed?

From his very first comments, it becomes evident that the father is unwilling to go any further into the matter: He will not permit a discussion of the diagnosis of Stefania's problems. The counselor therefore decides to explain and show just how difficult it is to give suggestions. On the computer she shows the father which educational software or educational projects might be proposed if Stefania's main problem is rooted in a cognitive impairment and what could be adopted if, on the contrary, the problem is mainly of linguistic and gnostic origin. To decide what to do, a diagnosis is needed.

It is only at this point that Stefania's father explains all the difficulties he and his wife have experienced over the years trying to get a clear diagnosis; physicians and experts had never been explicit on this topic. Unfortunately—the counselor says—the response in this clinical field may sometimes be uncertain. Perhaps, however, a highly specialized hospital can be found, one more suited to Stefania's need. The father willingly accepts the address of a university clinic that specializes in the study of neuropsychological developmental pathologies. Some time later, he calls the counselor to announce that clinical examinations of Stefania have begun.

This counseling session is to be classified at the level of goal definition. To define the work objectives, basic information is needed: A precise diagnosis is obviously a prerequisite. Sometimes, especially at the developmental level, the diagnosis might be uncertain or still ongoing. In these cases it may be very difficult to make decisions about the rehabilitation plan, or about the adoption of an AT device, because any decision is related to a diagnostic and prognostic hypothesis. Professionals in the field, as well as the systems involved in AT choice, should be aware of this connection. As to the case itself, is it really possible that none of the specialists had made a diagnosis of Stefania's impairment? Perhaps it is the modalities of the story, rather than its truthfulness, that are worthy of interest. The counselor faces a disoriented father whose main purpose is to seek, to experiment. The first important step in the counseling was the description of this wandering as research. The second step was the exemplification of the practical consequences of a correct diagnostic procedure, connecting diagnosis and rehabilitation. Afterward, the family members need help in finding their way toward a reliable clinical service. In this way, what was the umpteenth grope in the dark— the request for a computer—leads to the definition of a turning point.

What Kind of Future? Awareness of Disability

Oliviero, age 15, has Down's syndrome, a fairly serious cognitive impairment, and severe visual impairment. His teacher called the counselors at SIVA because she wanted to introduce computers into her teaching so that Oliviero's grades in reading and writing could improve.

In the first part of the conversation with the teacher, Oliviero's learning situation emerged: He is still unable to read more than a few letters of the alphabet (providing they are at least 3 cm high), but he cannot name them, neither can he copy them with a pen. He has memorized the spelling of his first name, and he is able to "write" it in a mechanical fashion using some wooden letters. Oliviero is completing his last year of compulsory schooling and will then attend a socioeducational residential center, where he will be mainly involved in recreational activities. He likes using the computer, especially the mouse: He clicks here and there to see what happens on the screen, without any clear plan in mind. According to the teacher, the computer might be useful in teaching Oliviero finally to read and write.

The teacher's ideas about Oliviero's learning abilities in reading and writing seem to clash with the clinical situation described to the counselor. He has not achieved any meta-linguistic awareness and seems to have only a perceptual command of some letters as shapes—a level of learning that, after all, is to be expected given his cognitive impairment. Using a computer doesn't seem a suitable way of compensating for this kind of impairment. During the subsequent conversation, the teacher is asked to put her ideas regarding Oliviero's future into practice. Does she believe that he will be able to read in a functional way during his life? No, she doesn't: The present results were achieved only after a great deal of difficulty. Does she believe that he will be able to recognize his own first name among other words? Perhaps he will, if the words are written in large letters. Does she believe that he will be able to recognize some shop signs, or the metro sign? Yes, perhaps he will; those signs are large enough for him, but the boy may need a long period of training before being able to walk in the street alone.

At this point, the teacher draws her own a conclusion: Perhaps the educational project should be more closely related to the real situation. In this case, the school's duty should be to transfer its knowledge about Oliviero's competence as well as possible to the educators at the socioeducational centre that Oliviero is soon to attend; a wide-ranging work program might be proposed for him, including personal autonomy, orientation, and understanding skills. A computer might be introduced into this program to fulfill different objectives, such as drawing lines and pictures; trying out a small creative project of his own; and then modifying, printing, and reproducing it. Such a project could be Oliviero's original contribution to the small printing office at the socioeducational center.

Sometimes, as in Oliviero's case, work objectives are incorrectly set, not because of a lack of a diagnosis but because of a lack of a proper prognosis. Awareness about the influence of impairment at different chronological ages is extremely important in setting objectives, hence the work project and AT choice. In this case there was some confusion in transposing a diagnosis onto an educational project. The question Oliviero's teacher put to the counselor during their conversation ("Will the computer help Oliviero to learn how to read and write?") can be broken down into two further questions: *Will Oliviero learn how to read and write?* (pertaining to clinical prognosis aspects), and *will the computer be useful in building this boy's future?* (pertaining to the educational project). Once the request has been correctly formulated, the solution lies just around the corner.

Which of Us Is Right? The Moment in Life When Counseling Takes Place

As a consequence of a road accident, Matteo, age 16, sustained tetraplegia, dysarthria, vision impairment, and difficulties in memory and language processing. He also has some behavioral disturbances. His mother asked for a meeting to speak about AT for her son at a general level, above all for home accessibility. She arrived at the meeting with Matteo. She is awaiting a divorce from her husband, but Matteo's father unexpectedly comes to the meeting, too.

Even if Matteo's situation seems difficult at the neuromotor level, it appears to be fairly standard. Matteo lives in an apartment block, so perhaps the situation regarding stairs, lift, bathroom, and furniture should be addressed. Car adaptation might also need to be considered.

During the meeting, Matteo looks indifferent to the events around him, lost in a world of thoughts that make him smile, alone. He answers when questioned but first needs to be shaken out of his torpor. While saying hello to the female counselors, he does not miss the opportunity to address some bawdy comments to them.

The mother presents her request, in the form of an action plan. There is a lift in the block of flats where they live; it is a little bit narrow, but it can be accessed by removing the wheelchair armrests. While she is speaking, her husband contradicts her, questioning her solutions. As a counterproposal, he suggests his own home, which can more easily be made accessible: Only in his house, he says, will Matteo be able to live autonomously. This time his wife abruptly interrupts him in a broken voice: He will never carry out those changes, she knows him all too well.

The dialogue becomes heated. On the pretext of discussing accessibility, Matteo's parents try to convince the counselors that each one's own home is more suitable for Matteo and try to get them to express an opinion: Which one of the two solutions, of the two ways of life, is the right one? The divorce case is under way, and the judge has yet to rule on the boy's custody.

The counselors do not take sides. They state that they understand how complex the situation is and how important the decisions are that the parents have to make. The best thing they can do, for the moment, is not to go ahead designing environmental changes but rather to give the parents all the necessary means of knowing what can be done so that they will be able to act in the right way at the right moment. Then the counselors give both parents a copy of the Italian law governing interventions for environmental accessibility.

More than a year later, Matteo's father asks for a meeting to evaluate the possibility of Matteo using a computer. The counselors are extremely curious. The father, Matteo, and Matteo's paternal grandfather come to the meeting. Matteo looks very different, more alert and collaborative. He tries to make some comments, but his father immediately hushes him.

Briefly, and proudly, the father tells us he has changed jobs and has moved to another town; he has bought a small house with a garden and has made it completely accessible. Matteo sees his mother on weekends, and the solution seems satisfactory for everybody. Now Matteo is going to attend a vocational course for which computer use is required. That is why his father requested this meeting.

The exact moment when the request is made explicit, when a counseling session is conducted, or both, is of the utmost importance. Ideas, values, feelings, and perceptions are inextricably linked to that particular moment. In this case the project is not firmly anchored, because nobody knows where, how, and when it will be accomplished. On this point there is total confusion. The counseling takes place at a moment in the family members' lives when important decisions and passionate feelings come into play. An opinion expressed by the counselor might be connoted as an untimely choice between two clashing systems, so the counselors decide to stay out of the fray, giving the parents some "work tools." These tools will be a useful starting point in the future when the parents' struggle is over: Only at that time will the parents, separately, be able to consider the question carefully and make the appropriate decision. By acting in this way, a counselor demonstrates firm trust (despite appearances) in the capacity of the system—or developing systems—to tackle and solve the matter.

To Whom Do I Belong? Relationships Within the Family

Mr. Antonio, age 32, has sustained hemiplegia on his left side and severe anarthria as a consequence of a brain injury. He does not have difficulties in memory and language comprehension. Although no longer able to draw or write with a pen, he has no apparent gnostic impairment, and he can read. His rehabilitation specialist asked for the technical opinion of the SIVA professionals; he thinks this might be the right moment to introduce a computer as an instrument for writing rehabilitation as well as a medium for interpersonal communication.

The outcome of the telephone interview supports the idea of using a computer. Obviously, Mr. Antonio will need somebody to support him in his daily exercises as well as a rehabilitation professional to outline and guide the whole project over time.

Mr. Antonio comes to the meeting a with his personal assistant. Trials demonstrate that he is able to use a traditional keyboard. He also tries to write something, but he makes a lot of spelling and syntax errors; it is evident that he needs psycholinguistic rehabilitation as well as specific exercises.

During the ensuing conversation the counselor discovers that Mr. Antonio had lived with his fiancée before the accident. Immediately afterward, one of his sisters requested a withdrawal of civil rights and was given care of him, with the approval of health department officers. She expected him to move in with her family. The sister pays for his personal assistant's salary, whom she asks to provide personal care and recreation; the fiancée has not given up and continues to look for rehabilitation possibilities. Thus, the counselor finds herself in the difficult position of asking help of a person who is willing to give it (i.e., the personal assistant) but who is paid by someone who disagrees with this proposal.

The counselor decides to question the specialist who asked for advice. He seems to be the key figure: He was favorable to the withdrawal of Mr. Antonio's civil rights and would like to introduce AT into his rehabilitation. Mr. Antonio leaves us for the moment, on the understanding that a further meeting will be needed. The counselor thinks that a computer might be useful for Mr. Antonio, but only if a way of getting him to learn its concrete use, for his life, and possibly for a new job, is found. Then, together with the specialist, the counselor decides to prescribe the computer and suggests that the sister buy one, too.

Almost a year later, Mr. Antonio's sister calls and demands the counselor tell her what she and Mr. Antonio must do with that computer. She is invited to the center, together with Mr. Antonio and his personal assistant. Then the counselor sums the whole story: She explains the reasons behind the choice and the professional possibilities the computer might open up for Mr. Antonio. But, the counselor reaffirms, someone must support Mr. Antonio in his daily work, following a precise rehabilitation protocol. The personal assistant—a new one—is familiar with PC use and would willingly cooperate in this project. The sister states that she is still perplexed; according to her, Mr. Antonio will never be able to rid himself of his disability.

Some months later, Mr. Antonio's fiancée calls and tells us they are now living together again and are starting to use the computer. She would like to check with us about a good way to start and requests regular meetings to verify the progress of their work.

In this case, the counseling discussion involves the decision-making level. Any decision that, as in the present case, involves a way of life or a global project requires either agreement or battle. Here the acquisition of a technical aid is equivalent to taking sides in an ideal choice: well-being–illness, autonomy–assistance. The outlined project requires daily exercise, as the counselor clearly underlined. A silent fight is taking place behind Mr. Antonio's back. It is a fight between his life systems, between ways of life. On the one hand, with a great spirit of sacrifice, the sister is ready to look after her brother forever: According to her, Mr. Antonio will remain definitively invalid; he will never become independent again. On the other hand, the fiancée does not want to give up the project of living together, so she is obviously inclined to look for a change. Mr. Antonio, held back by feelings, obligations, and impossibilities, has been cheated of his own right to decide. Even Mr. Antonio's rehabilitation specialist, for his part, has been trapped in this situation, because he actually made contradictory moves. The counselors could only lay the cards on the table, by explaining the impasse in which they too were trapped. By asking the specialist to take sides, the skein begins to unravel: The sister is forced to make a decision, which implies a different style of life. Perhaps this is one of the reasons why Mr. Antonio's life has radically changed direction. The various steps are not known, but all the systems involved contributed to produce an unexpected change.

It's Up to Me: Relationships Between the Family and the Rehabilitation Service

Veronica, age 20, has tetraplegia, severe dysarthria, and slight cognitive impairment as a consequence of cerebral palsy. Her mother called for a meeting. Veronica had completed her compulsory schooling and was attending a vocational course; the results would be more positive, and the professional prospects more promising, if the girl's communication were more fluent and intelligible. She makes use of Blissymbols on a table,[10] but in paper form, and using this communication system can be complicated for those who are unaccustomed to it. Veronica's mother wanted to know if there were any new technical instruments that might help her daughter.

The counselors decide to propose a portable communicator. The instrument's level of complexity will be decided during the counseling session, depending on Veronica's real cognitive possibilities. The meeting takes place as expected, without any surprise or snag. Veronica is a lively and resourceful woman. With her Bliss-table and her parents' help, she expresses opinions and wishes; the counseling session takes place in a climate of general cheerfulness. The family is in regular contact with a local rehabilitation center, which mainly keeps in touch with the social and health services; in the family's view, the center is not well informed about scientific developments and market innovations. A trial with a 20-box layout communicator proves

---

[10] Blissymbols is one of the existing systems in the field of augmentative alternative communication. They are mainly pictographic symbols, and they are always presented together with the corresponding word so that everyone can understand the message. They are drawn on a portable table, and the user can communicate by indicating the symbols in sequence. A European approach to augmentative alternative communication was presented by von Tetzchner and Jensen (1996).

satisfactory: Veronica immediately understands its use and, after a training period, will soon be able to exploit all its functions. Nevertheless, the counselors suggest involving her rehabilitation therapists in this activity, because careful construction of the basic messages is called for. These need to be related to her daily life and needs, and a set of specific messages suited to school activities must also be defined. The counselors give the parents a written report with the observation results so that they can present it, if they so desire, to the professionals at the rehabilitation center.

A short time later, Veronica's speech therapist called the counselors. She sounded resentful: Veronica's parents had gone to the rehabilitation center with a newly bought communicator in their hands. In addition, Veronica demanded to use it for communicating with the speech therapist, using messages she had already recorded with her mother's help. The speech therapist asked for details and explanations; she was not familiar with these new technical instruments at all. She was annoyed at the family's behavior: It is up to her to present innovations and to plan their use; it is during rehabilitation work that the most suitable messages should be recorded on the communicator.

The ensuing conversation was aimed at restoring the dialogue between the speech therapist and the family. The parents, the counselors assured the speech therapist, did not want to abuse their power or to encroach on the speech therapist's territory. They wished only to show off Veronica's new AT device, and they did so enthusiastically, because it might considerably enrich her life, work, and study. The speech therapist was unacquainted with alternative communication techniques and methodologies; therefore, the counselors gave her information on ongoing courses in Italy for professional in-service training in the field. They also invited the speech therapist to a meeting to be held shortly with Veronica and her family to discuss and verify their work.

The counseling session with Veronica and her family is a good illustration of the decision process, from needs definition to the choice of AT. But AT is meaningful only if it is actually used, and counseling sessions on AT are meaningful if they explore the concrete possibility of AT effectiveness. If the counselors had simply proposed the communicator to the family, its quality and frequency of use would have suffered. Veronica's life itself would have suffered. In fact, the device should become the medium of effective communication with a lot of people. The counseling session provided clear proof of the major role the rehabilitation center had played in safeguarding Veronica's important relationships. Consequently, the involvement of this system in the project is essential. Because of the difficult relationship between the family and the rehabilitation system it was not possible to involve the rehabilitation professionals from the very first meeting; they would probably have declined the invitation or would have felt they were under a sort of examination. In the end, the family's decision obliged them simply to take note of developments, even if they felt somewhat resentful. Starting from the very expression of the feelings stirred up by this difficult relationship, a new possibility for dialogue was built, and a window on the family's wishes was opened. These will provide a concrete possibility for a feasible future.

CONCLUSION

The cases reported here represent only an infinitesimal part of all the possible problem combinations with which an AT counseling service may have to deal. Some of these do not end, as might be expected, with the acquisition of a technical device but rather by adopting other remedial measures or by looking for solutions at a different level. By the same token, this chapter is intended to make as practical as possible the theoretical perspective adopted, namely the systemic approach. The cases have been used to illustrate some of the approach's main points.

1. There is no such thing as the problem of a sole individual; the situation must always be considered within a wider context, that of the system or systems to which that individual belongs. Only in this way can the real strengths, weaknesses, and goals be recognized.
2. There is no such thing as a neutral counselor able to judge, decide, and advise from the summit of an infallible science; rather, counselors are involved, together with the user and system, in finding solutions to the problem. They will be successful only if they are aware of this involvement and bring all their technical and methodological competence to the solution. Their achievement depends on awareness of their own work hypotheses, decisions, and attributions of meaning.
3. Because of the peculiarity of these two "systems," their meeting is unique and depends on the very moment of occurrence in the systems' reciprocal story. It is the counselor's task not only to analyze the request content but also to determine the moment at which it takes place.
4. The solution, or the group of possible solutions, is but the outcome of this meeting, the final result of a change planned in words. Because it depends on a cobuilding process, the solution can never be known or decided a priori but becomes evident—it has been said—as the conclusion of a dialogue between constraints and possibilities.

Renzo Piano, the eminent Genoese architect responsible for the famous Pompidou Centre in Paris and part of the Postdammerplatz project in Berlin, once demonstrated his working method on Italian television. Using a pencil, he sketched on a sheet of paper the topography of the territory on which the construction work was to be carried out; in a manner of speaking, he drew the "objective" situation, as it is. He then placed a transparency over this first sheet and, using an emerald green marker pen, outlined all the possible schemes he was able to imagine, to dream. He said he does this until he reaches the definitive plan, which, he hopes, will be approved by those who have the final word, and he'll fight for all he's worth to make sure that word is "yes."

Now, one might say that the topography of the territory corresponds to the user's "objective" situation (his or her constraints, as described by the counselor), for example, the data concerning impairment and disability or the existing technology available. Over this "scheme" the counselor can sketch possible future scenarios (his or her view of the user's possibilities), hypothesizing a plan of action. Only through dialogue with the user, with his or her description of the present and the future, will the counselor's sketch be modified, its lines redrawn, and the right placing found, until it has become a definite project.

To whom will the change belong? Certainly to the user, who has been drawn into somebody else's dream, to the point of modifying it for himself or herself, but also to the counselor, who will have gained greater understanding of the user's ideas and feelings, rearranged his or her working project to make it feasible, and have gained fresh insights into his or her own work and world of ideas (Cecchin, 1992).

REFERENCES

Andrich, R. (1993). Information/advice service on technical aids: SIVA's model. In *Proceedings of the ECART conference* (5.4, pp. 23–26). Stockholm: Swedish Handicapped Institute.

Andrich, R. (1996). *Consigliare gli ausili.* [Giving advce about technical aids]. Milan: Servizio Informazione Valutazione Ausili (SIVA), Fondazione "Pro Juventute" Don Gnocchi.

Andrich, R., & Porqueddu, B. (1990). Educazione all'autonomia: Esperienze, strumenti, proposte metodologiche. [Education to autonomy: Experiences, instruments, methodological proposals]. *Europa Medicophysica, 26,* 121–145.

Besio, S. (1997). The contribution of an AT consulting service to the construction of a disabled person's autonomy. In G. Anogianakis, C. Bühler, & M. Soede (Eds.), *Advancement of assistive technology: Proceedings of the 1997 AAATE Congress* (pp. 341–345). Amsterdam: IOS Press.

Besio, S., & EUSTAT Consortium. (1998). *Deliverable D04.2: Programs in assistive technology education for end-users in Europe.* Brussels, Belgium: European Commission DG XIII, Telematics Application Programme.

Boscolo, L., & Cecchin, G. (1981). *The flowering of family therapy.* Paper presented at "The Flowering of Family Therapy" conference, New York.

Boscolo, L., & Cecchin, G. (1988). Il problema della diagnosi da un punto di vista sistemico. [The problem of diagnosis from a systemic point of view]. *Psicobiettivo, 3,* 19–30.

Caillé, P. (1981). L'intervento terapeutico crea i presupposti per un cambiamento nelle relazioni umane. *Terapia famigliare, 9*(2), 73–86.

Cecchin, G. (1987). Hypothesizing, circularity, and neutrality revisited: An invitation to curiosity. *Family Process, 26,* 405–413.

Cecchin, G. (1992). The construction of therapeutic possibilities. In S. McNamee & K. J. Gergen (Eds.), *Therapy as social construction* (pp. 237–245). London: Sage.

Cecchin, G., Lane, G., & Ray, W. A. (1992). *Irreverence: A strategy for therapists' survival.* London: Karnac Books.

Cecchin, G., Lane, G., & Ray, W. A. (1994). *The cybernetics of prejudices in the practice of psychotherapy.* London: Karnac Books.

Ceruti, M. (Ed.). (1996). *Il vincolo e la possibilità.* [The constraint and the possibility]. Milan: Feltrinelli.

Dell, P. F. (1980). The Hopi family therapist and the Aristotelian parents. *Journal of Marital & Family Therapy, 6,* 42–54.

Duffy, T. M., Lowick, J., & Jonassen, D. (Eds.). (1993). Designing environments for constructive learning (*NATO ASI Series: F105*). Heidelberg, Germany: Springer-Verlag.

EUSTAT Consortium. (1998). *Deliverable D03.2: Critical factors involved in end-users' education in relation to assistive technology.* Brussels, Belgium: European Commission DG XIII, Telematics Application Programme.

Gadamer, H. G. (1994). *Dove si nasconde la salute.* [Where is health hidden]. Padua, Italy: Raffaello Cortina.

HEART Project Consortium, Line E—Rehabilitation Technology Training. (1994). *E.2.1. Report on job profile and training requirements for rehabilitation technology specialists and other related professions.* Brussels, Belgium: European Commission.

Hershenson, D. B. (1998). Systemic, ecological model for rehabilitation counseling. *Rehabilitation Counseling Bulletin, 42,* 40–50.

Hoffman, L. (1981). *Foundations of family therapy.* New York: Basic Books.

Malagoli Togliatti, M., & Telfener, U. (1983). *La terapia sistemica: Nuove tendenze in terapia della famiglia.* [Systemic therapy: New trends in family therapy]. Rome: Astrolabio.

Minuchin, S., & Fishman, C. H. (1982). *Guida alle tecniche della terapia della famiglia.* [A guide to family therapy techniques]. Rome: Astrolabio.

Neath, J. F., & Reed, C. A. (1998). Power and empowerment in multicultural education: Using the radical democratic model for rehabilitation education. *Rehabilitation Counseling Bulletin, 42,* 16–39.

Selvini Palazzoli, M., Prata, G., Boscolo, L., & Cecchin, G. (1975). *Paradosso e controparadosso.* [Paradox and counterparadox]. Milan: Feltrinelli.

Singers, G. H. S., & Powers, L. E. (Eds.). (1993). *Families, disability, and empowerment: Active coping skills and strategies for family interventions*. Baltimore: Paul H. Brookes.

Slavin, R. E. (1990). *Co-operative learning: Theory, research and practice*. Englewood Cliffs, NJ: Prentice Hall.

Swain, J., Finkelstein, V., French, S., & Oliver, M. (Eds.). (1993). *Disabling barriers, enabling environments*. London: Sage.

Thomas, K. M., & Velthouse, B. A. (1990). Cognitive elements of empowerment: An interpretative model of intrinsic task motivation. *Academy of Management Review, 2*, 666–681.

von Tetzchner, S., & Jensen, M. H. (Eds.). (1996). *Augmentative and alternative communication: European perspectives*. London: Whurr.

15

PARTNERSHIP AND ASSISTIVE TECHNOLOGY IN IRELAND

GERALD CRADDOCK

If you come to help me, you are wasting your time.
But, if you have come because your liberation is bound up with mine,
then let us work together. —Lila Watson

Assistive technology (AT) is moving beyond medical equipment to tools for independent living, from medical devices to common goods, from professionally driven choices to user-driven choices, from a patient status to a consumer status. It is no longer sufficient to look to AT to enhance individual functioning; it is more important to address whether AT helps the user achieve valued life roles and goals. To accomplish this, an educational continuum is advocated, one in which users and providers educate one another and work in true partnership, one in which AT practitioners learn to celebrate the diversities of people with disabilities and recognize their valued contribution to the process of lifelong learning. Assessing the outcomes of such collaboration requires thinking "outside the box" to use newer approaches as well as advocating and applying fundamental principles to a service delivery system on which I elaborate in this chapter.

Research in Europe has shown that success in AT is best achieved through stakeholder partnerships and a move away from the medical model of prescription toward a social model (Swedish Handicap Institute, 1993, 1995). It was on the basis of the social model and an educational continuum that the APHRODITE (A Partnership to Harness Resource Opportunities and Distribute Information and Technology Expertise) and STATEMENT (Systematic Template for Assessing Technology Enabling Mainstream Education) projects were initiated and successfully applied throughout Ireland. One of the central goals of APHRODITE was that people with disabilities would be trained to provide local support and information on AT in their own communities.

IRELAND: DISABILITY SERVICES IN CONTEXT

In Ireland the situation for people with disabilities is complex. Much of Ireland's social policy has come about through its membership in the European Council. Until 10 years ago, Ireland's economy was still developing, and there were neither the resources nor the social thinking to encompass the growing demand across Europe by people with disabilities for their rights and inclusion in society. The move toward a human rights approach to disability was explicitly endorsed by the European Council in its resolution of "Equality of Opportunity for People With Disabilities" (Commission of the European Communities, 1996). The council stressed the need for a renewed impetus toward the rights-based, equal-opportunities approach to disability, which focuses on the identification and removal of the many barriers preventing people with disabilities from achieving equality.

This approach is based on the notion of rights and entitlement rather than charity and an accommodation of differences. As a member of the European Union, Ireland had to initiate new legislation in regard to social policies. Throughout Europe, the European Union funded many projects that endorsed policy change in the member states; two of these funded projects were APHRODITE and STATEMENT. Both projects were based on the principles of inclusion and entitlement.

The majority of rehabilitation practitioners in Ireland involved in AT are professionals who are most likely to come from the paramedical field. In the public sector AT is funded through the health boards, and AT must be recommended by professionals such as physiotherapists, occupational therapists, or speech and language therapists. The focus is on the disability or functional limitation, which is in the clinical tradition and based on the medical model.

Because the area of disability is left to the health boards, the person with the disability is seen as a patient; therefore, once the diagnosis is identified, the intent is to try, through intervention, to find a cure. Mason (1995) described the medical model of disability as

> attacking one's relationship with oneself because the assumption is made that the impairment is the enemy. In reality the impairment is part of the person and only the person himself or herself can choose to separate them without feeling torn apart. So uninvited intervention, however well meaning, is a form of violence to the inner being. (pp. 3–8)

Mason is a woman with a disability and a trained artist who has written extensively on the oppression of disabled people and has been working with service providers to redesign their services to reflect the social model of disability.

Western culture celebrates the "body beautiful" (Stone, 1995); it places disability firmly within the "impaired body." The social model of disablement places disability firmly within the structures of society. Today, the focus must be increasingly on creating an environment in which people with disabilities are empowering themselves not only through participation but also through active partnership with others (professionals, peer support models, and so forth).

Some of the most important characteristics that make people human are choice, values, love, creativity, self-awareness, and potential. These are highly valued roles and goals of most people. Alderfer (1972) maintained that people's needs are on a continuum and that there are three sets of needs: (a) existence needs (the basics of life), (b) relatedness needs (social and interpersonal needs), and (c) growth needs (personal development needs). In applying AT, practitioners often need to be reminded to focus beyond the therapeutic or AT dimension to the human one and that these human needs do not differ regardless of whether a person has a disability. In essence, they need to be reminded that people with disabilities have the same desires for self-fulfillment as do nondisabled people.

Self-fulfillment is achieved in many ways; however, in Western civilization it tends to be marked by educational, vocational, economic, and social achievements; by being able to make life choices; and by being independent and in a position to make these self-directed choices. Historically, however, societal barriers have oppressed people with disabilities, and they have not been given life choices. Ruth (1996) argued that oppression is not random or accidental and that the experiences of mistreatment likely will be repeated. Every time this mistreatment occurs, the negative messages are reinforced. Over time, these negative messages gradually shape the self-image of the person and the group. If someone is told often enough that his or her needs are less important than the needs of others, then he or she will eventually feel less important and, ultimately, act less important. The crucial aspect of this process is that, over time, what begins as an external oppression becomes an internalized oppression. This is a key message for practitioners. It is not enough to work with people with disabilities, imparting knowledge; they must also constantly reassure and offer encouragement, hope, and opportunities for people to break out of their oppressed state. Society as a whole can play a valuable role in the liberation of an oppressed group through the celebration of diversity. It is possible to build strong bonds across different cultures by nurturing and celebrating differences instead of denigrating and oppressing them.

THE DISABILITY MOVEMENT IN IRELAND

The Centre for Independent Living (CIL) in Ireland, in the tradition of the independent-living movement, has begun to effect change in policy and practice. CIL's philosophy, like the independent-living philosophy in the United States, espouses consumer control, self-determination, environmental adaptation, community integration, access to ongoing support mechanisms, and freedom of choice for individuals with disabilities. The message is very clear: Disability is a social issue rather than a medical one.

In 1993, as a result of growing pressure from people with disabilities, the Irish government set up the Commission on the Status of People With Disabilities. The commission's task was to find out what life was like for people with disabilities in Ireland and to propose ways of making improvements. Commission members went out to meet people with disabilities, their families, and their caregivers all over the country. Public "listening meetings" took place at 30 venues around Ireland. The opening paragraph of the commission's report, published in 1995, read:

> People with disabilities are the neglected citizens of Ireland. On the eve of the 21st century, many of them suffer intolerable conditions because of outdated social and economic policies and unthinking public attitudes. Changes have begun to come about, influenced by international recognition that disability is a social rather than a medical issue, but many of those changes have been piecemeal. Public attitudes towards disability are still based on charity rather than on rights, and the odds are stacked against people with disabilities at almost every turn. Whether their status is looked at in terms of economics, information, education, mobility or housing they are seen to be treated as second-class citizens. (Commission on the Status of People With Disabilities, 1995, p. 1)

This report was a significant development in promoting how people with disabilities viewed themselves and the issues that were of most concern to them. A strategy for equality marks a discursive reframing of the concerns and aspirations of people with disabilities by placing their needs and aspirations within a social model of disability rather then within a medical interpretation of needs. The traditional dominance of medically oriented services for people with disabilities has to be seen within the context of the structure of health services in Ireland. A wide range of social welfare services have historically been encompassed by the Irish health services, which have given the Department of Health broader responsibilities than other comparative departments in other European countries (Department of Health, 1994). Disability services are part of these responsibilities and, as such, have favored the promotion of a medical understanding of disability over a more holistic view grounded in the everyday experiences of people with disabilities.

The historic background of disability services developed within a medical framework explains why the primary responsibility for the assessment and administration of grant-aided technologies (or AT) for people with disabilities lies within the local health services. However, the Commission for the Status of People With Disabilities has reported that AT was inappropriately placed within the context of health services. The commission strongly recommended that responsibilities should be transferred to the Department of Social Welfare and the Department of Transport, Energy, and Communications and that it should be these two departments that introduce legislation to ensure access to AT and telecommunications, in line with United Nations standard rules (Commission on the Status of People With Disabilities, 1995, p. 210). However, at this point in time neither of these departments views it as its responsibility to take on the area of AT. This debate needs to be broadened and to encompass the Department of Education and the Department of Health.

The Irish government has formed a new National Disability Authority, which will oversee legislation, but the responsibility for legislation at this time remains with the Department of Health until such time as the new authority is in place. The provision of AT, therefore, remains closely linked to health services. Thus, service providers must work in cooperation with the health care professionals who currently provide services to people with disabilities.

In 1994 Ireland's Department of Health published a document, titled *Shaping a Healthier Future*, that laid out a strategy for developing health services that were to be guided by three main principles: equity, quality of service, and accountability. These principles are aimed at the health needs of the sectors of society that are most in need. "Access to healthcare should be determined by actual need rather than by ability to pay or geographical location" (Department of Health, 1994, p. 10). The guiding principle of equity within the Department of Health's future policy has particular relevance for the Client Technical Services (CTS) department, based at the Central Remedial Clinic (CRC) in Dublin. The CRC provides clinical services for people with disabilities funded through the Department of Health. It has provided a national AT service for the last 17 years, and in 1991 it established CTS to further develop its services.

CTS developed an AT service based on a multidisciplinary team consisting of a manager–engineer, an occupational therapist, a speech and language therapist, and a technician. It used the recommendations of the HEART study to develop a service that would best facilitate the AT needs of people with disabilities. It was in keeping with this principle of equity outlined by the Department of Health that CTS looked for other ways to deliver service at a local level. CTS's approach was to go beyond providing an expert outreach service; it was also concerned with integrating this service into existing health, social, and vocational services at a local level. This was also in keeping with the new health strategy, which identified the need to improve linkages and cooperation between complementary services at a local level. The health strategy also stated that although health and social services existed to serve the client, there has been little emphasis on this in guiding policy and in addressing the practicalities of providing a consumer-oriented service.

DEVELOPING A SERVICE DELIVERY PROCESS

CTS recognized early in its development that an AT service could best be delivered when it was based on a social model. There was an increasing recognition that technology prescribed without user involvement and training and support at a local level often resulted in abandonment (Martin & McCormack, 1999). The HEART study had recommended seven fundamental steps in the service provision of AT:

1. *Initiative:* the importance of the first contact
2. *Assessment:* evaluation of needs
3. *Typology of the solution:* choosing the appropriate AT
4. *Selection:* selecting the specific device
5. *Authorization for financing:* obtaining funding
6. *Delivery:* getting the device to the user
7. *Management and follow-up:* continued support.

The initiative for obtaining AT is assumed to be taken by the person with the disability. CTS operates a self-referral system in which the client can contact CTS without a doctor's referral. However, through its experience, CTS recognized that a precursor to this model must be outreach. An outreach service creates an awareness about how using AT can have a very positive impact on people's lives. The key elements to outreach are demonstrations, workshops, media advertising and, above all, being able to collaborate with successful users of AT as role models. Role models have a major impact on demonstrating to people with disabilities how AT can help them achieve their dreams (Craddock & Whitton, 1997).

When discussing awareness campaigns about the impact of AT, CTS members found that it was vital that practitioners be sensitive to the fact that they are dealing with a disempowered population. Awareness campaigns can be delivered only in consultation with disability groups. Critical to this delivery is having role models who have themselves overcome societal barriers and have achieved or are achieving their own goals and roles within society. An example of this process was the TEST (Training, Employment &

Support Using Technology) project funded under the employment initiative (Employment Horizon 1995–1997; Craddock & Gunning, 1997), which was managed and led by CTS.[1] TEST brought together a group of young adults of both genders with mobility impairments throughout Ireland. These people were no longer receiving regular services, had left the education process, and had no real focus or purpose for using their AT. Part of the TEST team included an expert user, who uses an augmentative communication technology device and is attending a university full-time. After some discussion, the team members decided that this expert user would talk to the group about how he had used AT to achieve his goals. This had an immediate impact on the group. They saw for the first time one of their peers using AT to achieve a high quality of life that they had heretofore not thought possible. He immediately became a role model: He was the same age as themselves, and had significant physical difficulties, yet he was achieving his goals through the use of his AT. Within days the individuals were discussing their goals with their facilitators and how AT might best assist them. Some members of the group decided to return to school; others continued with the project with new enthusiasm.

It was this experience in TEST that led CTS to make outreach and the recruitment of role models central parts of its AT service provision. Further funding was subsequently sought from the European Council under a new round of the Horizon Employment initiative (1997–1999). The APHRODITE project went into a pilot phase as part of CTS services. The significant difference brought about by the APHRODITE project was that people with disabilities were partners in the project from its inception. The CIL, which has a national network of 18 offices throughout Ireland, was a key partner. One of the central goals of APHRODITE was that people with disabilities would become Technology Liaison Officers (TLOs) in their local areas. TLOs would provide people with disabilities who were interested in AT or were existing users with local training, support, and information. They also became data gatherers of relevant preassessment information on people who wished to use the CTS service.

TLOs were interested and motivated but did not have the experience in AT to support their members in CIL. All TLOs completed both a structured individual AT program and group training. This training has been ongoing over the 2 years of the project. With this training the TLOs have been able to put together an outreach program, provide demonstrations of a cross-section of AT products, visit people in their own environments,

---

[1] Employment Horizon is a European Union program that promotes labor market access for people with disabilities by means of innovative projects. For additional information, contact Employment Horizon Support Structure, European section, National Rehabilitation Board (NRB), 25 Clyde Road, Dublin 4, Ireland.

loan equipment, gather valuable information for CTS about each client before the client's evaluation, and provide vital training and support once the client has been given the appropriate ATs.

Having a good local support network is now considered the key to the successful use of AT. Nine TLOs are now located throughout Ireland. All (seven men and two women) use wheelchairs. They either have their own transport or access to private transport. All TLOs have taken the Certificate in Assistive Technology Applications (CATA) course and achieved their certificates from University College Dublin. The caliber of the candidates is extremely high, which means that a lot of skills as well as life experiences are brought to the project. The TLOs are located in both urban and rural areas. Because all TLOs have disabilities, they have firsthand experience of how to access local services. They also act as role models and provide peer support, which has been fundamental to the service now being delivered.

INVESTIGATION OF EVALUATION TOOLS

AT evaluation and assessment are parts of the process that CTS has studied in depth. This process consists of ascertaining people's needs and requirements in relation to AT. It has been shown that assessing people's needs cannot be done in isolation, because needs are complex, and all aspects of peoples' lives—that is, environmental, psychosocial, educational, and so on—must be considered.

Kotler (1997) found that studying target markets with traditional methods such as questionnaires and surveys was not sufficient. Even focus groups are often inadequate, because participants are not very good at explicitly stating what they require in respect to their use of technology, particularly when they are unaware of what exists. People's needs can be unconscious, and they may not be able to articulate them. People may also express solutions as needs, which can actually be better served in other ways and with other interventions. Kotler also highlighted the fact that human activity cannot be reduced into separate features of an individual. It is not possible to separate human characteristics from the context and situations of use; a wider, macrolevel perspective needs to be adopted. In this wider perspective it is noted that human and machine do not form a system that operates the same regardless of context (i.e., physical, organizational, and social environments). Nardi (1996) advocated that technology should remain people's tools and that the main aim of design is to provide people with useful tools that help them fulfill their goals. Inglis, Fleming, and Bassett (1989) further supported this from an adult education perspective when he wrote that "if we operate within an horizon of myths or a galaxy of assumptions, then our real needs will not be so easily identified" (p. 32).

CTS investigated a number of evaluation processes and decided to use the matching person and technology (MPT) model and accompanying assessment instruments (Scherer, 1991). This was chosen because the MPT process is consumer driven and client centered and follows the social model adopted by CTS. This enabled a uniform approach to the pre-evaluation, evaluation, and postevaluation phases of the overall service delivery process and allowed for the assessment of outcomes resulting from AT. The MPT model was modified for the Irish context, which was further developed and delivered within the STATEMENT project (a European Union-funded project under the employment initiative Horizon [January 1999–December 1999]).

Other supports that have been developed as part of the service delivery process is a talk shop (chat room) on the World Wide Web where the TLOs can communicate with each other and with CTS personnel for support and information. Such a chat room can also be a source of information and communication for consumers around the country. The TLOs have also held "information days" for both service providers and consumers in their local areas.

As a result of these efforts, put in place under the auspices of APHRODITE, the public profile of CTS has increased dramatically. An increased confidence in service has been noted, and it is perceived that the CRC is improving its services to rural consumers by providing services outside of Dublin. The project has allowed CTS to form positive working relationships with other service providers around the country.

CATA

A further core feature of the TEST project was providing a certification course for the TLOs; people with disabilities; and other stakeholders, such as caregivers, practitioners, and so on. CATA was developed following collaboration with California State University—Northridge, which had developed a similar course in the United States (Craddock & Murphy, 1998). CATA has been a tremendous success, and more than 60 participants have completed the course over the past 2 years. Critical to its success has been the fact that at least one third of the participants were people with disabilities. This created a dynamic that has enriched and educated not only the other participants (occupational therapists, speech and language therapists, physical therapists, information technology trainers, center managers, teachers, disability advisers, and so on), but also the program trainers. The core trainers of the course are the people comprising the evaluation team in CTS. The interactions among themselves and the participants have demonstrated the many benefits of a multidisciplinary team approach in action.

It has not been necessary to emphasize both how and why the team approach is the best option in AT; participants experience this firsthand in the program.

Another factor leading to the success of CATA is that the team uses a participative approach, which is a fundamental element of lifelong learning and adult education. In this approach each participant brings valid experiences to the course, which is duly recognized by the trainers, who see themselves as facilitators rather than experts. This is the educational continuum, where Ruth states that "practitioners leave their control and arrogance at the door" (Ruth, 1996). Practitioners and participants work together to share knowledge and in doing so empower and liberate one another.

THE KEYS TO APHRODITE'S SUCCESS

The positive outcomes of the APHRODITE project are due to critical elements that were built in from the beginning. The key elements essential to its success are

- Training the trainers to localize and deliver AT
- Strategic partnerships on both national and international levels
- Having people with disabilities (TLOs) trained in AT and being at the "coalface," or at the grassroots level, of service at the local community level
- Being able to provide a certified course in AT to people with disabilities and their caregivers as well as to service providers
- Providing a technology infrastructure that enables the TLOs to communicate with each other and with the national center
- Providing a loan library of AT equipment for the TLOs to give to people in their own environments for trial usage of such equipment
- Localizing the MPT process, which enables uniform information to be gathered about a particular individual consumer by the TLOs and the evaluation team
- Providing peer support and role models at a local level to people with disabilities.

STATEMENT PROJECT

The STATEMENT project was developed to respond to the identified need of students who required an effective evaluation service that would identify and advise them on available AT as they moved from second-level education on to further education, work, or vocational training. This project offers a proactive approach by evaluating and identifying the student's requirements in AT before he or she begins a course or enters work. From this evaluation, each student receives a written statement of need, which is then used to negotiate his or her AT requirements with the prospective college, training center, or employer. Where necessary, the student then receives training in whatever AT was recommended.

The stages of the overall assessment process used in STATEMENT are as follows:

- application and signing of consent form
- preassessment
- summary of AT need
- main assessment
- written "statement of need"
- training in identified AT
- postassessment.

The preassessment again uses the MPT process, which was adapted to fit the structures and situations as they exist in Ireland. Questions in the MPT model are both qualitative and quantitative and are focused very much on identifying needs and requirements as identified by students. A summary of the pre-evaluation stage is sent to the student to verify that the information is correct. This step has enabled students to spend additional time evaluating their situations before coming to the evaluation. What transpires as a result is a more educated and empowered consumer. These needs then become the focus in the main evaluation stage.

The STATEMENT project achieved the building of a formal relationship among the CRC, the National Association for Deaf People, the National Council for the Blind of Ireland, the Association for Higher Education Access and Disability, and the Association for Children and Adults With Learning Disabilities. At present there is no single service that provides advice and evaluations for visual, physical, hearing, and learning difficulties in the area of AT in Ireland. Any and all previous collaboration among the project partners was done on an ad hoc basis. For the first time, the STATEMENT project brought all the national service organizations together to provide a seamless service from the users' perspective.

The adaptation of the MPT model in the STATEMENT project provided the mechanism for achieving a client-focused evaluation service. The overwhelming positive reaction from participating students is illustrative of the effectiveness of this approach. Many have publicly described their experiences, something that has proved to be particularly effective in demonstrating the impact of the process and the value of the technology recommended on students' experiences in education. The students' testimony also points to the fact that the developments of effective evaluation systems are central to ensuring the maximum use of technology. The following excerpt is from one of the students. It shows the dramatic impact that her technology had on both her education and her well-being.

> Since I received [my AT] my life has become unbelievably easier. The Kurzweil 3000 reads the material I need out to me and . . . now instead of 3–4 hours, it takes me 45 minutes to an hour. . . The Dragon Naturally Speaking also saves me time, as usually I spend so much time concentrating on my spelling that I lose my train of thought and cannot focus on the correct way to phrase my words. . . . The pressure that I was under is practically gone. For the first time in my life I am interested and excited about reading and I am realising how restricted I was. As it would have made my life so much easier, I could never have believed that reading and studying could be this enjoyable.

OUTCOMES

The main focus of CTS over the past 6 years has been to pilot how best to deliver a client-centered service. Achievements include the following:

- Partnerships have been formed with key stakeholders in delivering AT.
- A structure has been established whereby people with disabilities can participate and be a service provider (TLO) in evaluating and supporting AT for other people with disabilities.
- An evaluation process has been developed and implemented that has the potential to provide a mechanism for measuring a quality service to people with disabilities.
- A benchmark (CATA) has been provided regarding quality assurance and qualification in AT service provision.
- A framework has been created for implementing individual AT plans for students and expanding this to all people with disabilities who are receiving services from CTS.

CONCLUSION

When one looks back at how AT and people with disabilities have moved forward in the past 10 years, one notes a sense of positive change and accomplishment. However, there still is a considerable way to go before universal design and service are part of everyday living. Rehabilitation professionals can move forward only by developing true partnerships and recognizing the abilities of all stakeholders. The European Union and the

Irish government must play a key role in providing the legislation and infrastructure to create a more inclusive society that celebrates diversity. This will enable researchers and developers in Ireland to view people with disabilities as a unique cultural group and will ensure that new developments in technology will consider the economical, political, social, and legal rights of people with disabilities in the new millennium. Efforts must be made within this new framework to influence, lobby, and infiltrate the power infrastructure to make significant changes throughout global society.

The services delivered by CTS and the two projects APHRODITE and STATEMENT are examples of how an AT service can be delivered within the framework of a social model. This model focuses on enabling and empowering people with disabilities, which leads to their inclusion in all aspects of community life. Systems change is a slow process; it can be achieved only by having fundamental principles that are adhered to and implemented. Heumann (1998) stated that a lot of effort has been put into system change in rehabilitation and AT service delivery without much reward. However, progress can often be slow at the beginning, and the liberation that is sought can be achieved only by working together. As a road sign in Africa says, "The road is too rough to drive slowly."

REFERENCES

Alderfer, C. (1972). *Personality and organisations*. New York: Harper & Row.

Commission of the European Communities (1996, July 30). A new European community disability strategy on equality of opportunity for people with disabilities. Presented by Commission of the European Communities, Brussels.

Commission on the Status of People With Disabilities. (1995). *Strategy for equality* (Issue Brief No. 0-7076-3739-2). Dublin, Ireland: Government Stationery Office.

Craddock, G., & Gunning, T. (1997). TEST—Integration in training. In G. Anogianakis, C. Buhler, & M. Soede (Eds.), *Advancement of assistive technology— Assistive technology research series* (Vol. 3, pp. 144–147). Washington, DC: IOS Press.

Craddock, G., & Murphy, H. J. (1998). Training under Project APHRODITE. In I. P. Porrero & E. Ballabio (Eds.), *Proceedings of the 3rd TIDE Congress: Improving the quality of life for the European citizen—Technology for inclusive design and equality* (pp. 131–134). Washington, DC: IOS Press.

Craddock, G., & Whitton, M. (1997, September). *Thinking globally, networking locally*. Paper presented at the meeting of the Communication Matters Conference, Lancaster University, Lancaster, England.

Department of Health. (1994). *Shaping a healthier future*. Dublin, Ireland: Government Stationery Office.

Heumann, J. (1998, August). *Human rights for persons with disabilities from a north and south perspective* [On-line]. Available: http://www.independentliving.org/LibArt/HumanRightsConf/Sem2.html

Inglis, T., Fleming, B., & Bassett, N. (1989). *For adults only—A case for adult education in Ireland*. Dublin, Ireland: AONTAS.

Kotler, P. (1997). *Marketing management, analysis, planning, implementation and control* (9th ed.). London: Prentice Hall.

Martin, B., & McCormack, L. (1999). Issues surrounding assistive technology use and abandonment in an emerging technological culture. In C. Buhler & H. Knops (Eds.), *Assistive technology on the threshold of the new millennium* (pp. 413–420). Amsterdam: IOS Press.

Mason, M. (1995, January). The breaking of relationships. *Present Time*, pp. 3–8.

Nardi, B. A. (Ed.). (1996). *Context and consciousness: Activity theory and human–computer interaction*. Cambridge, MA: MIT Press.

Ruth, S. (1996). *Self-esteem and the traveller child*. Paper presented at the annual meeting of the Association of Teachers of Traveller People, Dublin, Ireland.

Scherer, M. (1991). *Matching person and technology*. (Available from Marcia Scherer, 486 Lake Road, Webster, NY 14580 USA).

Stone, S. D. (1995). The myth of bodily perfection. *Disability and Society, 10*, 413.

Swedish Handicap Institute. (1995). *HEART (Horizontal European Activities in Rehabilitation Technology) study report: Line C-Service delivery* (Report No. C.5.1-C.6.1). Stockholm: Author.

IV

A LOOK AHEAD

16

FUTURE DIRECTIONS IN ASSISTIVE TECHNOLOGIES

ALBERT M. COOK

Future developments in assistive technologies (ATs) and the successful application of these technologies to meet the needs of people with disabilities will be driven by several factors. Rehabilitation practice is changing, and these changes will affect AT application. Technological advances are occurring quickly, and the capability of technologies to meet the needs of people with disabilities is growing daily. If these trends in rehabilitation and technology are to be exploited to the fullest in the development and application of ATs, then rehabilitation professionals must have a clear understanding of the underlying principles of AT application. I begin this chapter with a discussion of the changes occurring in rehabilitation practice and technology and then describe how those two forces, together with an understanding of AT application, determine future directions for AT development.

CHANGES IN REHABILITATION PRACTICE THAT AFFECT AT APPLICATIONS

Three key factors related to rehabilitation practice will have an impact on the future development and application of ATs: (a) the move from institutional to community-based services, (b) the change from a medical to a social model of disability, and (c) an increasingly active role for the AT consumer in selection and application of these technologies.

The move toward community-based services has been driven by many factors. Costs of institutional care are rising, and a major goal of health care administrators is to reduce these costs by shortening stays and transferring more care to the community. Early discharges from acute care facilities have resulted in patients being transferred to rehabilitation before they are ready. This has placed additional demands on rehabilitation providers, because the length of stays in rehabilitation also are being shortened. However, many services, including most AT services, are more appropriately delivered in the community where they will be used. Thus, service delivery programs now travel to schools, homes, or work settings to conduct AT assessments, to deliver technologies, and to train consumers in their use.

Fougeyrollas and Gray (1998) described changes in the classification of disability over the past 20 years. Classification schemes have moved away from a medical model of rehabilitation to a social model of disability. The former emphasizes repair of damaged tissues and organs and management of the "problem of disability." Although this approach is still important and essential in the early stages after injury leading to disability, it fails to recognize the social dimensions of disability. The social model, now incorporated into the World Health Organization's (2001) International Classification of Functioning, Disability, and Health, provides a richer and more complete view of both disability and the role of ATs in the lives of people who have disabilities. The most important implication of the emergence of the social model of disability is the recognition that the environment or context of use for these technologies is an important driving force for their development and application. It is no longer important to achieve success only in the clinic or laboratory: The real test is in daily community use of the technologies. The social model of disability has also spawned a wide range of studies of AT applications that focus on culture, discrimination, and social impact. These studies will help shape future developments in ATs.

Community-based services are also being driven by an emerging alliance between the largely institutionally based rehabilitation establishment and the largely community-based disability community. Lysack and Kaufert (1999) discussed the implications of this alliance for responsibility for care. This includes responsibility for choices of AT devices and services, and consumers are playing a larger role in the decisions made regarding what they receive and the evaluation of the quality of both the devices and services. For example, in Europe, the Empowering End-Users Through Assistive Technology (EUSTAT) project has developed guidelines for trainers, a set of critical factors for AT training and descriptive information on programs that provide AT training for consumers (see http://www.siva.it/research/eustat/index). One of the documents developed by EUSTAT is written for consumers of AT services and gives practical guidance regarding how to access these services. This is an example of the expanding collaboration between providers of AT services and the disability community that they serve.

In North America, Heerkens, Briggs, and Weider (1997) developed a peer-mentoring process using the matching person and technology model. This project, part of the New York State Technology Assistance initiative called *TRAID* (Technology-Related Assistance to Individuals with Disabilities), focuses on helping consumers identify the most appropriate ATs to meet their needs. A scenario is presented to illustrate both the process used in the peer mentoring and to describe a successful outcome.

CHANGES IN TECHNOLOGY THAT AFFECT AT APPLICATIONS

As the 21st century begins, the worldwide economy is changing from a machine-based economy to a knowledge-based one, from a regional–national scope to a global scope, from host-based to network-based systems, and from text-based to graphically based systems (Ungson & Trudel, 1999). Each of these trends has significant implications for individuals who have disabilities and, therefore, for the future of AT development and application. Workers will be connected not by physical location but by communication channels. Access to information will be increasingly obtained from Internet resources that are accessed through PCs. This raises the question of what the PC and Internet will look like in the future. The editors of PC Magazine identified 10 trends that are likely to occur over the next 10 years (Miller et al., 1999). Many of these, if they are realized, will have a profound impact both on ATs and on the individuals who use them.

One prediction Miller et al. (1999) made is that computers will become more "human." By this they meant that computers will have more human attributes, such as reacting to spoken words or handwritten instructions. In general, the emphasis is on making the user interface more "friendly." The use of natural language processing for input has its origins in automatic speech recognition (ASR), a technology used by people with disabilities. Telephone access to the Internet by means of ASR is already available. ASR will continue to improve, but a major challenge will continue to exist for people who have dysarthric speech. Current ASR systems do not provide good results for this population, and this is clearly an area in which ATs must be developed to allow people with speech disabilities to access the new user interfaces. Similar problems could occur if user interfaces require recognition of handwriting.

Another feature designed to make the user interface more humanlike is the concept of the *chaterbot*. This is a virtual character that responds to questions using voice synthesis. The questions are asked by the user in a particular subject area, and they are input by means of ASR. These user interfaces are "smart," that is, they are based on expected questions and answers in a given subject area. They are not intelligent in the way that humans are, that is, they can't reason or problem solve. The use of a natural-language interface of this type has great appeal for use by people who have intellectual disabilities. The question is this: How forgiving will these interfaces be if the user becomes confused or uses nonstandard forms of language and speech? Once again, AT practitioners must ensure that these general-purpose technologies are inclusive of all individuals. One possible approach to this problem, cited by Miller et al. (1999), is the inclusion of emotion in the user interface. Current work in this area includes cameras that monitor facial expressions and sensors that detect physiological changes. These signals provide the information necessary for an affective tutor to adjust a program to react to emotions. For example, if the tutor detects confusion, an alternative explanation could be offered. Researchers are also working on user interfaces that express emotion to the user as well. These are based on animated characters that change facial expressions to react to input questions. These advances could be of benefit to individuals who have intellectual disabilities and require more concrete interactions.

Two trends in networks have the potential to benefit individuals with disabilities. The first of these is the expansion of existing networks into home, work, and community environments. These networks will connect people in unique and powerful ways. For example, automobile networks will be connected to toll booths and automated fuel pumps. They will also make assisted driving possible, with a potential benefit to people with disabilities. Much of this network will become wireless in the future, and connectivity will be a function of local resources, not existing hard-wired communications providers. The good news in this is that people with disabilities can use their ATs to connect to the network. The bad news is that the ATs must keep pace with constant changes in the design of network configurations to ensure access for people with disabilities.

The second major trend is an increase in the intelligence of the Internet. Web browsers will be able to track sites by the characteristics for which the user typically looks. This might include styles, colors, and sizes of clothing and particular items of interest. Software will also determine a profile for the user based on these preferences and then compare the profiles with those of other users who have similar tastes and interests. The intelligent agent can then recommend products and services that match the profile. These changes require an enhanced programming language over HTML, the software language that is currently used to develop Internet applications. XML (for *eXtensible Markup Language*) provides the necessary capability. For individuals with disabilities to make maximum use of this new language, it must have accessibility guidelines. Fortunately, these are being developed by the World Wide Web Consortium Web Access Initiative (see http://www.w3.org/WAI). The enhancements provided by XML and other new software will make searches easier and more productive. This will benefit all users.

Along with expanded networks will come smarter appliances. From watches to dishwashers, all appliances will have embedded microcomputers. Some of these, such as cellular phones, will include access to the Internet and other computing functions. Others will merely make it possible to network a home and to control it remotely. For example, a meal can be started from work by remotely turning on the stove. One of the keys to these applications is the use of hardware and software that allow digitally controlled appliances to "self-organize" into a community without a desktop computer to manage the network. Appliances will be interconnected in many ways. For example, an image from a television can be e-mailed to a relative. This type of interconnectivity and remote control is ideal for individuals who have difficulties in manipulating or in seeing appliance controls. To ensure accessibility, the software and networks must be accessible and compatible with assistive devices used for input or output from the network.

Increasing realism in computer games will result in better graphics, digital characters, and 3-dimensional interaction. Virtual reality input and output devices, such as stereoscopic 3-dimensional glasses and "force feedback" joysticks, enrich the experience for the user. Primitive forms of these virtual input–output tools have already been applied to create virtual experiences for individuals who have disabilities. For example, children who have cerebral palsy can walk, run, and play with other children in a virtual world. Others have used virtual simulations of homes and business to evaluate the accessibility to wheelchairs prior to construction or modification.

There will also be major changes in e-mail and chat rooms. They will proceed beyond pure text to text linked to 3-dimensional graphics. E-mail and chat rooms have the advantage of anonymity, and this can be a major benefit to individuals who have disabilities (Blackstone, 1996). As Blackstone pointed out, the Internet allows a person who has a disability to communicate with others without his or her disability being immediately apparent. People who have disabilities report that they enjoy establishing relationships with people who experience them first as a person and later learn of their disability. As the ability of the Internet to connect people grows, the benefits to people who have disabilities will also increase. The challenge rehabilitation professionals face is to ensure that these individuals continue to have access to both input to and output from the Internet as this growth progresses.

Other trends cited by Miller et al. (1999) also would affect people with disabilities. There will be smarter and more powerful software. Computing hardware will continue to expand in speed, memory, and functionality, with decreasing or stable cost. The size of information-processing electronics will continue to shrink with greater and greater capability in smaller and smaller packages. This will have implications for ATs that depend on large amounts of signal processing with severe size and weight limitations, such as hearing aids and augmentative communication devices. Miniaturization and low power consumption will also allow major advances in portable systems, and these developments can be exploited to benefit people with disabilities. Much more business will be conducted over the Internet. This will reduce the need for transportation for errands, a major benefit to people who have disabilities.

Computing is not the only area in which changes that can benefit people with disabilities will be seen. Materials are becoming lighter while retaining or even increasing in strength. These materials can be used in products such as wheelchairs, seating systems, prosthetics, and orthotics. More sophisticated control systems are also leading to miniaturization of electromechanical components. This makes it possible to have greater functionality with lower weight and stable cost. This affects areas such as mobility for both individuals who are unable to walk and individuals who are blind.

ATS: GOING WITH THE FLOW OR BUILDING BRIDGES?

Several factors will affect the future design of ATs. The changes in rehabilitation and in technology will each help shape AT development. Products designed specifically for individuals who have disabilities are inherently more expensive because of low production volumes. The design of standard commercial products to include features that enhance their accessibility is termed *universal design*. This is much less expensive than modifying a product after production to meet the needs of a person with a disability, and federal regulations mandate this universal-design approach for certain types of equipment (e.g., telecommunications equipment). A large number of commercial products are being designed according to principles that ensure usability by all people, to the greatest extent possible, without the need for adaptation or specialized design (North Carolina State University, Center for Universal Design, 2001). Features are built into the product to make it more useful to people who have disabilities (e.g., larger knobs; a variety of display options, such as visual, tactile, and auditory; and alternatives to reading text, such as icons and pictures). In some countries, universal design is known as *design for all*. Professionals at the Center for Universal Design at North Carolina State University, in conjunction with advocates of universal design, have compiled a set of principles of universal design, shown in Exhibit 16.1. This center also maintains a Web site on universal design (see http://www.design.ncsu.edu/cud).

On the basis of the previous discussion, one can define the infrastructure for future accessibility as consisting of the following elements: (a) an expanded, smarter, and more available "real" and "virtual" Internet; (b) home automation systems that are smarter and have greater interconnectivity; (c) universal design principles that are applied more widely;

EXHIBIT 16.1
Principles of Universal Design

1. *Equitable Use*—The design is useful and marketable to people with diverse abilities.
2. *Flexibility in Use*—The design accommodates a wide range of individual preferences and abilities.
3. *Simple and Intuitive Use*—Use of the design is easy to understand, regardless of the user's experience, knowledge, language skills, or current concentration level.
4. *Perceptible Information*—The design communicates necessary information effectively to the user, regardless of ambient conditions or the user's sensory abilities.
5. *Tolerance for Error*—The design minimizes hazards and the adverse consequences of accidental or unintended actions.
6. *Low Physical Effort*—The design can be used efficiently and comfortably and with a minimum of fatigue.
7. *Size and Space for Approach and Use*—Appropriate size and space are provided for approach, reach, manipulation, and use regardless of user's body size, posture, or mobility.

Note. Adapted from *Principles of Universal Design.* Copyright 1997 NC State University, The Center for Universal Design. For complete guidelines, visit http://www.design.ncsu.edu:8120/cud/univ_design/princ_ overview.htm

(d) alternative approaches for accessing information technologies; and (e) special-purpose ATs.

If people who have disabilities are to keep pace with the move to a knowledge-based economy, they must continue to have access to the Internet. However, as the Internet becomes more and more dependent on multimedia representations involving complex graphics, animation, and audible sources of information, people who have disabilities have greater challenges in the retrieval of information. The most obvious barriers are for those who are blind. However, as the amount of auditory Web content increases, people who are deaf and cannot access this auditory information are also placed at a significant disadvantage. People who have learning disabilities and dyslexia also find it increasingly difficult to access complicated Web sites that may include flashing pictures, complicated charts, and large amounts of audio and video data. Individuals who have physical disabilities may also find it difficult to use standard keyboard and mouse input modes. Because as many as 40 million people in the United States have physical, cognitive, or sensory disabilities (Lazzaro, 1999), the importance of making the Internet accessible to all is very high. The World Wide Web Consortium's Web Access Initiative project (see http://www.w3.org/WAI) has developed a set of guidelines for developing accessible Web pages. Their "quick tips" for making accessible Web sites are shown in Exhibit 16.2. Vanderheiden (1998) provided an overview of both current approaches to

- *For images and animations:* Use the alt attribute to describe the function of all visuals.
- *For image maps:* Use client-side MAP and text for hotspots.
- *For multimedia:* Provide captioning and transcripts of audio and descriptions of video.
- *For hypertext links:* Use text that makes sense when read out of context. For example, avoid "click here."
- *For page organization:* Use headings, lists, and consistent structure.
- Use CSS for layout and style where possible.
- *For graphs and charts:* Summarize or use the longdesc attribute.
- *For scripts, applets, and plug-ins:* Provide alternative content in case active features are inaccessible or unsupported.
- *For frames:* Use NOFRAMES and meaningful titles.
- *For tables:* Make line-by-line reading sensible. Summarize.
- Check your work. Validate. Use tools, a checklist, and guidelines at http://www.w3.org/TR/WAI-WEBCONTENT

Internet access by people with disabilities and prospects for future developments based on emerging technologies.

One of the principles of Internet access is that users must be able to interact with a user agent (and the document it renders) using the supported input and output devices of their choice and according to their needs (*see* http://www.w3.org/wai). The user agent is the software used to access Web content. This includes desktop graphical browsers, text and voice browsers, mobile phones, multimedia players, and software ATs used with browsers (e.g., screen readers, magnifiers, adapted input devices). Mouse and mouse alternative pointing devices; head wands; keyboards and keyboard alternatives, such as on-screen keyboards and Braille input keyboards, switches and switch arrays, and microphones can all serve as input devices for user agents. Output devices for Internet access for people who have disabilities, in addition to the typical computer monitor and audible output, are often provided by screen magnifiers or screen readers used in conjunction with Braille displays and speech synthesizers.

Several types of alternative input modes are used for computer access (Cook & Hussey, in press). Keyboard entry can be replaced by enlarged or contracted keyboards, automatic speech recognition, on-screen keyboards (e.g., an image of the keyboard is placed on the screen, and a pointer is directed to cells representing individual keys), and indirect selection methods. *Indirect selection* includes scanning (choices are presented to the user sequentially, and the user chooses the one he or she wants through a single switch activation) and coded access (a code, such as Morse code, is used to represent each key on the keyboard). Mouse alternatives include adaptation such as trackballs (large and small), joysticks, and head-controlled pointers. These approaches work well when the input required is text. However, if the person with a disability is to have access to the virtual worlds and smart Web browsers described earlier, this simple access may not be sufficient. For example, some of the virtual reality software requires specially designed controls. Will these be usable by people who have disabilities? Will the "standard" AT input alternatives be usable with the virtual reality and Web access software of the future? Likewise, the increasing use of portable devices will require that input of information be made using devices other than a keyboard or a mouse. Will these be accessible to individuals who have manipulation disabilities? Ensuring access to these portability technologies is essential if the community-based social model of disability is to become a reality. This model requires increased mobility for people with disabilities, increasing the need for access to the technologies being developed. Thus, there are many issues raised for people with disabilities by the advances forecast for information technologies.

There will also be challenges for people who are blind or have low vision. Screen magnifiers are adaptations that allow people with low vision to access the computer screen, and they may be built into the operating system provided by the computer manufacturer or purchased as separate products (Lazzaro, 1999). Because it is difficult for the user to know where he or she is on the screen once it is enlarged, navigational aids are important. The most common navigational aid is to have the viewing window follow (i.e., move the viewing window to that location) mouse cursor movement, follow any text editing that is done, or follow keyboard entry. In addition, both inverted (e.g., white letters on a black background) and high-contrast modes are available. As software for accessing the Internet becomes more sophisticated, the demands placed on screen magnifiers may also increase. For example, enlarging animated characters that move quickly across the screen will require more sophisticated tracking features. Enlarging displays on small portable devices used for Internet access will also present major challenges for AT developers.

A *screen reader* is a software program that converts on-screen information to a form that can be spoken through a speech synthesizer or displayed on a refreshable Braille display. For text information this is a straightforward task. However, conversion of graphical information is much more difficult. Currently, good practice dictates that all graphics characters have a description that can be read through a speech synthesizer. For static characters this works well. When the characters move (as in video or animation), then a running description is required. When the characters are three-dimensional objects, such as the affective tutor or chaterbot described earlier, then the task of portraying these graphical characters is significantly more difficult. For example, how can an emotional facial response be represented in speech or Braille form?

CONCLUSION

On the basis of the discussion in this chapter, anticipated changes in technologies, coupled with the focus on the social aspects of disability, provide a significant opportunity for major advances in the degree to which individuals with disabilities can participate in all aspects of life, including work, school, leisure, and self-care.

These advances will be particularly important as the percentage of the population that is elderly rises. Concepts from universal design will be important in ensuring that this segment of the population remains active and is able to participate in society. This new group of elderly individuals will also be more experienced with computers and other technologies than their predecessors, and they may well demand greater performance and adaptability from both ATs and mainstream devices such as appliances, automobiles, and communications equipment (e.g., telephones, Internet communication). There will also be a greater percentage of individuals with long-term disabilities who join the over-65 age group. These individuals may be among the first large group to be long-term users of ATs, and their experience may have both positive and negative implications. Certainly their extensive experience with the use of ATs will make them a rich source of information regarding effective design and application of these technologies. However, the negative aspects of this use of technologies in the long run are unknown. For example, what will be the effects of vocal stress from use of ASR, or repetitive strain injury from keyboard use, or shoulder problems from manual wheelchair propulsion? It is also impossible to forecast what will be the new problems arising from the extensive use of technology.

Although much of what I have described is conjecture, it is based on modest extrapolation from the current state of the art. There are some things that are known with a high degree of certainty: For example, computer systems will be faster, have more memory, be smaller, and be less expensive for the same or greater functionality. Materials will continually be improved to be lighter, stronger, and more durable. It also is known that the communication channel bandwidth will continue to rise, allowing much more information and much more sophisticated information processing. Finally, it is clear that people with disabilities will continue to assert their right to fully participate in society.

These advances also raise questions for people who have disabilities. The most important of these is whether accessibility will keep pace with technological developments. For example, will ATs for input and output be compatible with the user agents and operating systems of tomorrow? A second major question is whether the needs of people with disabilities will be a driving force in future technological developments. Will people who have disabilities have to adapt to the existing technologies based on characteristics for nondisabled people, or will universal design become a greater reality? In the latter case, adaptations will become less important, and accessibility will become the rule rather than the exception. As I discussed earlier in the chapter, there are significant implications of emerging information-processing technologies for people who have disabilities. If not closely monitored, these could result in less rather than more access to the new information economy for people with disabilities.

Despite the wider use of universal design principles, there will still be a need for effective AT design and application if individuals with disabilities are to realize the full potential of the new information age.

REFERENCES

Blackstone, S. (1996). The Internet: What's the big deal. *Augmentative Communication News, 9*(4), 1–5.

Cook, A. M., & Hussey, S. M. (in press). *Assistive technologies: Principles and practice* (2nd ed.). St. Louis. MO: Mosby YearBook.

Fougeyrollas, P., & Gray, D. B. (1998). Classification systems, factors and social change: The importance of technology. In D. B. Gray, L. A. Quatrano, & M. L. Lieberman, (Eds.), *Using, designing and assessing assistive technology* (pp. 13–28). Baltimore: Brookes.

Heerkens, W. D., Briggs, J., & Weider, T. G. (1997). Using peer mentors to facilitate the match of person and technology. In *Proceedings of the 1999 RESNA conference* (pp. 484–486). Arlington, VA: RESNA Press.

Lazzaro, J. L. (1999). Helping the Web help the disabled. *IEEE Spectrum, 36*(3), 54–59.

Lysack, C., & Kaufert, J. (1999). Disabled consumer leaders' perspectives on provision of community rehabilitation services. *Canadian Journal of Rehabilitation, 12,* 157–166.

Miller, M. J., Kirchner, J., Derfler, F. J., Grottesman, B. Z., Stam, C., Metz, C., Oxer, J., Rupley, S., Willmott, D., & Hirsch, N. (1999, June 22). Future technology. *PC Magazine,* pp. 100–148.

North Carolina State University Center for Universal Design. (2001). *Principles of Universal Design.* Raleigh, NC: Author.

Ungson, G. R., & Trudel, J. D. (1999). The emerging knowledge-based economy. *IEEE Spectrum, 36*(5), 60–65.

Vanderheiden, G. C. (1998). Cross-modal access to current and next-generation Internet: Fundamental and advanced topics in Internet accessibility. *Technology and Disability, 8,* 115–126.

World Health Organization. (2001). *International classification of functioning, disability, and health.* Geneva, Switzerland: Author.

World Wide Web Consortium Web Access Initiative. (1999, May). Web content accessibility guidelines 1.0, Web Accessibility Initiative (WAI). Retrieved from http://www.w3.org/WAI

APPENDIX:
TOOLS FOR ENHANCING THE SKILLS OF REHABILITATION PROFESSIONALS: PROFESSIONAL TRAINING AND CERTIFICATION OF OCCUPATIONAL THERAPY PRACTITIONERS

AIMEE J. LUEBBEN

Occupational therapy is a profession that has been at the forefront of the growth of assistive technology (AT) as a field in its own right. The evolution of the occupational therapy profession, along with the education of its practitioners, serves as a model for related professions.

Occupational therapy is grounded in social and philosophical movements of the 18th, 19th, and early 20th centuries. The occupational therapy profession officially began on March 15, 1917, in Clifton Springs, New York, when the founders—who had such diverse backgrounds as social work, vocational education, nursing, psychiatry, teaching, and art—met to form the National Society for the Promotion of Occupational Therapy. This society was renamed the American Occupational Therapy Association (AOTA) 4 years later.

Occupational therapy is sometimes misunderstood, because the popular meaning of the word *occupation* has changed over the years to become very narrowly defined. The profession uses the following broad, historic definition: "Occupations are the ordinary and familiar things people do every day" (AOTA, 1995, p. 1015). Employment-related words (e.g., *job*, *trade*, and *career*) comprise an integral aspect of occupational therapy but are considered a subset of occupations.

One of the original function-based professions, occupational therapy is essential for people who have difficulty with one or more everyday life tasks. Occupational therapy practitioners believe each person to be a unique, active, and complex being of worth and dignity; they provide holistic services under the assumption that an individual's occupational performance is a unique interplay of three aspects (areas, components, and contexts), defined in the "Uniform Terminology for Occupational Therapy—Third Edition" (UT III; AOTA, 1994). It is interesting that the final draft of the revised

World Health Organization's (2001) classification system—the *ICF*—parallels much of the language in UT III, the occupational therapy taxonomy. For occupational therapy practitioners a person's performance areas (also called *occupations*) include three broad categories of human activity: (a) activities of daily living (e.g., eating, dressing, community mobility); (b) work and productive activities (e.g., shopping, money management, educational activities, job acquisition); and (c) play or leisure activities. The corresponding components within the *ICF* are designated as activities and participation. According to UT III, occupations are further subdivided into components— those sensorimotor, psychosocial, and cognitive elements required for successful participation in performance areas. The *ICF* labels the corresponding components "body functions and structures," with body functions similar to the three UT III performance components. Contexts have similar names and subdivisions in both classification systems. In occupational therapy, *contexts* are situations and factors that influence an individual's participation in performance areas and consist of temporal aspects (chronological, developmental, life cycle, disability status) and environmental aspects (physical, social, political, and cultural), whereas contextual factors in the *ICF* include personal and environmental components.

Because the primary focus of the profession is enhancement of occupational performance, occupational therapy practitioners are concerned with factors that promote, influence, or enhance occupational performance as well as with those factors that serve as barriers, limiting and restricting a person's ability to function across the life span. Thus, AT has been an integral aspect of the occupational therapy practitioner's domain of concern since the beginning of the profession, playing a major role in the occupational therapy profession's unique contribution of maximizing "the fit between what it is the individual wants and needs to do and his or her capabilities to do it" (Baum, 1997, p. 40).

Of the four intervention approaches (remediation/restoration, compensation/adaptation, disability prevention, and health promotion) listed in *The Guide to Occupational Therapy Practice* (Moyers, 1999), AT is instrumental in successful provision of services under the compensation/adaptation approach. The focus of the compensation/adaptation approach includes changing the task; altering the task method; adapting the task object; changing the context; educating the family, caregiver, or both; or providing environmental adaptation.

In occupational therapy, as in most professions, the purpose of professional training and certification is to protect the public by assuring practitioner competence. The word *competence* derives from *competo*, a Latin word that means "to be suitable" or "to be adequate" and implies meeting minimum standards but not a particular position along an excellence continuum. Minimum standards, therefore, protect the public but do not ensure quality. Generally, competence exists at two levels: (a) initial competence for practitioners just entering the occupational therapy profession and (b) continuing competence for occupational therapy practitioners beyond the entry level. The occupational therapy profession is composed of two practitioner types: (a) occupational therapists who are initially trained in professional-level programs and (b) occupational therapy assistants who complete technical-level programs.

INITIAL COMPETENCE

With a strong tradition of assuring entry-level practitioner competence, the occupational therapy profession formalized initial competence by accrediting preservice training programs first, followed closely by certifying individual practitioners. In addition, occupational therapy was one of the first professions to establish competencies related strictly to AT service provision.

Accreditation

Although founding members of the profession began discussing educational training requirements during that first 1917 meeting, AOTA adopted the first minimum training standards in 1923, and in 1931 occupational therapy became the first profession to seek a cooperative accreditation process with the American Medical Association (AMA). Two years later, the AMA formalized the collaboration and began inspecting occupational therapy programs, a cooperative process that continued until 1994, when the Accreditation Council for Occupational Therapy Education (ACOTE) was created within AOTA. In 1995, ACOTE received recognition by the U.S. Department of Education as the first agency in full compliance with new Department of Education regulations.

Although AOTA had established minimum preservice training program requirements 12 years before, the *Essentials of an Acceptable School of Occupational Therapy*—the first formal accreditation document, developed in 1935 in collaboration with the AMA—was based on results of early joint inspections of occupational therapy schools. The *Standards for an Accredited Educational Program for the Occupational Therapist* (ACOTE, 1998a), which became effective in 2000, replaced the *Essentials and Guidelines of an Accredited School for the Occupational Therapist*, which was revised in 1943, 1949, 1973, 1983, and 1991. According to the standards (ACOTE, 1998a), to graduate from an accredited educational program that trains occupational therapists, a student must demonstrate competence in various curriculum content areas, including theory, evaluation, intervention planning, models of service provision, research, ethics, and management, as well as communication, governmental and policy issues, lifestyle planning, diversity, and advocacy matters.

The occupational therapist was the sole type of occupational therapy practitioner until the profession began discussing the training of assistants in 1949. Seven years later, AOTA approved a plan to recognize a second level of occupational therapy personnel, designed to cover one area: psychiatry (Cottrell, 2000). The minimum educational program requirements for the training of occupational therapy assistants, *Essentials and Guidelines of an Accredited School for the Occupational Therapy Assistant,* was initially adopted in 1958 and revised in 1962, 1967, 1970, 1975, and 1991. The most recent iteration of this accreditation document, *Standards for an Accredited Educational Program for the Occupational Therapy Assistant* (ACOTE, 1998b), became effective in 2000.

Currently, ACOTE is the official accrediting agency for entry-level educational programs for occupational therapists and occupational therapy assistants in the United States and its territories. Because of requests to expand geographically, however, the influence of ACOTE reaches beyond the United States, with a university in Scotland first to seek ACOTE accreditation.

Although an entry-level training curriculum is the commonality among occupational therapy educational programs, credentials awarded to students by institutions of higher education vary. Most institutions that offer educational programs for occupational therapy assistants award associate's degrees to graduates; however, some training programs award certificates or diplomas. As of 2001, the graduate of an entry-level educational program for occupational therapists emerges with one of the following credentials: (a) baccalaureate degree, (b) postbaccalaureate certificate, (c) certificate in partial fulfillment of a master's degree, (d) professional master's degree, (e) combined baccalaureate–master's degrees, or (f) entry-level doctoral degree. The first three options will cease to exist on January 1, 2007, when the postbaccalaureate degree is established as the new entry level for occupational therapists. Practicing occupational therapists also have opportunities for advanced graduate study in occupational therapy through postprofessional master's and doctoral degrees. As of 2001, however, occupational therapy accreditation does not exist for postprofessional graduate degrees for advanced study in occupational therapy.

Certification

In addition to the strong foundation of credentialing educational training programs, the occupational therapy profession has enjoyed a long history of credentialing individual practitioners. Registration came first, and in the beginning credentialing of individuals was tied to AOTA membership. Although AOTA resolved to establish a national registry of qualified occupational therapists in 1926, the first *National Registry of Occupational Therapists* was published in 1932. The following year, AOTA determined that credentialing of individuals be coupled with credentialing of educational training programs; however, the decision to register only individuals who had graduated from accredited educational programs was not enforced until 1939. Credentialing individuals became a hot topic again in 1945, when the first national registration examination was introduced. The initial essay format lasted for 2 years, until 1947, when the registration examination was redesigned with multiple-choice questions, a format that continues in current certification examinations.

AOTA controlled both types of credentialing (for educational programs and for individual practitioners) for decades. To avoid potential antitrust-related litigation, AOTA created the American Occupational Therapy Certification Board (AOTCB), an autonomous unit within the professional organization in 1986. AOTCB was incorporated as a separate, independent entity in 1988.

Until AOTCB was created, maintaining practice credentials was a matter of paying AOTA annual membership fees. AOTCB, however, was designed to administer the practitioner examinations and grant initial certification on a one-time-only basis to successful examination candidates. In other words, the intention of AOTA was that the person who received initial certification from AOTCB would pay the fee one time and became a certified occupational therapy practitioner for life. The year 1996 signaled a significant time for the profession when AOTCB (a) changed its name to the National Board for Certification in Occupational Therapy (NBCOT), (b) trademarked the names Occupational Therapist Registered OTR and Certified Occupational Therapy Assistant COTA, and (c) unveiled a certification renewal process to be completed every 5 years. To practice occupational therapy at the entry level a prospective practitioner must successfully complete four requirements. The occupational therapist must (a) graduate from an ACOTE-accredited entry-level professional educational program, (b) complete a minimum of 6 months of supervised internships, (c) pass NBCOT's *Certification Examination for Occupational Therapist Registered OTR*, and (d) comply with the statues and regulations related to the occupational therapist in the practice location. On the other hand, a prospective occupational therapy assistant must (a) graduate from an ACOTE-accredited entry-level technical educational program, (b) complete a minimum of 4 months of supervised internships, (c) pass NBCOT's *Certification Examination for Occupational Therapy Assistant COTA*, and (d) comply with the statues and regulations related to the occupational therapy assistant in the practice location.

As a result of NBCOT's changes, many occupational therapists and occupational therapy assistants, once initially credentialed (through AOTA, AOTCB, or NBCOT), opted not to participate in the certification renewal process. After consulting statutes and regulations of governmental entities in which they practiced, some occupational therapy practitioners found they could continue practicing without NBCOT certification. Because practitioners who successfully complete the NBCOT renewal process are eligible to use the NBCOT trademarked phrases (including initials) that designate the two types of occupational therapy practitioners, occupational therapists and occupational therapy assistants who do not renew through NBCOT drop one letter from the credentials that follow their names (i.e., OT or OTA, rather than OTR and COTA, respectively).

Governmental regulation of occupational therapy practitioners became an issue in the 1960s. Opposed at first to the concept of potential external constraints on the profession, AOTA later supported the movement for governmental regulation by developing an initial model for licensure in 1969. By the 1970s and 1980s, occupational therapy practitioners became proactive in seeking governmental regulation, resulting in 53 jurisdictions that currently regulate occupational therapy practitioners. Although most governmental entities offer licensure, some jurisdictions have certification, registration, or trademark laws. Requirements vary across jurisdictions; however, most governmental entities require occupational therapy practitioner applicants to provide evidence of passing scores on the NBCOT examination.

Technology Competence

For years, occupational therapy practitioners have been expected to enter the field with competence in technology. In fact, both agencies responsible for assuring initial competence have listed technology requirements in official documents: Preservice programs must be compliant with ACOTE's accreditation standards, which include technology requirements, and NBCOT tests entry-level practitioners on AT-related questions. In other words, entry-level expertise in AT is assumed for practitioners who graduate from an ACOTE-accredited educational program and pass the NBCOT examination.

In the early 1990s, the occupational therapy profession began the formal process of formulating technology competencies, resulting in preliminary technology competencies, training guidelines, and areas of technology content (Hammel & Smith, 1993). The competencies related to technology were refined in Hammel and Angelo's (1996) document, which included two levels: general technology information and AT. For the AT level, this document lists 39 competencies across three areas (evaluation, intervention, and resource coordination), for three stages (entry, intermediate, and advanced) and for both types of occupational therapy practitioners.

Occupational therapy practitioners are expected to graduate from their preservice educational training at the beginning AT stage. At this stage, entry-level occupational therapists and occupational therapy assistants are expected to show the same 5 (63%) intervention competencies and 12 (75%) resource coordination competencies. Only in evaluation competencies do the two occupational therapy practitioner types differ: The occupational therapist demonstrates 11 (73%) competencies, whereas the occupational therapy assistant achieves 1 (7%) competency.

CONTINUING COMPETENCE

To practice occupational therapy, entry-level requirements are clear-cut; however, requirements at this time related to continuing practice after initial credentialing are indefinite and somewhat confusing, particularly to people outside the profession. For years, competence beyond the entry level was considered an internal aspect of professionalism: Individual occupational therapy practitioners were expected to ensure they were keeping current in the field. In the early days, AOTA offered members various methods of maintaining and developing new knowledge and skills. Meetings and conferences were the primary methods of assuring continuing competence, with the first meeting occurring in 1917, within 6 months after occupational therapy became a profession.

The year 1922 was significant because of two events related to continuing competence. The first event was the decision to offer the annual conference in conjunction with the American Hospital Association. The reasoning behind this decision was twofold: AOTA members could choose from the offerings of two associations, and American Hospital Association members could learn about occupational therapy. The second event was the creation of the first professional occupational therapy journal. Named *Archives of Occupational Therapy*, the privately owned journal was first available by subscription, separate from AOTA membership. In 1925, the journal was renamed *Occupational Therapy and Rehabilitation* and offered as an AOTA member benefit until 1946. The following year, AOTA began publishing the *American Journal of Occupational Therapy*, still a membership benefit and one of many AOTA continuing education options, which include annual conferences, self-paced clinical courses, workshops on disk, Internet-based on-line workshops, and telephone seminars.

Competency has been addressed in the *Occupational Therapy Code of Ethics*, adopted first in 1977 and revised in 1979, 1988, 1994, and 2000. One of the seven principles of the *Occupational Therapy Code of Ethics*,

Principle 4, is that "Occupational therapy practitioners shall achieve and continually maintain high standards of competence" (AOTA, 2000, p. 615). Specific duties for occupational therapy practitioners listed under this fourth principle include

- holding appropriate credentials,
- using procedures that conform to AOTA documents relevant to practice,
- maintaining and documenting competence by participating in professional development and educational activities,
- critically examining and keeping current with emerging knowledge,
- protecting service recipients,
- providing supervision, and
- referring to or consulting with other service providers.

More recently, the profession has become interested in more formal methods of assuring as well as documenting continuing competence. In 1991, AOTA began looking at competency issues related to just one narrow area, physical agent modalities, and then broadened the view by addressing competence all levels and settings of the profession. AOTA's approach was to provide structure for the internal process of assuring continuing competence; the first document was a self-appraisal guide (Thomson et al., 1995). According to Thomson et al. (1995),

> Maintaining and updating one's skills is a developmental and ongoing process throughout one's career. There are a variety of methods to achieve competency, and many measures of competency are used to document one's knowledge and performance skills. Ensuring competence is the responsibility of everyone, including the individual practitioner, employers, professional associations, and regulatory boards. The key, however, rests with the individual who must be self-directed to attain and maintain competence. (p. 4)

This self-appraisal guide (Thomson et al., 1995, pp. 6–8) lists 13 methods to achieve competency, including

- independent study,
- academic coursework,
- continuing education,
- teaching activities,
- presentations,
- publications,
- research activities,
- professional certification,
- specialty certification,

- recertification and relicensure,
- preceptor–supervisor–mentor relationship,
- peer review, and
- on-the-job training and experience.

More important, the Thomson et al. (1995) publication provides 10 methods of documenting competency, including

- written examinations,
- self-appraisal tools,
- competency checklists or rating forms,
- evaluation by clients–students or participants–employees,
- continuing education credits or contact hours,
- years of experience or direct treatment hours,
- presentations and publications,
- academic degrees,
- awards and honors, and
- quality management activities.

The remainder of this document is a competency self-appraisal tool.

To develop additional AT competence many occupational therapy practitioners work to achieve Hammel and Angelo's (1996) competencies at the intermediate stage or advanced stage. At the intermediate stage occupational therapists and occupational therapy assistants are expected to show the same 5 (63%) intervention competencies and 14 (88%) resource coordination competencies. Only in the evaluation competencies do the two types of occupational therapy practitioner differ: The occupational therapist will have achieved 11 (73%) competencies for a total of 30 (77%) competencies, whereas the occupational therapy assistant will show 6 (40%) competencies for a total of 25 (74%) competencies. Both types of occupational therapy practitioners are expected to demonstrate the maximum eight intervention competencies at the advanced AT stage. As for the other areas in the advanced stage, occupational therapists are expected to demonstrate 15 in evaluation and 16 in resource coordination, a maximum of 39 competencies. At the advanced stage occupational therapy assistants are expected to show 9 (60%) competencies in the evaluation area and 14 (88%) competencies in the resource coordination area for a total of 29 (74%) competencies.

For occupational therapy practitioners, methods of achieving competence in AT vary. Some occupational therapists and occupational therapy assistants use continuing education, independent study, teaching activities, academic coursework, presentations, publications, and research activities as means of achieving competency in AT, whereas other occupational therapy practitioners have taken the specialty certification route. The Rehabilitation

Engineering and Assistive Technology Society of North America (RESNA) provides specialty certification in AT, offering written examinations for AT practitioners and AT suppliers. Passing either examination and using the credentials provide a readily recognizable measure of documenting AT competence.

DECIPHERING THE "ALPHABET SOUP" OF CREDENTIALS

Although wording of titles may vary in other countries (e.g., *ergotherapist* in France), occupational therapists exist throughout the world. The United States, however, is the only country with the other occupational therapy practitioner type: the occupational therapy assistant. As in other countries, occupational therapy practitioners in the United States sometimes bear the brunt of gentle ribbing for the "alphabet soup," or the string of initials they carry after their names. Deciphering the alphabet soup can, however, provide information regarding an occupational therapy practitioner's education, specialty certifications, and national honors, as well as whether the occupational therapist or occupational therapy assistant opted to renew his or her credentials through NBCOT. In the United States, the order of initials for an occupational therapy practitioner is not absolute; however, by convention most practitioners place only the highest earned degree first, directly after the name. Occasionally, an occupational therapist lists a doctorate followed by a master's degree, especially if the latter degree indicates educational training in another profession. By convention, a national honor is placed last in the alphabet soup, and all other initials are placed are located between. When the alphabet soup for some practitioners became lengthy, the occupational therapy profession outlawed the use of periods to save space in publications. Before moving to the individual descriptions that follow, try to decipher the alphabet soup of the following fictitious occupational therapy practitioners:

- Sarah Coggins, OTR-C, CHT, BCP, ATP, BCN
- Nikki Mercer, COTA/L
- Dorothy Powers, PhD, OT/L, FAOTA
- Sam Routt, OTR, ATS, RTS
- Ben Takacs, MBA, OTA, AP, ROH

Sarah Coggins, OTR-C, CHT, BCP, ATP, BCN, is an occupational therapist whose designation shows she has chosen to renew her credentials through NBCOT (OTR) and that she works in a state that regulates occupational therapy practitioners through certification (-C). Having practiced for more than 20 years across multiple areas, she has chosen the external credentialing route to add to her occupational therapy background. First practicing in orthopedics, she became a certified hand therapist (CHT), a credentialing process offered by the American Society of Hand Therapists to occupational therapists and physical therapists. When she wanted to have the same holidays and vacations as her children, she began contracting with a special education cooperative to serve on the multidistrict AT team and provide occupational therapy services. After several years in this position, she successfully completed the process to become board certified in pediatrics (BCP), which is offered by AOTA to occupational therapists. In addition, she completed the credentialing process offered by RESNA to become an AT practitioner (ATP). Her most recent success in external credentialing is reflected in the initials BCN, which indicate that she is board certified in neurorehabilitation, a specialty credentialing process offered by AOTA to occupational therapists.

Nikki Mercer, COTA/L, just graduated from an occupational therapy assistant program in a community college, passed the certification examination, and received her initial designation of certified occupational therapy assistant (COTA) from NBCOT. She works in a community-based center for adults with brain injuries. Because her workplace is in a state in which occupational therapy practitioners are licensed, and she has complied with the state's credentialing requirements, she carries the designation /L.

Dorothy Powers, PhD, OT/L, FAOTA, practiced full time for 29 years before entering higher education. An associate professor in a master's entry level occupational therapy curriculum on the West Coast, she teaches all content related to AT. According to the initials that follow her name, (a) the PhD shows she has completed a doctorate, but content area of this graduate degree is not specified; (b) the OT/L indicates she carried the initials OTR (occupational therapist) at the time of her initial certification, but changed to the OT designation when she chose not to renew her certification with NBCOT, whereas the /L shows that she has complied with the credentialing requirements in a state that offers licensure; and (c) the FAOTA designates her as a Fellow of the American Occupational Therapy Association, an award bestowed on occupational therapists by AOTA indicating leadership in the profession.

Sam Routt, OTR, ATS, RTS, is a seating and mobility specialist who became interested in the occupational therapy profession through his work on AT evaluation teams. Recently, he graduated from a weekend baccalaureate degree program in occupational therapy and passed the NBCOT examination. He is now the southeast regional manager of a brand of wheelchairs made in the United States. The initials that follow his name indicate that he (a) is an occupational therapist who is initially certified (OTR) by NBCOT, (b) successfully completed the credentialing process through

RESNA to be called an AT supplier (ATS), and (c) completed the credentialing process through National Registry of Rehabilitation Technology Suppliers (NRRTS) that designates him as a rehabilitation technology supplier (RTS).

Ben Takacs, MBA, OTA, AP, ROH, is an occupational therapy assistant. Before completing a baccalaureate degree in business and a graduate degree in business administration (MBA), he was trained in a diploma-level occupational therapy assistant program in a technical school. His occupational therapy practitioner designation (OTA) indicates that he chose not to renew his credentials with NBCOT. In addition, his other initials indicate he successfully completed the advanced practice (AP) credentialing process offered by AOTA to occupational therapy assistants and is enrolled on the Roster of Honor (ROH), an AOTA leadership award bestowed on occupational therapy assistants.

CURRENT TRENDS AND ISSUES

Methods of assuring practitioner competence, professional training, and certification have re-emerged as two of the hottest issues in occupational therapy today. One issue, assuring the initial competence of entry-level occupational therapists, has resulted in a trend toward postbaccalaureate entry with a recent decision to move the entry level for the occupational therapist beyond the baccalaureate degree. Assuring the continuing competence of occupational therapy practitioners beyond the entry level is the second issue. This second issue culminated in a battle for control, litigation, and, finally, a renewed effort to cooperate for the good of the occupational therapy profession.

Issue 1: Postbaccalaureate Degree Entry

In April 1999, the occupational therapy profession took the first step in moving entry level to beyond the baccalaureate degree. This is not a new idea in the occupational therapy profession; the "great entry-level debate" actually began in 1958 when occupational therapy leaders advocated moving to a master's entry level. With the baccalaureate degree mandated as entry level for occupational therapists at that time, the United States set the standard for other countries in which curricula to train occupational therapists consisted of 3-year diploma programs. In the 1980s, when other professions (e.g., physical therapy) were considering raising their entry levels, this issue was hotly debated again in occupational therapy. At that time, AOTA conducted an extensive study and recommended that moving to master's degree entry would be in the best interest of occupational therapy; however, the profession did not act.

Recently the debate resumed, but terminology changed. No longer using the word *master's* to indicate entry level, the occupational therapy profession began using the phrase *postbaccalaureate degree entry* to reflect approval of the first entry-level doctoral curriculum in occupational therapy as well as current entry-level changes in the pharmacy and audiology professions, both of which have moved to doctoral entry level. The occupational therapy profession finally resolved this initial competence issue when Resolution J: Movement to Required Postbaccalaureate Level of Education (Commission on Education & Commission on Practice, 1999) was adopted during the 1999 session of AOTA's Representative Assembly, the national association's legislative body.

In August 1999, ACOTE mandated that only curricula awarding postbaccalaureate degrees in occupational therapy will be eligible for accreditation after January 1, 2007. As of 2001, educational programs that train occupational therapists and currently award the baccalaureate degree are redesigning their existing baccalaureate degree curricula into (a) combined baccalaureate–master's degrees curricula, (b) professional (basic) master's degree programs, or (c) entry-level clinical doctorates. Universities continuing to offer only the baccalaureate degree in occupational therapy beyond January 1, 2007, will lose their accreditation status from ACOTE, and their students will be ineligible to sit for the NBCOT certification examination.

Issue 2: Continuing Competence

To provide external assurances of occupational therapy practitioner competence, NBCOT started a certification renewal process in 1996. The first phase of the renewal process consisted of NBCOT requiring occupational therapy practitioners to respond to a self-attestation form and notifying them that a plan for continuing competence would be developed for future renewal cycles. Arguing that recertification was outside NBCOT's purview and that competence was a matter of professional responsibility, AOTA (1999) set forth five continuing competence standards including knowledge, performance skills, interpersonal abilities, critical reasoning, and ethical reasoning.

In May 2001 representatives from the boards of AOTA and NBCOT met in an effort to develop an understanding of participance in a national program for continuing competence and certification renewal. The representatives agreed to incorporate AOTA's (1999) Standards for Continuing Competence and self-assessment tool as integral aspects of NBCOT's certification renewal program. As of June 2001, the outcome of this meeting was awaiting approval by each organization's board.

REFERENCES

Accreditation Council for Occupational Therapy Education. (1998a). *Standards for an accredited educational program for the occupational therapist.* Bethesda, MD: Author.

Accreditation Council for Occupational Therapy Education. (1998b). *Standards for an accredited educational program for the occupational therapy assistant.* Bethesda, MD: Author.

American Occupational Therapy Association. (1994). Uniform terminology for occupational therapy—Third edition. *American Journal of Occupational Therapy, 48,* 1047–1054.

American Occupational Therapy Association. (1995). Position paper: Occupation. *American Journal of Occupational Therapy, 49,* 1015–1018.

American Occupational Therapy Association. (1999). Standards for continuing competence. *American Journal of Occupational Therapy, 53,* 599–600.

American Occupational Therapy Association. (2000). Occupational Therapy Code of Ethics (2000). *American Journal of Occupational Therapy, 54,* 614–616.

Baum, C. M. (1997). The occupational therapy context: Philosophy, principles, practice. In C. H. Christiansen & C. M. Baum (Eds.), *Occupational therapy: Enabling function and well-being* (2nd ed., pp. 26–45). Thorofare, NJ: SLACK.

Commission on Education & Commission on Practice. (1999). *Resolution J: Movement to required postbaccalaureate level of education* (Item 1999R9). Bethesda, MD: American Occupational Therapy Association.

Cottrell, R. P. F. (2000). OTA education and professional development: A historical review. *American Journal of Occupational Therapy, 54,* 407–412.

Hammel, J., & Angelo, J. (1996). Technology competencies for occupational therapy practitioners. *Assistive Technology, 8,* 34–42.

Hammel, J., & Smith, R. O. (1993). Development of technology competencies and training guidelines for occupational therapists. *American Journal of Occupational Therapy, 47,* 970–979.

Moyers, P. A. (1999). The guide to occupational therapy practice. *American Journal of Occupational Therapy, 53,* 247–322.

Thomson, L. K., Lieberman, D., Murphy, R., Wendt, E., Poole, J., & Hertfelder, S. D. (1995). *Developing, maintaining, and updating competency in occupational therapy: A guide to self-appraisal.* Bethesda, MD: American Occupational Therapy Association.

World Health Organization. (2001, June 15). *ICF: International classification of functioning, disability, and health, Final draft* (English full version) [On-line]. Retrieved from http://www.who.int/icidh/ICIDH-2%20Final%20Draft%ENG%20Website%2022_04.pdf

AUTHOR INDEX

Numbers in italics refer to listings in reference sections.

SUBJECT INDEX

satisfaction and, 35–36
from user's perspective, 32
Assessment modifications
as consumer right, 194
Asset values
and adaptation to disability, 135
Assistive devices (ADs)
in common use, 5
definition of, 5–6, 110–111, *169*
description of, 4–5
in educational access, 194
evaluation of
consumer-based criteria in, 77
consumer participation in, 77
sensory, 186–187
Assistive Technology Act of 1998, 23–24
funding for individualized legal advocacy, 24
Assistive technology (AT)
changes and future directions in
accessibility and, 274–278
computer interface, 271–272
in design and access, 274–278
in e-mail and chat rooms, 273
in information-processing electronics, 273–274
interconnectivity and remote control of appliances, 272–273
Internet intelligence increase, 272–273
materials, 274
in materials, 274
miniaturization of electromechanical components, 274
network expansion, 272
in rehabilitation practice, 269–271
in software, 273
in software and hardware, 273–274
technological, 271–274
design of, 274, 275
devices in (*See* Assistive devices (ADs))
in improvement of everyday competencies, 111–112
integration of devices and, 24
interventions for life domains, 112
for long-term care, 113, 114
nomenclature in, 110–111

nonuse of
disability within culture, 171
factors associated with, 170
self-concept in, 170
stigma in, 170
origin of term, 17
for prevention, 112–113, 114
for rehabilitation, 113, 114
role of, 110–113
skills retraining in
for rehabilitation psychologist, 187–188
strategies in, 110–111
structures of, 110
as tool and symbol, 173
universal design of, 274
use of
benefits of, 117–118
biographical consequences and, 118–119
and personal control theory, 116–117
principles for, 113–116
Assistive technology (AT) service
definition of, 6
in social model of rehabilitation
environments in, 7
primary factors in, 7–8
Assistive technology (AT) service provider
to aging population, 10–11
credentialing of, 11
informational role of, 11
partnership with user, 10
roles and characteristics of, 8
Assistive Technology Device Predisposition Assessment (ATDPA)
matching person and device
adolescents through adults, 33
Assistive technology outcomes measurement (ATOM) model
components of, 91
determinants in, 91
domains in, 90, 91
flexibility of, 91
as future framework, 90
AT. *See* Assistive technology (AT)
Attitudes
toward AT ownership and use
gender, race, ethnicity, culture effects on, 104–105

Family
    acceptance of AT, 10
    in counseling process, 236
        in two case histories, 245–249
    in education of consumers, 158, 159
    feelings of, 176
    involvement of
        in AT for children, 36–37
        in instruction of older member,
            120, 121
        in rehabilitation, 158–159
        in service delivery, 157–158
    and ownership and use of assistive
        equipment, 104
    in training for AT use, 159
Federal agencies
    research agendas
        for AT-related issues, 179
Feelings
    caregiver and family respect for, 176
    of control, 176
    of guilt or shame, 175, 176

Gender differences
    in activities of daily living aid use,
        99
    in assistive devices and personal care
        devices use
        Medical Expenditure Panel Sur-
            vey, 98
    in assistive devices used in social set-
        tings, 99–100
        by professionals in science and en-
            gineering, 99–100
    in assistive device use
        persons with cerebrovascular acci-
            dent, orthopedic deficits,
            lower limb amputation, pre-
            and post-discharge, 100
    in assistive technology use
        study variation and, 100–101
    in cognitive device use, 100
    in health and health care use, 95
    in-home grab bars, shower seats, spe-
        cial railings and wheelchair
        access
        Asset and Health Dynamics of
            the Oldest survey, 98
    in mobility, vision, hearing aids use
        Canadian study, 99

    in mobility aid use, 98–99
    in mobility and ADL aid use
        Netherlands study, 98
        Wales, 98–99
    in ownership and use of assistive de-
        vices, 97–101
        Canadian study, 97
        Medicare enrollees, Long-Term
            Care Survey, 97
        Swedish study, 97
        U.S. National Health Interview
            Study, 97–98
    in walking aid ownership and use,
        100
Guilt
    feelings of, 175, 176

Hasssles Scale
    of situational stressors
        in chronic pain assessment, 68
Hearing impairment
    hearing aid use in, 99
    telecommunication display devices
        for, 200
Hispanic Americans
    acceptance of disabilities and adapta-
        tion to AT, 160
Home environment
    and ownership and use of assistive
        equipment, 103–104
Home modification
    functional–environmental need
        model for, 113–114
Hope
    in disability acceptance, 136
Human activity assistive technology
    model, 77
Human environment/technology model,
    77

ICF. *See International Classification of
    Functioning, Disability, and Health:
    Final Draft*
Identity confusion
    in acceptance of disability, 135–136
Illness Behavior Questionnaire
    in chronic pain assessment, 68
Impairment(s)
    cognitive

in continuing education of rehabilitation professional, 193
Individuals With Disabilities Education Act Amendments of 1990,
36
Individuals With Disabilities Education Act (IDEA) of 1975 and
amendments, 21
Rehabilitation Act of 1973, 18,
19–20
rehabilitation professional and
knowledge of, 192
Social Security Act Amendments of
1972, 18
Technology-Related Assistance for
Individuals With Disabilities Act
of 1988, 5, 17
Telecommunications Act of 1996,
25
Workforce Investment Act of 1988,
20
Life Experiences Survey
of situational stressors
in chronic pain assessment, 68
Life span planning
by rehabilitation professional,
193–194
Life-threatening conditions
Comprehensive Health Enhancement Support System in, 204
Long-term care
AT in, 113, 114

Master's degree
for occupational therapist
entry level, 292–293
Master's degree program
distance learning in, 217–218,
226–227
Matching
of client and service, 104, 159
Matching Assistive Technology and
CHild (MATCH) system, 33
in assessment, families in, 36–37
Matching person and technology (MPT)
model, 77
as basis for outcomes measurement
of consumer satisfaction, 81
family in, 36–37
incorporation of user in, 33–34, 35

in Ireland, 261
multidimensional screening of person–device match in, 42
satisfaction outcome in, 42
Material adjustments
definition of, 111
Meaning
of assistive technology and devices
in ethnic minorities, 171, 190
of comfort
patient/nurse, 85
of AT and devices
in progressive disorders, 132–
133
of satisfaction, 78
in AT use, 136–137
Mediated learning. See Distance learning
Medical Outcomes Survey Symptom–
Function Checklist (SF–36)
health quality of life and, 68
Medical patients
emotional disorders in, 48
Millon Behavioral Health Inventory
in chronic pain assessment, 68
Minnesota Multiphasic Personality Inventory (MMPI)
in chronic pain assessment, 67
Minnesota Multiphasic Personality Inventory–2 (MMPI–2)
in chronic pain assessment, 67
Premorbid Somatic Complaint Questionnaire and, 51
Mobility aids
self-concept and, 170
use of, 99
Motivation
in disability acceptance
and AD use, 136
in learner-centered education, 221
and use, 135, 171–172
Motor function deficits
pain assessment in
adaptive devices in, 70–71
eyeblinks in, 71
numerical rating scales in, 70
Mouse
alternatives to, 277
Multicultural issues
belief about disability, 189–190
cultural syntonicity, 190
disability as culture, 189

Multicultural issues, *continued*
  in retraining of rehabilitation psychologist, 189–191

National Board for Certification in Occupational Therapy (NBCOT)
  certification renewal and, 285–286
  creation of, 285
National Institute on Disability and Rehabilitative Research (NIDRR),
  156
Native Americans
  acceptance of disabilities and adaptation to AT, 160
Networks
  expansion of, 272
  telecommunication
    in videoconferencing, 202–203
    in telehealth delivery, 202–203
Nociception
  in pain, 60

Occupational therapist
  accreditation of
    American Medical Association collaboration in, 283
    historical, 283–284
  accreditation of training programs for, 283–284
  certification of
    history of, 284–285
    renewal of, 285, 286, 293
  continuing competence of
    achievement of, 288–289
    annual conference in, 287
    documentation of, 289
    Occupational Therapy Code of Ethics and, 287–288
    professional journals in, 287
    self-appraisal guide to, 288–289
  credential acronyms for
    examples and designations of, 290–292
  entry level
    baccalaureate degree, 292
    master's degree, 292–293
    postbaccalaureate degree requirement, 293
  government regulation of, 286

  in AT instruction, 120
  licensure *vs.* certification of, 286
  technology competence of
    continuing, 289–290
    initial, 286–287
Occupational therapy
  AT in, 282
  assistants in, 283
  competence in
    continuing, 287–290
    initial, 283–287
  contexts in, 282
  definition of, 281
  history of, 281
  intervention approaches in, 282
  occupational performance in, 281–282
  person in, 281
  practitioners in, 283
  professional journals for, 287
  taxonomy in, 281–282
  training and certification in
    purpose of, 282–283
Occupational therapy assistant
  accreditation of
    credentials in, 284
    entry-level educational requirements for, 284
  certification of, 285
  continuing competence of, 289
  entry-level competence of
    AT competence in, 287
    educational program requirements for, 284
Occupational Therapy Code of Ethics, 287–288
On-line learning. *See* Distance learning
Orientation and awareness
  AT interventions in, 112
Outcomes
  comparative studies in videoconferencing, 206–207
  measurement of
    assistive technology outcomes measurement model in, 90–91
    domains in, 78
  successful
    evaluation, selection, use, satisfaction in, 161
  in telehealth research, 203–209

Pain
    assessment of
        for affect, 64–65
        assistive technology in, 70
        behavioral observations in, 71
        in children, 70
        disability and, 69–71
        in disabled persons, 69–71
        in elderly, 70
        for intensity, 61–64
        for pain behaviors, 65–67
        physiological measures in, 71
        psychological, 67–69
        self-report scales in, 61–64
    association with AT use, 70
    chronic
        psychological assessment of,
          67–69
    comorbidity in, 67
    definition of, 59
    multilayered model of, 60
    self-report scales in, 60–67
Pain affect
    McGill Pain Questionnaire, 64
    measurement of
        Descriptor Differential Scale of
          Pain Affect in, 65
        Pain Discomfort Scale in, 65
        verbal rating scale in, 64
        visual analogue scales in, 64–65
Pain behavior
    assessment of
        continuous observation in, 66
        duration measures in, 66
        frequency counts in, 66
        functional analysis in context, 65
        interval recording in, 67
        as isolated phenomenon, 65
        options available in, 65–67
        time sampling in, 66–67
    in multilayered model of pain, 60
Parents
    involvement in child's individualized
        education plan, 158
Participation
    consumer
        in rehabilitation practice
          changes, 270–271
        in evaluation of assistive device, 77,
          178
        in service delivery

        of caregiver, 157
        of consumer, 157
        of family, 157–158
Partnership
    of consumer and rehabilitation psy-
        chologist, 186
    in disabilities services in Ireland,
        253–254, 259, 262
    of AT provider and user, 10
    in social model of rehabilitation,
        255
Personal assistance
    use of
        gender differences in, 97
        with AT use, 97
Personal care attendants
    in cerebral palsy, 129–130
    in congenital disabilities, 128
    decrease in use of
        AT ownership and, 125
Personal control theory
    primary mechanisms in, 116
    secondary mechanisms in, 116
    and AT use, 116–117
Personality
    assessment of
        comparison of pathological and
          nonpathological measures, 50
        historical overview of, 48–49
        interpretation of results, 51
        nonpathological and pathological
          devices for, 50–51
        recommendations for AT, 50–51
        selection of measures for, 50
    Assistive Technology Device Predis-
        position Assessment and, 31
    evaluation for AT, 49–53
    influence on use, 33
    nonpathological measures of
        NEO Personality Inventory/
          NEO Five Factor Inventory,
          50
        utility of, 51
    pathological measures of
        Million Clinical Multiaxial Inven-
          tory-III, 50
        Minnesota Multiphasic Personal-
          ity Inventory–2, 50, 67
    and use or nonuse, 51–52
Personal relationships
    among on-line course students, 225

mechanism for client-focused
evaluation, 263–264
needs and requirements identification in, 263
purpose of, 262–263

Technical Liaison Officer (TLO, Ireland)
APHRODITE project and, 259, 262
certification of, 260
training of, 259
work of, 259–260
Technology-Related Assistance for Individuals With Disabilities
(TRIAD) Act of 1988, 5–6
AD definition in, 169
AT as term in, 5, 17
consumer selection and, 270–271
Telecommunication display devices
(TDDs)
in telehealth for deaf persons, 200
Telecommunication networks
integrated service digital network,
203
Internet IP-based, 202–203
local area, 202
plain old telephone (POTS), 202
in telehealth delivery, 202–203
wide area, 202
Telecommunications-mediated health services (TMHS)
efficacy and cost effectiveness issues
in, 197
growth of, 197
Telecommunication technologies
comparative studies of, 207–209
video vs. speakerphone vs. face-to-
face counseling study
assessment scales and findings in,
208
comfort with equipment in, 208
cost estimates for, 209
distraction in, 208
in rural teenagers with seizure disorders, 207–209
therapy homework assignments
and, 208–209
Telehealth
asynchronous communication in,
200
cost effectiveness of

for homebound or rural population, 199–200
definition of, 198
growth of
rationale for, 199–200
outcomes research in, 203–209
comparative studies of telecommunication technologies,
207–209
for cost effectiveness, 210
Internet studies, 203–204
need for, 209
telephone studies, 204–206
vidoconferencing studies,
206–207
process studies of, 210
relation to AT services, 198
research in
for client training material,
210–211
for practice guidelines, 210–211
synchronous communication in
examples of, 200
networks in, 202–203
telephone in, 200–201
vidoconferencing in, 201–203
telecommunication display devices
in, 200
telecommunications systems and,
200–203
use of information technology in,
198
Telephone
comparative outcome studies of
in adherence to treatment, 205
in blood pressure improvement,
205–206
in counseling, 204
in telecommunication, 200–201
in telecommunication networks,
202
TEST. See Training, Employment &
Support Using Technology
(TEST)
The Guide to Occupational Therapy Practice, 282
Training
client
telehealth materials for, 210–211
of consumer
goals in, 177

ABOUT THE EDITOR

Marcia J. Scherer is director of the Institute for Matching Person and Technology in Webster, NY. She also is associate professor of Physical Medicine and Rehabilitation, University of Rochester Medical Center, and senior research associate, International Center for Hearing and Speech Research (a joint program of the University of Rochester and the National Technical Institute for the Deaf/Rochester Institute of Technology). She received a PhD and an MPH from the University of Rochester.

Dr. Scherer is author of *Living in the State of Stuck: How Assistive Technology Impacts the Lives of People With Disabilities* (3rd ed., 2000) and coeditor (with Jan Galvin) of *Evaluating, Selecting, and Using Appropriate Assistive Technology* (1996). She also coedited (with Laura Cushman) *Psychological Assessment in Medical Rehabilitation* (1995, American Psychological Association), which is Volume 1 in the APA series "Measurement and Instrumentation in Psychology."

Dr. Scherer has written widely on technology use and is on the editorial boards of the journals *Disability and Rehabilitation, Assistive Technology,* and *Home Health Care Dealer/Provider.* She is a Fellow of the APA in the divisions of Rehabilitation Psychology (Division 22) and Applied Experimental and Engineering Psychology (Division 21). She is a member of the American Association of Spinal Cord Injury Psychologists and Social Workers, the American Educational Research Association, the American Congress of Rehabilitation Medicine, the Rehabilitation Engineering and Assistive Technology Society of North America, the Council for Exceptional Children, and the New York Academy of Sciences.